Health Informatics

This series is directed to healthcare professionals leading the transformation of healthcare by using information and knowledge. For over 20 years, Health Informatics has offered a broad range of titles: some address specific professions such as nursing, medicine, and health administration; others cover special areas of practice such as trauma and radiology; still other books in the series focus on interdisciplinary issues, such as the computer based patient record, electronic health records, and networked healthcare systems. Editors and authors, eminent experts in their fields, offer their accounts of innovations in health informatics. Increasingly, these accounts go beyond hardware and software to address the role of information in influencing the transformation of healthcare delivery systems around the world. The series also increasingly focuses on the users of the information and systems: the organizational, behavioral, and societal changes that accompany the diffusion of information technology in health services environments.

Developments in healthcare delivery are constant; in recent years, bioinformatics has emerged as a new field in health informatics to support emerging and ongoing developments in molecular biology. At the same time, further evolution of the field of health informatics is reflected in the introduction of concepts at the macro or health systems delivery level with major national initiatives related to electronic health records (EHR), data standards, and public health informatics.

These changes will continue to shape health services in the twenty-first century. By making full and creative use of the technology to tame data and to transform information, Health Informatics will foster the development and use of new knowledge in healthcare.

More information about this series at http://www.springer.com/series/1114

Homero Rivas • Katarzyna Wac

Editors

Digital Health

Scaling Healthcare to the World

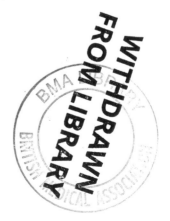

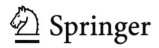

Springer

Editors
Homero Rivas
Stanford University School of Medicine
Stanford, CA
USA

Katarzyna Wac
University of Copenhagen
Copenhagen
Denmark

ISSN 1431-1917   ISSN 2197-3741   (electronic)
Health Informatics
ISBN 978-3-319-61445-8   ISBN 978-3-319-61446-5   (eBook)
https://doi.org/10.1007/978-3-319-61446-5

Library of Congress Control Number: 2017963147

This Springer imprint is published by Springer Nature
The registered company is Springer International Publishing AG
The registered company address is: Gewerbestrasse 11, 6330 Cham, Switzerland

Foreword

Prepare for a new digital era of medicine. In 2017, millions of people are collecting their vital signs, such as blood pressure and respiratory rate, on everyday devices like smartwatches and iPhones. Surgeons are leveraging advanced robotics in the operating room and live-streaming their most challenging cases via virtual reality headsets. Primary care practitioners are capturing patient data in real time without glancing once at a screen, thanks to their augmented reality "smart" glasses. And medical records, once stacked in filing cabinets at hospitals and clinics across the country, are now being stored electronically (http://www.modernhealthcare.com/article/20160531/NEWS/16053999).

Many of these technological advancements were subsidized into existence through the major health reforms of the past decade, which should not be overlooked—notably the Affordable Care Act and the Health Information Technology for Economic and Clinical Health ("HITECH Act"). These legislative changes inspired venture investors in Silicon Valley and other tech hubs to open their checkbooks to health technology entrepreneurs, and for the world's most valuable companies like Apple, Amazon, and Google to begin eyeing opportunities in the $3 trillion medical sector for the first time. Healthcare is an "enormous" opportunity, Apple chief executive Tim Cook recently told the television news network CNBC in a revealing interview. "You can have patients that really feeling like customers… and can have systems and applications that bring out the best in medical professionals." Imagine a health system that could deliver an experience on par with one that consumers expect in every other industry from retail to financial services.

But before all this technology can deliver on its potential to transform the health experience for the better, a deeper change is required. Incentives need to shift from older financial models that reward hospitals and clinics for expensive procedures and tests, rather than on keeping their patients healthier for longer. The United States spends twice as much as any other developed country on healthcare, but this investment has not resulted in improved health outcomes (http://www.pbs.org/newshour/bb/u-s-pays-health-care-rest-world/). This nation surpasses the rest of the world on cutting-edge research and basic science, but it has failed to provide a path for ordinary Americans to access these innovative therapies at an affordable price tag. Former US Vice President Joe Biden considered selling his home to pay for his son's cancer treatment. If the country's leaders can barely afford life-saving treatment, just imagine the plight faced by ordinary Americans.

Shifting these incentives will be the task of policymakers, but it also presents an opportunity for the exploding crop of health technology start-ups in Silicon Valley and beyond. The emerging category known as digital health, which broadly refers to the convergence of digital tools with health and healthy living, raised a mammoth $4.2 billion in 2016 alone (https://rockhealth.com/reports/2016-year-end-funding-report-a-reality-check-for-digital-health/). Other upcoming areas include digital therapeutics, which involve computer-based interventions to replace or augment drugs, and computational biology, such as machine learning tools to parse through miles of medical images and scans.

Many of these companies make their money by propping up the status quo. But a select few are attempting to forge a new path, that is, to down health costs by providing people with digital services to manage their own care preventatively and to avoid expensive medicines and emergency room visits. Such companies are producing simple apps and messaging tools that are designed to provide pertinent health information to low-income communities that lack reliable access to care. Or the companies that are connecting people in rural areas, located many miles from a hospital, with a new way to consult with a physician via video chat. A category called "liquid biopsies" are developing tests to screen for diseases like cancer that can be treated in the early stages. Vijay Pande, appointed to run the new bio fund for the well-known technology investment fund Andreessen Horowitz, has gone as far as to describe this whole transformation as the "industrial revolution for biology" (https://a16z.com/2015/11/18/bio-fund/).

Amid all this excitement, these technologies will need to be evaluated in three key ways: Can they improve overall health outcomes for patients, enhance the quality of care, and reduce health costs? This framework for optimizing health system performance is known as the "triple aim."

In healthcare, many new technologies will initially add cost to the system. But the hope is that such advancements are laying the groundwork for potential cost savings. The promise of electronic medical record systems, for instance, is improved care coordination and disease management between physicians and their patients, as well as reduced errors. But before that dream can become a reality, it will need to be far easier for these electronic medical record systems to aggregate and share data.

Indeed, the next phase of medicine will require integration or interoperability of health information in support of a new style of medicine based on data and evidence. Some of the world's most valuable companies, including Apple, Amazon, and Google, have all taken on this challenge in different ways. These companies are betting on health hardware, such as wearable technologies and medical devices, machine learning and artificial intelligence as applied to medical specialties like radiology, telemedicine or virtual care, and software tools for users to view their personal medical information. However, before any of these services are truly valuable, it will be necessary to aggregate medical information from charts, labs, devices, health apps, and so on.

From Silicon Valley to Washington D.C. and beyond, a movement is underway backed by government officials, nonprofits, and patient advocates for patients to access their medical information in a user-friendly format. One of the most successful efforts is a nonprofit organization called OpenNotes, which advocates for patients to access their physicians' notes. Despite ongoing resistance from the medical community that patients would misinterpret this information, some 14 million people have accessed these notes electronically—with little confusion and few mishaps (https://patienten-gagementhit.com/news/using-opennotes-for-positive-impact-on-patient-data-access).

The winners that emerge in healthcare in the coming years have a choice: Do they build tools for healthcare as it is today? Or are they building for a future that is both patient-centered and evidence-based? The latter option represents a windier, longer, and more challenging path, but it's the right one.

CNBC, San Francisco   Christina Farr
CA, USA

References

http://www.modernhealthcare.com/article/20160531/NEWS/16053999.

http://www.pbs.org/newshour/bb/u-s-pays-health-care-rest-world/.

https://rockhealth.com/reports/2016-year-end-funding-report-a-reality-check-for-digital-health/.

https://a16z.com/2015/11/18/bio-fund/.

https://patientengagementhit.com/news/using-opennotes-for-positive-impact-on-patient-data-access.

Contents

Contributors

Mussaad Al-Razouki Kuwait Life Sciences Company, Sharq, Kuwait

Dan E. Azagury Stanford University School of Medicine, Stanford, CA, USA

Stanford Byers Center for Biodesign, Stanford, CA, USA

Thomas Boillat Stanford University, Stanford, CA, USA

University of Lausanne, Lausanne, Switzerland

David Bychkov InHealth, Johns Hopkins University, Baltimore, MD, USA

Carlo V. Caballero-Uribe Associated Professor of Medicine, Universidad del Norte, Barranquilla, Colombia

Larry F. Chu Stanford School of Medicine, Stanford, CA, USA

Matthew Cooper Stanford University School of Medicine, Stanford, CA, USA

Nathan Cortez Dedman School of Law, Southern Methodist University, Dallas, TX, USA

Lyn Denend Stanford Byers Center for Biodesign, Stanford, CA, USA

Jamison G. Gamble Stanford School of Medicine, Stanford, CA, USA

Michael Gelinsky Centre for Translational Bone, Joint and Soft Tissue Research, University Hospital and Medical Faculty, Technische Universität Dresden, Dresden, Germany

Mitchell G. Goldenberg Keenan Centre for Biomedical Science, International Centre for Surgical Safety, St. Michael's Hospital, University of Toronto, Toronto, ON, Canada

Pishoy Gouda Division of Internal Medicine, Foothills Medical Centre, University of Calgary, Calgary, AB, Canada

Maurits Graafland Department of Surgery, Academic Medical Centre, Amsterdam, The Netherlands

Teodor P. Grantcharov Keenan Centre for Biomedical Science, International Centre for Surgical Safety, St. Michael's Hospital, University of Toronto, Toronto, ON, Canada

Bronwyn Harris Stanford University School of Medicine, Stanford, CA, USA

J.P. van der Heijden Research and Development, KSYOS TeleMedical Center, Amsterdam, The Netherlands

Alain Labrique Department of International Health, Johns Hopkins Bloomberg School of Public Health, Baltimore, MD, USA

Department of Epidemiology, Johns Hopkins Bloomberg School of Public Health, Baltimore, MD, USA

Global mHealth Initiative, Johns Hopkins Bloomberg School of Public Health, Baltimore, MD, USA

Pedro Matabuena Unmanned Aerial Vehicle Systems, Instituto Tecnológico Autónomo de México and Aidronix, CDMX, Mexico

Bertalan Mesko Semmelweis University, Budapest, Hungary

Arlen Meyers Society of Physician Entrepreneurs, South Norwalk, CT, USA

Ian Miller Virtual Reality Medical Center, Interactive Media Institute, San Diego, CA, USA

John Morton Stanford University School of Medicine, Stanford, CA, USA

Sara Riggare Karolinska Institutet, Stockholm, Sweden

Homero Rivas Stanford University School of Medicine, Stanford, CA, USA

Stanford University, Stanford, CA, USA

Carolina Garcia Rizo Roche Molecular Systems, San Francisco, CA, USA

Dara Rouholiman Stanford School of Medicine, Stanford, CA, USA

Marlies Schijven Department of Surgery, Academic Medical Centre, Amsterdam, The Netherlands

Ashish G. Shah Stanford School of Medicine, Stanford, CA, USA

Steve Steinhubl Scripps Translational Science Institute, La Jolla, CA, USA

Nick van Terheyden Gaithersburg, MD, USA

Lavanya Vasudevan Center for Health Policy and Inequalities Research, Duke Global Health Institute, Durham, NC, USA

Department of International Health, Johns Hopkins Bloomberg School of Public Health, Baltimore, MD, USA

Global mHealth Initiative, Johns Hopkins Bloomberg School of Public Health, Baltimore, MD, USA

Katarzyna Wac Stanford University, Stanford, CA, USA

Department of Computer Science, University of Copenhagen, Copenhagen, Denmark

Quality of Life Technologies Lab, University of Geneva, Geneva, Switzerland

Brenda K. Wiederhold Interactive Media Institute, Virtual Reality Medical Center, San Diego, CA, USA

Mark D. Wiederhold Interactive Media Institute, Virtual Reality Medical Center, San Diego, CA, USA

L. Witkamp Department of Medical Informatics, KSYOS TeleMedical Centre, Academic Medical Centre Amsterdam, Amsterdam, The Netherlands

Sharon Wulfovich Stanford University, Stanford, CA, USA

Sean D. Young Department of Family Medicine, Center for Digital Behavior, University of California Institute for Prediction Technology, University of California, Los Angeles, CA, USA

Hubert Zajicek Health Wildcatters, Dallas, TX, USA

Kelsey Zeller Department of International Health, Johns Hopkins Bloomberg School of Public Health, Baltimore, MD, USA

Global mHealth Initiative, Johns Hopkins Bloomberg School of Public Health, Baltimore, MD, USA

Chapter 1
Creating a Case for Digital Health

Homero Rivas

Abstract The central paradigm in medicine is based on the patient–provider relationship. In these times, previously unheard diseases are being described every day while novel therapies for previously uncured diseases are introduced along with novel state-of-the-art diagnostic and therapeutic technologies. These developments alter the patient–physician relationship, which has remained largely unchanged for thousands of years. *Digital Health* represents an evolutionary adaptation of the art and science of medicine to pervasive information and communication technologies (ICTs). Without a doubt, this represents a phenomenal opportunity for us to scale access to care to any area in the world where connectivity may be available. This chapter reviews the ways that healthcare has evolved and its conceivable opportunities, challenges, and socioeconomic consequences.

Keywords Digital Health • Medicine • ICTs • Patient–Provider Relationship • Social Media • Wearables • 3D Printing • Augmented and Virtual Reality • Economics

1.1 Evolution of Medicine and Delivery of Healthcare

The practice of medicine goes back thousands of years. There is enough evidence to show that stone-age humans practiced some type of medicine and even developed primitive instrumentation to perform surgery such as cranial trepanation (Fig. 1.1). While modern medicine and surgery have evolved dramatically during the last hundred years, with many breakthroughs such as antisepsis, anesthesia, analgesia, antibiotics, endoscopic, robotic and even scar-less surgery among many others, the

H. Rivas, M.D., M.B.A.
Stanford University School of Medicine,
300 Pasteur Ct, Suite H3680H, Stanford, CA 94305, USA
e-mail: hrivas@stanford.edu

© Springer International Publishing AG 2018
H. Rivas, K. Wac (eds.), *Digital Health*, Health Informatics,
https://doi.org/10.1007/978-3-319-61446-5_1

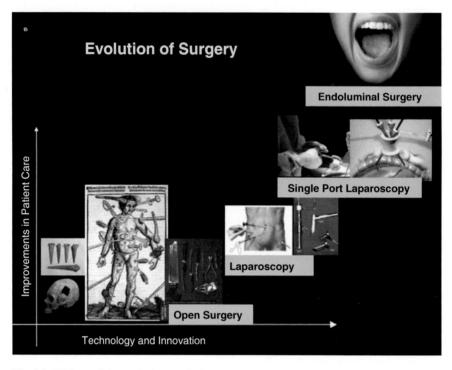

Fig. 1.1 While medicine and other specialties such as surgery have evolved dramatically, the practice of medicine cannot be scaled as it still depends on a one-to-one patient-provider relationship

essence of the business model of medicine has changed very little if any (Neuburger 1910; Kelly et al. 2003; Schlich 2007). The practice of medicine remains very artisanal, requiring at least a one-to-one ratio of medical provider to patient for a single medical encounter, thus preventing the scalability of healthcare delivery. With higher standards of care almost universally available and resulting longer life spans and prevalence of more chronic diseases, there is a shortage of medical providers for the continuously larger surplus of patients (Petterson et al. 2012; Sheldon et al. 2008). Conventional medicine, unlike technology industries such as software, hardware, semiconductors, microcontrollers, etc., cannot scale production from day to day. Conversely, if a company such as Google or Facebook decides to change basic or complex software algorithms, a logo design, color, fonts, etc., they can do it immediately and have an impact on masses of users (Rogers 2003; Moore 2014). On the other hand, practicing medicine usually relies on one-to-one patient–provider encounters/relationships; hardly scalable if any potential implementation would be needed to include large groups of people. Medicine itself can only scale to a degree by medical education, rendering new doctors who will see more people, or by implementation of public health through preventive medicine strategies. Both efforts will still have severe constraints and neither can achieve the technological scalability of the industries described before.

1.2 Digital Health as an Opportunity and Challenge in the Twenty-First Century

Digital health bases itself on the implementation and leverage of information and communication technologies (ICTs) to deliver and scale healthcare to the masses. Throughout this book, we will discover many of the technologies that are being implemented with great success in healthcare to make this a reality.

Presently in the USA, nearly 20% of the gross domestic product is used for healthcare. This represents more than three trillion US dollars per year spent for healthcare (Centers for Disease Control and Prevention n.d.; Centers for Medicare and Medicaid Services 2015). Certainly this will not be sustainable in the near future unless cost containment strategies are widely implemented. During the recent past, former US Secretary of Health and Human Services, Kathleen Sebelius, referred to mHealth as "the biggest technology breakthrough of our time" and maintained that its use would also "address our greatest national challenge" (Sebelius 2011; Steinhubl et al. 2013). Without a doubt, this is not only applicable to the USA, but also to the rest of the world. Nathan Cortez et al. recently published a review of the FDA regulation on mobile healthcare technologies where they identified at least 97,000 available health apps (Cortez et al. 2014). This number has grown exponentially over the last couple of years to be approximately 250,000 health apps available online and/or in the healthcare market (McCarthy n.d.). Unfortunately, this truly represents an enormous challenge as the FDA has approved much less than 1% of those apps for clinical use. Furthermore, there is a forecast of 1.7–2 billion users of digital health by 2018 (Cortez et al. 2014). In addition, as with many other disruptive technologies, it is unclear if many have been responsibly created or if they are inclusive of all critical stakeholders in this market (care providers, patients, administrators, computer scientists, behavioral scientists, entrepreneurs, investors, etc.) as they likely are underrepresented by patients and care providers or led by technologists and entrepreneurs. Historically there is a great disconnect between those two polarized groups of people, and while physicians claim to embrace innovation, their ecosystem has great limitations to innovate in comparison to technologists and others. In general, no formal medical school curriculum includes digital health, and physicians and healthcare systems would rarely embrace innovative ways to take care of patients due to a lack of scientific evidence, potential liability, and red tape among many others (Beck 2015; Asch and Weinstein 2014; Armstrong and Barsion 2013; Woods and Rosenberg 2016). The profile of a successful physician usually includes being extremely risk-averse and having a low tolerance for failure. Although not extensively talked about, physicians are known to engage in secrecy in research, cost insensitivity, and other behaviors. Conversely, very successful innovators and entrepreneurs (i.e., founders of major media conglomerates such as Google, Facebook, YouTube, etc.) have a very opposite profile of success to that of physicians. They usually have a high tolerance for failure, a great enthusiasm for risk, and embrace crowd-source collaboration, etc. (Rogers 2003; Moore 2014; Chamorro-Premuzic 2013.). Finding a middle ground to merge successful physician and innovator profiles into one represents a big and very ambitious challenge. However, once achieved, this could lead to the successful implementation of digital technologies in healthcare. For this to be sustainable, a culture of innovation must be nurtured to become pervasive throughout basic and advanced medical education curricula. Interestingly, while there are several hurdles for innovation adoption; including the nature of technologies themselves, regulation, cost, universal availability, etc., historically the biggest barrier is professional inertia. This is likely a result of a fixed mindset that most physicians have not to change the way they have learned and practiced medicine for a very long time. During the last few years, the widespread use of mobile phones, patient social communities, telemedicine, consumer driven health, low-cost commercially available wearable technologies, the Quantified Self movement, low-cost 3D printers, virtual and augmented reality, artificial intelligence engines, among several others are rapidly sculpting the way new generations will practice medicine and, certainly, how patient expectations will likely be in the near future (Sweeney 2011; Turner-McGrievy et al. 2013; Spring et al. 2017; McConnell et al. 2017; Spring et al. 2013; Case et al. 2015; Mackillop et al. 2014; Smith 2013; Turakhia and Harrington 2016; Sinnenberg et al. 2016; Eichstaedt et al. 2015; Patel et al. 2015a; Logghe et al. 2016; Flynn et al. 2017; Pew Research Center 2013; Chung et al. 2017; Farmer and Tarassenko 2015; Patel et al. 2015b; Bassett et al. 2010; Rosenberger et al. 2016; Walsh et al. 2014; Jakicic et al. 2016; Troiano et al. 2014; Shull et al. 2014; Schreinemacher et al. 2014; Pagoto et al. 2014; The Independent 2015; Zheng et al. 2016; Lim et al. 2016; Biglino et al. 2015; Randazzo et al. 2016; Giannopoulos et al. 2016; Wengerter et al. 2016; Burn et al. 2016; AlAli et al. 2015; Hong et al. 2017; Ng et al. 2016; Preis and Öblom 2017; Morrison et al. 2015; Wiederhold 2016; Lafond et al. 2016; Mosso-Vázquez et al. 2014; Wiederhold et al. 2014; Zhu et al. 2017; Bernhardt et al. 2017; Lyon 2017; Rochlen et al. 2017; LeBlanc and Chaput 2016; Lister et al. 2014; Esteva et al. 2017; Rumsfeld et al. 2016; He et al. 2017; Ashley 2015) (Figs. 1.2–1.5).

Throughout the world, digital health is being implemented in daily clinical practice. From simple software algorithms utilized in feature phones to improve adherence to tuberculosis medication, to very interactive software applications used in smart phones to evaluate heart rhythm (Sweeney 2011; Turner-McGrievy et al. 2013; Spring et al. 2017; McConnell et al. 2017; Spring et al. 2013; Case et al. 2015; Mackillop et al. 2014; Smith 2013) (Fig. 1.6). The low cost of many of these digital health innovations makes them very attractive to emerging markets. In fact, most emerging markets commonly have prevalent needs and constraints that usually result in unique creativity (Lewis et al. 2012; The Economist 2010). The social and economic impacts that some of these digital health implementations could be dramatic even in the developed world, like in the USA, where the medication adherence market represents at least 300 billion US dollars (P&S Market Research 2016). Even very modest mHealth strategies could have dramatic returns on investment. This has attracted many entrepreneurs to this market segment.

In addition, an overall lower cost of digital health technologies and less regulation in such emerging markets may result in a very fertile ecosystem for them to thrive and, thereby, expand and accelerate their adoption. The same has been experienced in other

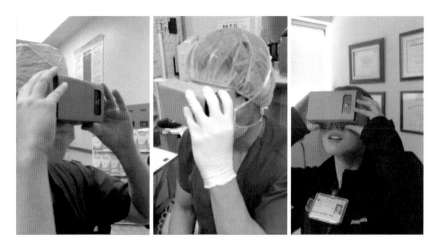

Fig. 1.2 This is an example of a very low cost cardboard device used with a mobile phone that allows a virtual reality experience. This can be used for teaching purposes on patients, students, providers, etc. Additionally it can be used to improve patient experience by distracting patients from an otherwise unpleasant experience

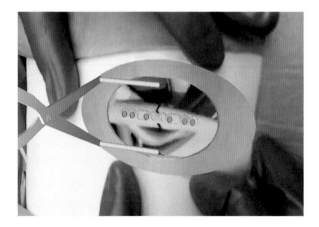

Fig. 1.3 Augmented reality obtained through head mounted displays, merging reality and suspended holograms which can be interactive

arenas, such as banking, where a few years ago, in places like Kenya, near to 80% of transactions were done by mobile phone versus in places like in the USA where they would have a market share less than 10% (The Economist 2010). Already in places like Gaza, innovators are using 3D printing to print very simple, low cost medical instruments and devices such as stethoscopes, needle drives, oxymeters, among others

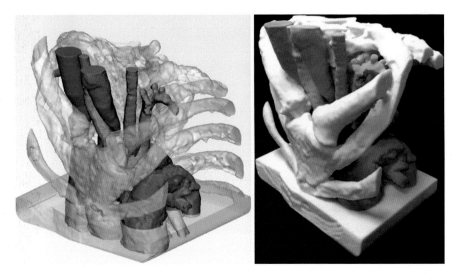

Fig. 1.4 3D Printing can produce low cost replicas of exact anatomical models used for teaching, simulation, surgical planning, among others. More costly materials can be used to print exact implants (i.e. joint implants, etc.)

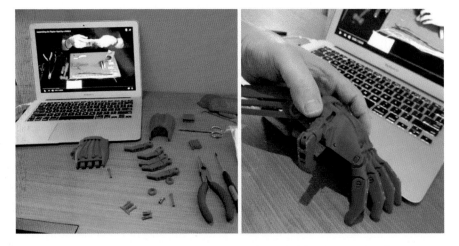

Fig. 1.5 Low cost 3D printers can print on low cost materials, highly functional prosthesis, which otherwise would have a prohibitive cost to many around the world. Social media and crowd-source learning platforms can be used to obtain free blue prints of such prosthesis

(The Independent 2015). Presently, the USA and other developed countries are implementing very strict regulations to any 3D printing done for medical purposes, even when this might not even be bio-printing yet (Morrison et al. 2015). With no doubt, such regulations will maintain safety; however, they also may hinder innovation and rapid adoption.

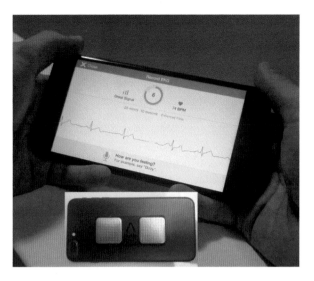

Fig. 1.6 This is an example of a low cost, FDA device and software, that allows to obtain and to share, medical grade EKG monitoring at anytime, anywhere. Additionally and through an artificial intelligence engine, it can assess for common hearth rhythm pathologies

1.3   The Economics of Digital Health

In general, the economics of digital health seem very conducive for the universal adoption of many of its value propositions. Usually, for a given innovation to be massively adopted it must be simple in nature, simple to use, easily reproducible or scalable, cost-effective, make sense, have relative advantage(s), low cost, and be safe among other features (Rogers 2003; Moore 2014). In general, in conventional medicine, many of these features cannot be easily matched and often times, innovative diagnostic or therapeutic modalities are complex in nature, not user-friendly or highly operator-dependent, of questionable value/benefit, and very expensive to say the least.

Economic opportunities have been already identified by major venture capitalists in healthcare as investment in digital health has dramatically peaked over the last few years. In the USA alone, about 55% of all digital health investments since 2011 have been in companies whose technologies interface with the consumer in some manner [76, 77]. This reflects the convergence of technologies to drive and measure improved health outcomes and cost savings, and funding has followed. In general, most stakeholders acutely identify great strengths and opportunities in less-regulated areas, such as fitness and wellness, through the implementation of numerous wearable devices that can monitor most body functions, vital signs, biometric parameters, physical activity, posture, etc. (Farmer and Tarassenko 2015; Patel et al. 2015b; Bassett et al. 2010; Rosenberger et al. 2016; Walsh et al. 2014; Jakicic et al. 2016; Troiano et al. 2014; Shull et al. 2014; Schreinemacher et al. 2014). By encouraging consumers and patients to change health-related behaviors through personal accountability, many propose their use is not only for prevention, but also for clinical diagnosis and management of disease. This has been, in fact, the strategy that many have utilized to enter the medical market as it follows the shifts toward clinically driven consumer health not only for prevention and wellness, but also (and very attractively) for the management of numerous chronic diseases (high blood pressure, diabetes, obesity, asthma, etc.). While entering a more regulated market represents the need for formal clinical studies, only a few highly compelling technologies have undertaken formal randomized clinical trials. This would only lead to support from the medical community and more universal adoption if such studies show beneficial results. Clinically proven software and hardware would be integrated to drive better health outcomes and cost savings not only in clinical care, but also in research and education.

Additionally, very innovative research is being done thanks to nearly universal access to information and communication technologies, through the use of crowd-sourced recruitment of patients, and/or crowd-sourced funding in research. Investigational technologies, such as the SCANADU™, have leveraged their micro-investor crowd base to also become investigational subjects once they have received their device for personal use (Fig. 1.7). Only then, and after signing an informed

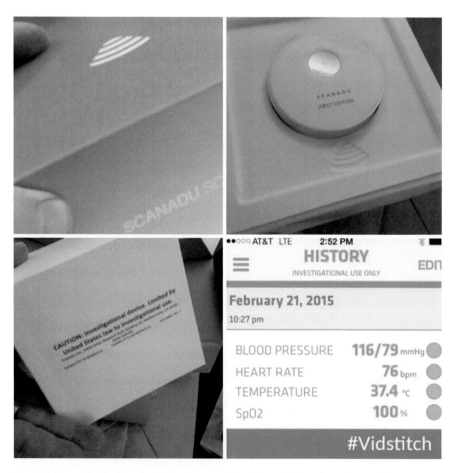

Fig. 1.7 Innovative business models using crowd funding and micro investing are being successfully used in digital health. Additionally some groups are using models of crowd source research, where all micro investors also become research subjects

consent form to be part of the study, could they use such devices. This will crystalize into a complete clinical study lead by Scripps Clinic in San Diego, CA, USA, which may be finished soon. Even if such devices do not prove any individual clinical benefit to prevention, prompt diagnosis, and/or offer more efficient management of disease, many of these digital health technologies can greatly improve the efficiencies and logistics of clinical research with great economic saving during conventional clinical trials. Often times, patients have to travel great distances just for simple evaluations done through interviews, basic assessments of physical signs and/or biometrics, and other methods. Many of these clinical parameters can be easily attained through telemedicine, medical grade wearable devices, or other means. Undoubtedly, digital health allows access not only to care but also to research of people even in remote locations.

1.4 Crowdsourcing Healthcare, Artificial Intelligence and Final Thoughts

Lastly, but perhaps of greater importance, digital health can be greatly utilized in educating patients, medical students, physicians, allied personnel, and also in communicating among themselves and with others. Crowd-sourced knowledge that patients share through online patient communities is truly priceless and was impossible to attain only a few years ago. Now through some of these communities, patients suffering rare diseases can leverage on the experience of many other similar people throughout the world regarding symptoms, diagnosis, and treatment. The same can be experienced with widely prevalent diseases such as obesity, diabetes, etc. Most disease management and remote monitoring companies are shifting their focus to specific diseases to help patients and providers better manage the condition as opposed to providing general solutions aimed at patients facing different diseases. In addition, many have proposed that through engines of artificial intelligence, algorithms could soon evaluate mass data and propose more educated diagnosis and treatment than what many experienced physicians could offer themselves.

Envisioning an ideal patient-centered framework, we could conclude that knowledge, engagement, and consumer friendliness can be improved through digital health. Providing ready access to education and relevant and personalized health information, could improve health literacy. Engaging and affecting behavioral change in healthcare consumers to better manage their own health could provide them with better tools to manage their health and wellness. Lastly, by improving consumer-friendliness, we could greatly improve consumers' access to healthcare and their user experience. Patients' choices can be improved and better price transparency is expected. User experience, in general, is critical when implementing any innovation universally as successful innovations must be easy to use, have great incentives—like improvement of health—and must make economic sense. Digital health shares all of these qualities.

References

AAMC. Releases physician workforce projection report. Significant primary care, overall physician shortage predicted by 2025. 2015. http://www.aafp.org/news/practice-professional-issues/20150303aamcwkforce.html.

AlAli AB, Griffin MF, Butler PE. Three-dimensional printing surgical applications. Eplasty. 2015;15:e37.

Armstrong EG, Barsion SJ. Creating "innovator's DNA" in health care education. Acad Med. 2013;88(3):343–8.

Asch DA, Weinstein DF. Innovation in medical education. N Engl J Med. 2014;371:794–5.

Ashley EA. The precision medicine initiative: a new national effort. JAMA. 2015;313(21):2119–20.

Bassett DR Jr, Wyatt HR, Thompson H, Peters JC, Hill JO. Pedometer-measured physical activity and health behaviors in U.S. adults. Med Sci Sports Exerc. 2010;42(10):1819–25.

Beck, Melinda. Innovation is sweeping through U.S. medical schools. WSJ, Feb 16, 2015. https://www.wsj.com/articles/innovation-is-sweeping-through-u-s-medical-schools-1424145650.

Bernhardt S, Nicolau SA, Soler L, Doignon C. The status of augmented reality in laparoscopic surgery as of 2016. Med Image Anal. 2017;37:66–90.

Biglino G, Capelli C, Wray J, et al. 3D-manufactured patient-specific models of congenital heart defects for communication in clinical practice: feasibility and acceptability. BMJ Open. 2015;5:e007165. doi:10.1136/bmjopen-2014-007165.

Burn MB, Ta A, Gogola GR. Three-dimensional printing of prosthetic hands for children. J Hand Surg Am. 2016;41(5):e103–9. doi:10.1016/j.jhsa.2016.02.008.

Case MA, Burwick HA, Volpp KG, Patel MS. Accuracy of smartphone applications and wearable devices for tracking physical activity data. JAMA. 2015;313(6):625–6.

Centers for Disease Control and Prevention. National Center for Health Statistics. https://www.cdc.gov/nchs/fastats/health-expenditures.htm.

Centers for Medicare & Medicaid Services. National Health Expenditures 2015 highlights. https://www.cms.gov/Research-Statistics-Data-and-Systems/Statistics-Trends-and-Reports/NationalHealthExpendData/Downloads/highlights.pdf. 2015.

Chamorro-Premuzic T. The five characteristics of successful innovators. Harv Bus Rev. https://hbr.org/2013/10/the-five-characteristics-of-successful-innovators. 2013;

Chung AE, Skinner AC, Hasty SE, Perrin EM. Tweeting to health: a novel mHealth intervention using Fitbits and twitter to Foster healthy lifestyles. Clin Pediatr (Phila). 2017;56(1):26–32.

Cortez NG, Cohen IG, Kesselheim AS. FDA regulation of mobile health technologies. N Engl J Med. 2014;371(4):372–9.

Eichstaedt JC, Schwartz HA, Kern ML, et al. Psychological language on twitter predicts county-level heart disease mortality. Psychol Sci. 2015;26(2):159–69.

Esteva A, Kuprel B, Novoa RA, Ko J, Swetter SM, Blau HM, Thrun S. Dermatologist-level classification of skin cancer with deep neural networks. Nature. 2017; doi:10.1038/nature21056.

Farmer A, Tarassenko L. Use of wearable monitoring devices to change health behavior. JAMA. 2015;313(18):1864–5.

Flynn S, Hebert P, Korenstein D, Ryan M, Jordan WB, Keyhani S. Leveraging social media to promote evidence-based continuing medical education. PLoS One. 2017;12(1):e0168962.

Giannopoulos AA, Mitsouras D, Yoo SJ, Liu PP, Chatzizisis YS, Rybicki FJ. Applications of 3D printing in cardiovascular diseases. Nat Rev. Cardiol. 2016;13(12):701–18. doi:10.1038/nrcardio.2016.170.

He KY, Ge D, He MM. Big data analytics for genomic medicine. Int J Mol Sci. 2017;15:18(2).

Hong N, Yang GH, Lee J, Kim G. 3D bioprinting and its in vivo applications. J Biomed Mater Res B Appl Biomater. 2017;20 doi:10.1002/jbm.b.33826.

Jakicic JM, Davis KK, Rogers RJ, King WC, Marcus MD, Helsel D, Rickman AD, Wahed AS, Belle SH. Effect of wearable technology combined with a lifestyle intervention on long-term weight loss. The IDEA randomized clinical trial. JAMA. 2016;316(11):1161–71. doi:10.1001/jama.2016.12858.

Kelly N, Rees B, Shuter P. Medicine through time: Heinemann; 2003. isbn:978-0-435-30841-4.

Lafond E, Riva G, Gutierrez-Maldonado J, Wiederhold BK. Eating disorders and obesity in virtual reality: a comprehensive research chart. Cyberpsychol Behav Soc Netw. 2016;19(2):141–7.

LeBlanc AG, Chaput JP. Pokémon Go: A game changer for the physical inactivity crisis? Prev Med. 2016. pii: S0091–7435(16)30365–6.

Lewis T, Synowiec C, Lagomarsino G, Schweitzer J. E-health in low- and middle-income countries: findings from the center for health market innovations. Bull World Health Organ. 2012;90(5):332–40. doi:10.2471/BLT.11.099820.

Lim KH, Loo ZY, Goldie SJ, Adams JW, McMenamin PG. Use of 3D printed models in medical education: a randomized control trial comparing 3D prints versus cadaveric materials for learning external cardiac anatomy. Anat Sci Educ. 2016;9(3):213–21.

Lister C, West JH, Cannon B, Sax T, Brodegard D. Just a fad? Gamification in health and fitness apps. JMIR Serious Games. 2014;2(2):e9.

Logghe HJ, Boeck MA, Atallah SB. Decoding twitter: understanding the history, instruments, and techniques for success. Ann Surg. 2016;264(6):904–8.

Lyon J. Augmented reality goes bedside. JAMA. 2017;317(2):127. doi:10.1001/jama.2016.20270.

Mackillop L, Loerup L, Bartlett K, Farmer A, Gibson OJ, Hirst JE, Kenworthy Y, Kevat DA, Levy JC, Tarassenko L. Development of a real-time smartphone solution for the management of women with or at high risk of gestational diabetes. J Diabetes Sci Technol. 2014;8(6):1105–14. doi:10.1177/1932296814542271.

McCarthy J. How many health apps actually matter? http://www.healthcareitnews.com/news/how-many-health-apps-actually-matter.

McConnell MV, Shcherbina A, Pavlovic A, Homburger JR, Goldfeder RL, Waggot D, Cho MK, Rosenberger ME, Haskell WL, Myers J, Champagne MA, Mignot E, Landray M, Tarassenko L, Harrington RA, Yeung AC, Ashley EA. Feasibility of obtaining measures of lifestyle from a smartphone AppThe MyHeart counts cardiovascular health study. JAMA Cardiol. 2017;2(1):67–76. doi:10.1001/jamacardio.2016.4395.

Moore, Geoffrey. Crossing the chasm: marketing and selling high-tech products to mainstream customers (1991, revised 1999 and 2014). 2014.; ISBN 0-06-051712-3.

Morrison RJ, Kashlan KN, Flanangan CL, Wright JK, Green GE, Hollister SJ, Weatherwax KJ. Regulatory considerations in the design and manufacturing of implantable 3D-printed medical devices. Clin Transl Sci. 2015;8(5):594–600.

Mosso-Vázquez JL, Gao K, Wiederhold BK, Wiederhold MD. Virtual reality for pain management in cardiac surgery. Cyberpsychol Behav Soc Netw. 2014;17(6):371–8.

Neuburger M. History of medicine . Translated by Ernest Playfair. London.: H. Frowde: Oxford Medical Publications; 1910.

Ng WL, Wang S, Yeong WY, Naing MW. Skin bioprinting: impending reality or fantasy? Trends Biotechnol. 2016;34(9):689–99. doi:10.1016/j.tibtech.2016.04.006.

Global medication adherence market size, share, development, growth and demand forecast to 2022- industry insights by product, by class or medication. P&S Market Research. April 2016. http://www.reportlinker.com/p03861584-summary/Global-Medication-Adherence-Market-Size-Share-Development-Growth-and-Demand-Forecast-to-Industry-Insights-by-Product-Hardware-Centric-Offering-and-Software-Only-Offering-by-Class-or-Medication-Cardiovascular-Diabetes-Oncology-CNS-Respir.html.

Pagoto S, Schneider KL, Evans M. Tweeting it off: characteristics of adults who tweet about a weight loss attempt. J Am Med Inform Assoc. 2014;21:1032–7.

Patel R, Chang T, Greysen SR, Chopra V. Social media use in chronic disease: a systematic review and novel taxonomy. Am J Med. 2015a;128(12):1335–50.

Patel MS, Asch DA, Volpp KG. Wearable devices as facilitators, not drivers, of health behavior change. JAMA. 2015b;313(5):459–60. doi:10.1001/jama.2014.14781.

Petterson SM, Liaw WR, Phillips RL Jr, Rabin DL, Meyers DS, Bazemore AW. Projecting US primary care physician workforce needs: 2010-2025. Ann Fam Med. 2012;10(6):503–9.

Pew Research Center. Social networking fact sheet. http://www.pewinternet.org/fact-sheets/social-networking-fact-sheet/. 2013. Accessed 2 May 2016.

Preis M, Öblom H. 3D–printed drugs for children-are we ready yet ? AAPS PharmSciTech. 2017;18(2):303–8.

Randazzo M, Pisapia JM, Singh N, Thawani JP. 3D printing in neurosurgery: a systematic review. Surg Neurol Int. 2016;7(Suppl 33):S801–9.

Rochlen LR, Levine R, Tait AR. First-person point-of-view-augmented reality for central line insertion training: a usability and feasibility study. Simul Healthc. 2017;12(1):57–62.

Rogers E. Diffusion of innovations. 5th ed: Simon and Schuster; 2003. isbn:978-0-7432-5823-4.

Rosenberger ME, Buman MP, Haskell WL, McConnell MV, Carstensen LL. Twenty-four hours of sleep, sedentary behavior, and physical activity with nine wearable devices. Med Sci Sports Exerc. 2016;48(3):457–65.

Rumsfeld JS, Joynt KE, Maddox TM. Big data analytics to improve cardiovascular care: promise and challenges. Nat Rev. Cardiol. 2016;13(6):350–9.

Schlich T. Contemporary history of medicine: issues and approaches. Med J. 2007;42(3–4):269–98.

Schreinemacher MH, Graafland M, Schijven MP. Google glass in surgery. Surg Innov. 2014;21(6):651–2.

Sebelius K. mHealth summit keynote address. NCI Cancer Bullet 2011. http://www.cancer.gov. laneproxy.stanford.edu/ncicancerbulletin/121311/page4. Accessed 31 Aug 2013.

Sheldon GF, Ricketts TC, Charles A, King J, Fraher EP, Meyer A. The global health workforce shortage: role of surgeons and other providers. Adv Surg. 2008;42:63–85.

Shull PB, Jirattigalachote W, Hunt MA, Cutkosky MR, Delp SL. Quantified self and human movement: a review on the clinical impact of wearable sensing and feedback for gait analysis and intervention. Gait Posture. 2014;40(1):11–9.

Sinnenberg L, DiSilvestro CL, Mancheno C, Dailey K, Tufts C, Buttenheim AM, Barg F, Ungar L, Schwartz H, Brown D, Asch DA, Merchant RM. Twitter as a potential data source for cardiovascular disease research. JAMA Cardiol. 2016;1(9):1032–6. doi:10.1001/jamacardio.2016.3029.

Smith A. Smartphone ownership 2013. Washington, DC: Pew Research Center; 2013.

Spring B, Gotsis M, Paiva A, Spruijt-Metz D. Healthy apps: mobile devices for continuous monitoring and intervention. IEEE Pulse. 2013;4(6):34–40.

Spring B, Pfammatter A, Alshurafa N. First steps into the brave new Transdiscipline of mobile health. JAMA Cardiol. 2017;2(1):76–8. doi:10.1001/jamacardio.2016.4440.

Steinhubl SR, Muse ED, Topol EJ. Can mobile health technologies transform health care? JAMA. 2013;310(22):2395–6. doi:10.1001/jama.2013.281078.

Sweeney C. How text messages could change global healthcare [Internet]. Popular Mechanics. 2011. Availablefromhttp://www.popularmechanics.com/science/health/med-tech/how-text-messages-could-change-global-healthcare.

Out of thin air: the behind-the-scenes logistics of Kenya's mobile-money miracle. The Economist 10 June 2010. http://www.economist.com/node/16319635.

Gaza doctor Tarek Loubani creates 3D printed stethoscopes to alleviate medical supply shortages caused by blockade. The Independent, London, 2015. http://www.independent.co.uk/news/world/middle-east/gaza-doctor-tarek-loubani-creates-3d-printed-stethoscopes-to-alleviate-medical-supply-shortages-10495512.html.

Troiano RP, McClain JJ, Brychta RJ, Chen KY. Evolution of accelerometer methods for physical activity research. Br J Sports Med. 2014;48(13):1019–23.

Turakhia MP, Harrington RA. Twitter and cardiovascular disease. Useful chirps or noisy chatter? JAMA Cardiol. 2016;1(9):1036–7. doi:10.1001/jamacardio.2016.3150.

Turner-McGrievy GM, Beets MW, Moore JB, Kaczynski AT, Barr-Anderson DJ, Tate DF. Comparison of traditional versus mobile app self-monitoring of physical activity and dietary intake among overweight adults participating in an mHealth weight loss program. J Am Med Inform Assoc. 2013;20:513–8.

Walsh JA 3rd, Topol EJ, Steinhubl SR. Novel wireless devices for cardiac monitoring. Circulation. 2014;130(7):573–81.

Wengerter BC, Emre G, Park JY, Geibel J. Three-dimensional printing in the intestine. Clin Gastroenterol Hepatol. 2016;14(8):1081–5.

Wiederhold BK. Lessons learned as we begin the third decade of virtual reality. Cyberpsychol Behav Soc Netw. 2016;19(10):577–8.

Wiederhold BK, Gao K, Sulea C, Wiederhold MD. Virtual reality as a distraction technique in chronic pain patients. Cyberpsychol Behav Soc Netw. 2014;17(6):346–52.

Woods M, Rosenberg ME. Educational tools: thinking outside the box. Clin J Am Soc Nephrol. 2016;11(3):518–26.

Zheng YX, Yu DF, Zhao JG, Wu YL, Zheng B. 3D printout models vs. 3D-rendered images: which is better for preoperative planning? J Surg Educ. 2016;73(3):518–23.

Zhu M, Liu F, Chai G, Pan JJ, Jiang T, Lin L, Xin Y, Zhang Y, Li Q. A novel augmented reality system for displaying inferior alveolar nerve bundles in maxillofacial surgery. Sci Rep. 2017;7:42365.

Chapter 2
Mobile Health

Lavanya Vasudevan, Kelsey Zeller, and Alain Labrique

Abstract Rapid innovations in digital communications technologies have fueled the use of mobile phones for delivering health services and information—a phenomenon termed mobile health (mHealth). Current mHealth strategies for health service delivery range from the implementation of simple text message reminders to complex clinical decision support algorithms, and extending in recent years to connect mobile phones to sensors and other portable devices for diagnosis at the point-of-care. This chapter summarizes the current state of mHealth, important strides that have been made in strengthening the global mHealth evidence base, and key 'best practices' in scaling mHealth for achieving universal healthcare.

L. Vasudevan
Center for Health Policy and Inequalities Research, Duke Global Health Institute,
Durham, NC, USA

Department of International Health, Johns Hopkins Bloomberg School of Public Health,
Baltimore, MD, USA

Global mHealth Initiative, Johns Hopkins Bloomberg School of Public Health,
Baltimore, MD, USA

K. Zeller
Department of International Health, Johns Hopkins Bloomberg School of Public Health,
Baltimore, MD, USA

Global mHealth Initiative, Johns Hopkins Bloomberg School of Public Health,
Baltimore, MD, USA

A. Labrique (✉)
Department of International Health, Johns Hopkins Bloomberg School of Public Health,
Baltimore, MD, USA

Department of Epidemiology, Johns Hopkins Bloomberg School of Public Health,
Baltimore, MD, USA

Global mHealth Initiative, Johns Hopkins Bloomberg School of Public Health,
Baltimore, MD, USA
e-mail: alabriqu@jhsph.edu, alabriqu@gmail.com

© Springer International Publishing AG 2018
H. Rivas, K. Wac (eds.), *Digital Health*, Health Informatics,
https://doi.org/10.1007/978-3-319-61446-5_2

Keywords Mobile health • mHealth • Digital health • 12 common mHealth and ICT applications • Universal health care

2.1 Introduction

No other technological innovation has diffused through human society as rapidly as mobile phones. Mobile-cellular network infrastructure has seen an exponential growth in the last decade, reaching almost 95% of the world's population in 2016 (International Telecommunications Union 2016). Some of the most rapidly growing regions of mobile phone ownership and use are in the developing world, including countries in the Asian and sub-Saharan African continents. In concert with this growth in infrastructure, ownership, and use, the rapid evolution of mobile devices has fostered new opportunities to address information and communication challenges that previously did not exist (Qiang et al. 2012). While phone calls and short messaging service (SMS) continue to remain the most common modes of communication, mobile phones present a novel modality for internet access not previously possible in rural, hard to reach areas or for individuals without a means of accessing traditional fixed broadband connections. Currently, close to 3.6 billion people are anticipated to be reached by mobile internet services (International Telecommunications Union 2016). Massive infrastructural investments by mobile network operators in extending the reach of mobile network coverage, along with the accessibility, portability, and connectivity-on-the-go offered by mobile phones make them a widely-appealing communication medium for the delivery of information and services (World Health Organization 2009). Not surprisingly, several areas of innovation leveraging mobile phones have emerged in the last decade, including mHealth, mAgriculture, mGovernance and mFinance (Kelly et al. 2012). Increasingly, the power of mobile network connectivity is being harnessed within these mDomains to improve service delivery, user experience, and coverage, supplementing the basic phone call and text messaging services utilized by individuals in their daily lives (Kelly et al. 2012).

One area where the utilization of mobile phones has garnered much attention is health care. The use of mobile phones to optimize the delivery and receipt of health information and services, also referred to as mobile health or mHealth, is innovative for several reasons. First, the ubiquity of mobile phones makes the concept of remote health care a viable and scalable reality. No longer is health care tethered to facilities as mHealth pushes these bounds further to the communities, and in many cases to the individual themselves. Unlike prior generations of digital innovation such as telemedicine and eHealth, there has been little to no investment by the Public Health community to build this global infrastructure. Second, the fact that most mobile phone owners carry the device with them where they go, we now have the unprecedented ability to deliver health services and information to individuals where they are and when they want or need it. Third, mobile phones have allowed users of healthcare to seek information and connect to providers with ease. In many developing countries, people are using mobile phones as the preferred medium to access the internet. Consequently, their ability to seek health information-on-demand is very high, even in the absence of formalized mHealth programs. As phones incorporate increasing computational power, while becoming cheaper and sleeker, the opportunities for health service delivery via these devices are tremendous. Current mHealth strategies for health service delivery range from the implementation of simple text message reminders to complex clinical decision support algorithms, and extending in recent years to connect to sensors and other portable devices to aid diagnosis at the point-of-care (Labrique et al. 2013a).

In this chapter, we will describe the 12 key applications of mHealth that have categorized how this technology has been used in mitigating the key constraints to health systems. We will use real-world implementations of mHealth to illustrate how these technologies function across the three layers of healthcare, namely at the patient, provider and health system-level. We will briefly review the current evidence base and highlight areas where more rigorous evaluations are warranted to establish the impact of mHealth. Finally, we will close with recommendations for researchers new to mHealth on currently available resources to help plan research and implementation of these technologies.

2.2   mHealth and Its Public Health Appeal

Numerous constraints and barriers exist to providing high quality, accessible, and timely health services, especially in low-resource settings (Labrique et al. 2013a; Mehl and Labrique 2014; Agarwal et al. 2015). These health constraints impede optimal health promotion, diagnosis, and care, and can be described as barriers to (1) information, (2) availability, (3) quality, (4) acceptability, (5) utilization, (6) efficiency, or (7) cost related to health or health services (Mehl and Labrique 2014; Mehl et al. 2015). The "bottom billion", representing the world's poorest populations, receives health care predominantly from low trained, non-facility based frontline health workers (Agarwal et al. 2015; Kallander et al. 2013). Equipping these frontline health workers with mHealth solutions helps bring these clients under the umbrella of the traditional health system, allowing them to be counted and enumerated, which builds accountability for frontline health workers to their supervisors. mHealth interventions capitalize on key features inherent in mobile technologies to bridge these constraints. In settings where women frequently give birth at home, the decision to seek medical help during delivery can be a difficult one (Kim et al. 2012; Kruk et al. 2016; Sikder et al. 2011). In many cases, women require family approval and input before such a decision is made. Even without the need for co-decision making, the choice to move to a health facility is complicated, weighing the potential financial costs and/or difficulty of reaching the facility in light of the woman's obstetric risks during childbirth (Sikder et al. 2014). mHealth interventions may act in several ways to reduce these barriers. In a more robust system, where frontline health workers have registered every pregnancy and are aware of impending births, they can be held accountable for attending these births, advocating for women, and helping the family make the decision when it is time to go to a health facility. Several mHealth interventions aim to compress this delay, using methods ranging from digital population registries to SMS-based labor and birth notification (Kruk et al. 2016; McNabb et al. 2015). In the event an extensive registry system like this is not available, provision of one simple thing-the emergency contact number of the designated frontline health worker to the woman and her family-enables the family to connect with a supportive decision-maker. Leveraging simple SMS-based delivery of health information leading up to childbirth about reasons for delays/danger signs can also help women and other key members of her family make a decision to seek medical attention in a timely manner (Lund et al. 2012).

2.3   The 12 Common mHealth and ICT Applications

The 12 common mHealth and ICT applications are currently the most widely adopted categorization of the ways in which mobile technologies are used for the delivery of health services and information (Fig. 2.1) (Labrique et al. 2013a).

The 12 applications are cross-cutting—extending across the three layers of the healthcare system—patient, provider and broader system. At the client level, there are extensive examples for the use of mHealth as a medium to deliver behavior change communication in a variety of health domains. Current implementations focus on leveraging simple communication modalities such as phone calls and text messaging to reach a broad audience—especially for those without access to smartphone technologies and 'apps'. Examples include the use of text messaging services or interactive voice response systems for the delivery of health information related to family planning, pregnancy and newborn care, immunizations, and management of chronic illnesses. In South Africa, the national Ministry of Health has capitalized

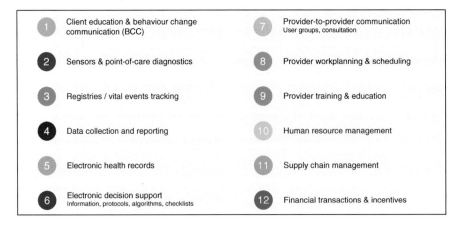

Fig. 2.1 Twelve common mHealth and ICT applications (Labrique et al. 2013a)

on high mobile phone ownership among pregnant women to register them and provide age and stage-appropriate messages related to their health and the health of their babies (Department of Health, Republic of South Africa 2014; Johnson and Johnson 2014). Similarly, the Mobile 4 Reproductive Health (m4RH) program provided family planning information on demand in Kenya and Tanzania. In a randomized control trial in Kenya, individuals accessing m4RH had 13% higher family planning knowledge compared to control individuals (FHI360 2017; L'Engle et al. 2013; Willoughby and L'Engle 2015). Other examples include the provision of mobile phone-based reminders, either for upcoming clinical visits or for adherence to medication regimens. The mTika project in Bangladesh was successful in improving timely vaccination coverage in rural areas as well as urban slums in Dhaka through text message reminders to mothers about upcoming vaccination appointments (Uddin et al. 2016). In rural Kenya, mobile phone text messaging promoted adherence to antiretroviral therapy in HIV patients (Chang et al. 2012). At their very core, mHealth deployments facilitate communication between patients and providers as well as within peer groups (Rotheram-Borus et al. 2012). This improved access to a clinical or non-clinical support network alone may impact the ability of individuals to monitor their own health.

In contrast to the simple modes of communication on client-focused mHealth deployments, implementations of mHealth for streamlining health service delivery by providers may be more complex, often leveraging smartphone technology. This means providers using mobile phones have the ability to collect, manage, and longitudinally track patient data on mobile phones. The Open Smart Register Platform (OpenSRP) is a tablet-based data management system for frontline health workers to register and track their community-based clients longitudinally (THRIVE consortium 2017). OpenSRP includes several features such as automated scheduling to prioritize services to clients, risk profiling to prioritize clients in need for immediate attention, dynamic patient look ups that facilitate the ability to pull up relevant patient records, and automated reporting to improve timeliness of data use and reduce the reporting burden for the frontline health worker. Finally, multimedia integration abilities support provider-initiated counseling using OpenSRP. Advanced clinical decision-support algorithms may be programmed into the phone such that health providers may be guided in clinical decision-making. For instance, D-Tree's electronic integrated management of childhood illness (eIMCI) application promoted higher adherence to the IMCI protocol by health providers compared to a paper version of the protocol (Mitchell et al. 2012; Derenzi et al. 2008). Mobile phones also enable providers to connect to each other, enhancing the ability to seek expert support for complex cases, make referrals, and coordinate care. Closed user groups such as that managed by Switchboard in Ghana allow trained health workers to call within their network at no cost (Kaonga et al. 2013a; b). This encourages peer-problem solving and communication. Several portable point-of-care diagnostic devices such as ultrasounds, heart monitors, and glucometers now come with the ability to connect wirelessly to mobile devices such that readings are automatically processed, captured, and displayed in meaningful ways. The portability of these devices implies that preventive screening and diagnostics can be conducted at the point-of-care or in community-based settings such that the coverage of preventive programs is maximized. Examples include AlivCor Heart Monitor, MobiUS SP1 ultrasound and the Pocket Colposcope (Lam et al. 2015; MobiSante 2016.; AliveCor 2016).

At the health system-level, mHealth-facilitated data collection ensures that health management information is available in a reliable and timely manner to support decision-making and resource allocation. Web-based dashboards and analytics support meaningful visualization of health determinants, health status, and human resources, making it easier for the district or national-level health managers to make informed decisions and prioritize areas of need. The District Health Information System (DHIS 2) is currently used in over 40 countries to monitor health and human resource performance at the district and national levels (Health Information Systems Programme, University of Oslo 2017). Platforms such as iHRIS are customized for tracking and managing health worker performance and training (Intrahealth 2017). mHealth deployments can be used to track and manage the supply chain for essential commodities and medicines, reducing incidences of stock-outs. SMS for Life used text message-based check-ins with hospital pharmacies about essential commodity levels to reduce stock-outs of anti-malarials (Barrington et al. 2010). Other supply tracking systems such as cStock include performance planning for district product availability teams, thereby building capacity while supporting logistics management (Dimagi 2016). Health management systems also allow surveillance of diseases and can be used to pre-empt outbreaks, thereby reducing delays in response (Vasudevan et al. 2016).

Complex health systems require multiple solutions to address equally complex constraints. With the recent establishment of new global health targets under the sustainable development goals, universal health care (UHC) has emerged as a key area of focus. UHC encompasses three key concepts—equitable access, quality healthcare, and protection from financial risk (World Health Organization 2017). In this context, the domain of mHealth has seen a renewed interest based on recognition by global stakeholders that it represents a comprehensive strategy addressing these key concepts—the use of mHealth for client enumeration, development of registries to track patient care, and coverage of essential interventions can be leveraged to facilitate and monitor achievement of UHC (Mehl and Labrique 2014; Labrique et al. 2012). Digital patient records using systems such as OpenMRS promote continuity in care and informed clinical decision-making that was previously challenging in the era of fragmented paper-based recordkeeping systems (Regenstrief Institute 2017). In parallel, mHealth interventions that take advantage of mobile financial transactions to promote savings, health insurance payments or provide reimbursements for health services can make healthcare costs more affordable, reducing the financial burden on clients (Wakadha et al. 2013).

2.4   Evidence for mHealth Impact

The term, mHealth, was first coined by Istepanian in 2004. With the emergence of smartphone technologies from 2006–2010, the field of mHealth entered a phase of rapid innovation and, in parallel, unfettered proliferation. The rampant duplication of mHealth projects led to the coining of the term, "pilotitis", highlighting the frequent failure of mHealth projects to translate beyond small-scale (i.e., pilot) implementations (Labrique et al. 2013b). The 2011 Bellagio eHealth declaration warned that mHealth implementation must be guided by evidence, going as far as stating that 'if used improperly, (e)Health may divert valuable resources and even cause harm' (Fraser et al. 2011). Tomlinson and others offered strategies to streamline efforts in mHealth—encouraging innovative research designs, interoperability, and a focus on the scalability and sustainability (Tomlinson et al. 2013). During this time, we reported that mHealth evidence was emerging and that there were ongoing research studies that would enrich our understanding of the impact these technologies have on health and service delivery. Currently, there are several systematic reviews that describe the growing evidence base for strategies of mHealth. (Agarwal et al. 2015; Free et al. 2013a; b; Beratarrechea et al. 2014; Bloomfield et al. 2014; Watterson et al. 2015; L'Engle et al. 2016).

There is also a growing recognition that mHealth projects have a unique project maturity pathway. As mHealth projects evolve from pilot to scale, evaluations must be tailored to ask relevant questions at different time points—ranging from feasibility and usability at earlier time points to efficacy and cost-effectiveness at later stages. A recent 2017 WHO toolkit reviews the range of stage-appropriate methods of evaluation and program monitoring from observational studies to randomized trials (see Box 2.1).

Box 2.1 Useful Resources and Tools for mHealth Researchers

1. ASH compendia	http://www.africanstrategies4health.Org/Mhealth-database.Html
2. mHealthknowledge	http://www.Mhealthknowledge.Org/Resources/Mhealth-Compendium-Database
3. K4Health mHealth planning guide	https://www.k4health.Org/toolkits/mhealth-planning-guide
4. mFHW report	https://media.Wix.Com/ugd/f85b85_cc8c132e31014d91b108f8dba524fb86.Pdf
5. MAPS toolkit—readiness for scale	http://www.Who.Int/reproductivehealth/topics/mhealth/maps-toolkit/en/
6. mERA guidelines for reporting	http://www.Who.Int/reproductivehealth/topics/mhealth/mERA-checklist/en/
7. Monitoring and evaluating digital health interventions: A practical guide to conducting research and assessment	http://www.Who.Int/reproductivehealth/publications/mhealth/digital-health-interventions/en/
8. PMNCH country readiness for ICT/RMNCH	http://www.Who.Int/pmnch/knowledge/publications/ict_mhealth.Pdf
9. eHealth strategy—enabling environment (WHO-ITU toolkit)	http://www.Itu.Int/pub/D-STR-E_HEALTH.05-2012
10. A practical guide for engaging with mobile operators in mHealth for RMNCH	http://www.Who.Int/reproductivehealth/publications/mhealth/mobile-operators-mhealth/en/

2.5 New Frontiers in mHealth

Important, across the examples presented in this chapter, is the recognition of inherent diversity in the emergent field of mHealth. Digital solutions, or strategies, align to the need or problem being addressed. The importance of clarity in describing the form and function of specific mHealth solutions cannot be undervalued, and forms a key point of the 2016 mHealth Evaluation Reporting and Assessment (mERA) guidelines (Agarwal et al. 2016). Disambiguation is critical to promotion the sharing of experiences and to reducing redundancy and re-invention in this field.

Over the past 5 years, important strides have been made in recognizing the existence of key 'best practices' in this space, enshrined in the ICT4D principles (Fig. 2.2).

Many are also acknowledging the importance of donor and government investments in the ecosystem and information systems architecture to promote more robust and scalable innovations, reducing the risk of "pilotitis". Most importantly, it is critical to keep in mind the importance of a systems approach to health problem solving, where mHealth strategies are one facet of a complex solution addressing the multidimensional root causes of the problem. mHealth strategies, derived from the information and communications revolution, solve problems which are inherently information and communications obstacles. Improved information and communications in the hands of the patient, the provider and the health system policy makers can help catalyze programs with known efficacy and impact potential. In thinking about the role of mHealth as part of a complex solution, it is best to view it as a catalyst, or digital "adjuvant", helping to improve the coverage, quality or demand for public health interventions we know can save or improve lives. Whether these are vaccine programs or nutritional interventions, mHealth strategies might be, in some cases, the missing ingredient to achieve the levels of effective or universal coverage so sought after in global health.

[AU6]

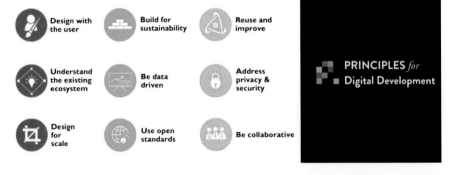

Fig. 2.2 The ICT4D (Information Communication Technologies for Development) principles endorsed by many development organizations, including USAID, World Bank, DFID, UNICEF and others (http://digitalimpactalliance.org/why-the-world-bank-endorses-the-principles-for-digital-development/)

References

Agarwal S, Perry HB, Long LA, Labrique AB. Evidence on feasibility and effective use of mHealth strategies by frontline health workers in developing countries: systematic review. Tropical Med Int Health. 2015;20(8):1003–14.

Agarwal S, LeFevre AE, Lee J, et al. Guidelines for reporting of health interventions using mobile phones: mobile health (mHealth) evidence reporting and assessment (mERA) checklist. BMJ. 2016;352:i1174.

AliveCor. Take control of your heart health; 2016.

Barrington J, Wereko-Brobby O, Ward P, Mwafongo W, Kungulwe S. SMS for life: a pilot project to improve anti-malarial drug supply management in rural Tanzania using standard technology. Malar J. 2010;9(1):298.

Beratarrechea A, Lee AG, Willner JM, Jahangir E, Ciapponi A, Rubinstein A. The impact of mobile health interventions on chronic disease outcomes in developing countries: a systematic review. Telemed J e-Health. 2014;20(1):75–82.

Bloomfield GS, Vedanthan R, Vasudevan L, Kithei A, Were M, Velazquez EJ. Mobile health for non-communicable diseases in sub-Saharan Africa: a systematic review of the literature and strategic framework for research. Glob Health. 2014;10:49.

Chang LW, Arem H, Ssempijja V, Serwadda D, Quinn TC, Reynolds SJ. Impact of a mHealth intervention for peer health workers on AIDS care in rural Uganda: a mixed methods evaluation of a cluster-randomized trial. AIDS Behav. 2012;15(8):1776–84.

Department of Health, Republic of South Africa. MomConnect. 2014. http://www.health.gov.za/index.php/mom-connect. Accessed 14 Mar 2017.

Derenzi B, Mitchell M, Schellenberg D, Lesh N, Sims C, Maokola W. e-IMCI: improving pediatric health care in low-income countries. 2008.

Dimagi. cStock: supply chains for community case management; 2016.

FHI360. Mobile for Reproductive Health (m4RH). 2017.; http://m4rh.fhi360.org/. Accessed 14 Mar 2017.

Fraser H, Bailey C, Sinha C, Mehl G, Labrique AB. Call to action on global eHealth evaluation. Consensus statement of the WHO Global eHealth Evaluation Meeting, Bellagio, Italy. 2011.

Free C, Phillips G, Watson L, et al. The effectiveness of mobile-health technologies to improve health care service delivery processes: a systematic review and meta-analysis. PLoS Med. 2013a;10(1):e1001363.

Free C, Phillips G, Galli L, et al. The effectiveness of mobile-health technology-based health behaviour change or disease management interventions for health care consumers: a systematic review. PLoS Med. 2013b;10(1):e1001362.

Health Information Systems Programme, University of Oslo. District Health Information System 2 (DHIS2): collect, manage, visualize and explore your data. 2017. https://www.dhis2.org/. Accessed 14 Mar 2017.

International Telecommunications Union. ICT facts and figs. 2016.

Intrahealth. iHRIS: open source human resources information solution. 2017.; https://www.ihris.org/. Accessed 14 Mar 2017.

Johnson and Johnson. MomConnect: Connecting Women to Care, One Text at a Time. 2014. https://www.jnj.com/our-giving/momconnect-connecting-women-to-care-one-text-at-a-time. Accessed 14 Mar 2017.

Kallander K, Tibenderana JK, Akpogheneta OJ, et al. Mobile health (mHealth) approaches and lessons for increased performance and retention of community health workers in low- and middle-income countries: a review. J Med Internet Res. 2013;15(1):e17.

Kaonga NN, Labrique A, Mechael P, et al. Mobile phones and social structures: an exploration of a closed user group in rural Ghana. BMC Med Inform Decis Mak. 2013a;13:100.

Kaonga NN, Labrique A, Mechael P, et al. Using social networking to understand social networks: analysis of a mobile phone closed user group used by a Ghanaian health team. J Med Internet Res. 2013b;15(4):e74.

Kelly T, Friederici N, Minges M, Yamamichi M. Information and communications for development. The World Bank. 2012: maximizing mobile. Washington DC. 2012.

Kim JM, Labrique A, West KP, et al. Maternal morbidity in early pregnancy in rural northern
Bangladesh. Int J Gynaecol Obstet. 2012;119(3):227–33.

Kruk ME, Kujawski S, Moyer CA, et al. Next generation maternal health: external shocks and
health-system innovations. Lancet. 2016;

Labrique AB, Pereira S, Christian P, Murthy N, Bartlett L, Mehl G. Pregnancy registration systems can enhance health systems, increase accountability and reduce mortality. Reprod Health
Matters. 2012;20(39):113–7.

Labrique AB, Vasudevan L, Kochi E, Fabricant R, Mehl G. mHealth innovations as health system
strengthening tools: 12 common applications and a visual framework. Glob Health Sci Pract.
2013a;1(2):160–71.

Labrique A, Vasudevan L, Chang LW, Mehl G. H_pe for mHealth: more "y" or "o" on the horizon?
Int J Med Inform. 2013b;82(5):467–9.

Lam CT, Krieger MS, Gallagher JE, et al. Design of a novel low cost point of care tampon
(POCkeT) Colposcope for use in resource limited settings. PLoS One. 2015;10(9):e0135869.

L'Engle KL, Vahdat HL, Ndakidemi E, Lasway C, Zan T. Evaluating feasibility, reach and potential impact of a text message family planning information service in Tanzania. Contraception.
2013;87(2):251–6.

L'Engle KL, Mangone ER, Parcesepe AM, Agarwal S, Ippoliti NB. Mobile phone interventions for
adolescent sexual and reproductive health: a systematic review. Pediatrics. 2016;138(3). http://
pediatrics.aappublications.org/content/138/3/e20160884.long

Lund S, Hemed M, Nielsen BB, et al. Mobile phones as a health communication tool to improve
skilled attendance at delivery in Zanzibar: a cluster-randomised controlled trial. BJOG.
2012;119(10):1256–64.

McNabb M, Chukwu E, Ojo O, et al. Assessment of the quality of antenatal care services provided
by health workers using a mobile phone decision support application in northern Nigeria: a pre/
post-intervention study. PLoS One. 2015;10(5):e0123940.

Mehl G, Labrique A. Prioritizing integrated mHealth strategies for universal health coverage.
Science. 2014;345(6202):1284–7.

Mehl G, Vasudevan L, Gonsalves L, et al. Harnessing mHealth in low-resource settings to overcome health system constraints and achieve universal access to health. In: Marsch LA, Lord
SE, Dallery J, editors. Behavioral health care and technology: using science-based innovations
to transform practice. Oxford: Oxford University Press; 2015. p. 239–64.

Mitchell M, Getchell M, Nkaka M, Msellemu D, Van Esch J, Hedt-Gauthier B. Perceived
improvement in integrated management of childhood illness implementation through use of
mobile technology: qualitative evidence from a pilot study in Tanzania. J Health Commun.
2012;17(Suppl 1):118–27.

MobiSante: Imaging at the point of c. Smartphone Ultrasound: The MobiUS SP1 system; 2016.

Qiang CZ, Yamamichi M, Hausman V, Miller R. Mobile applications for the health sector.
Washington DC: The World Bank; 2012.

Regenstrief Institute, Partners in health. Open Medical Record System (OpenMRS). 2017.; http://
openmrs.org/. Accessed 14 Mar 2017.

Rotheram-Borus MJ, Tomlinson M, Gwegwe M, Comulada WS, Kaufman N, Keim M. Diabetes
buddies: peer support through a mobile phone buddy system. Diabetes Educ. 2012;38(3):357–65.

Sikder SS, Labrique AB, Ullah B, et al. Accounts of severe acute obstetric complications in rural
Bangladesh. BMC Pregnancy Childbirth. 2011;11:76.

Sikder SS, Labrique AB, Shamim AA, et al. Risk factors for reported obstetric complications and
near misses in rural northwest Bangladesh: analysis from a prospective cohort study. BMC
Pregnancy Childbirth. 2014;14:347.

THRIVE consortium. Open Smart Register Platform (OpenSRP). 2017. http://smartregister.org/
index.html. Accessed 14 Mar 2017.

Tomlinson M, Rotheram-Borus MJ, Swartz L, Tsai AC. Scaling up mHealth: where is the evidence? PLoS Med. 2013;10(2):e1001382.

Uddin MJ, Shamsuzzaman M, Horng L, et al. Use of mobile phones for improving vaccination coverage among children living in rural hard-to-reach areas and urban streets of Bangladesh. Vaccine. 2016;34(2):276–83.

Vasudevan L, Ghoshal S, Labrique A. mHealth and its role in disease surveillance. In: Blazes DL, Lewis SH, editors. Disease surveillance: technological contributions to global health security. Boca Raton, FL: CRC Press; 2016.

Wakadha H, Chandir S, Were EV, et al. The feasibility of using mobile-phone based SMS reminders and conditional cash transfers to improve timely immunization in rural Kenya. Vaccine. 2013;31(6):987–93.

Watterson JL, Walsh J, Madeka I. Using mHealth to improve usage of antenatal care, postnatal care, and immunization: a systematic review of the literature. Biomed Res Int. 2015;2015:153402.

Willoughby JF, L'Engle KL. Influence of perceived interactivity of a sexual health text message service on young people's attitudes, satisfaction and repeat use. Health Educ Res. 2015;30(6):996–1003.

World Health Organization. mHealth: New horizons for health through mobile technologies. Switzerland. 2009.

World Health Organization. What is universal health coverage? 2017. http://www.who.int/health_financing/universal_coverage_definition/en/. Accessed 14 Mar 2017.

Chapter 3
Redesigning Healthcare Systems to Provide Better and Faster Care at a Lower Cost

J.P. van der Heijden and L. Witkamp

Abstract The use of information and communication technologies in the healthcare industry has been referred to as "telemedicine" or "e-health." Our healthcare systems are facing big increases in demand due to growing elderly populations, rising chronic diseases, and the rapid development of new treatments; thus, the use of telemedicine is believed to be a part of the solution in restructuring and redesigning our healthcare systems. Despite often positive results, many telemedicine services remain stuck in a pilot or experimental phase and never make it to a larger implementation. The most important obstacle is the lack of structural financial reimbursement and available budget. In The Netherlands, we have developed and successfully applied our Health Management Practice (HMP) Model on a large number of telemedicine services using the "start small, think big" approach, leading to fully integrated telemedicine services. Results show a 70–96% reduction in hospital visits in dermatology and ophthalmology, which translates into an immediate cost reduction of 18%. Response times of 4–5 working hours and the learning effect have a high impact on the quality of care delivered. Telemonitoring programs in mental health have shown that involving the patient as an active actor can result in more motivation and ownership of their own health. Telemedicine also allows hospitals to remain focused on delivering high-quality specialized care. In many peripheral centers in residential areas, more routine care services will be delivered close to the patient by paramedics, caregivers, and patients themselves under the direction and supervision of a general practitioner and medical specialist at a distance.

J.P. van der Heijden, Ph.D. (✉)
Research and Development, KSYOS TeleMedical Center, Amsterdam, The Netherlands
e-mail: j.vanderheijden@ksyos.org

L. Witkamp, Ph.D., M.D.
Department of Medical Informatics, KSYOS TeleMedical Centre, Academic Medical Centre Amsterdam, Amsterdam, The Netherlands

© Springer International Publishing AG 2018
H. Rivas, K. Wac (eds.), *Digital Health*, Health Informatics,
https://doi.org/10.1007/978-3-319-61446-5_3

Keywords Telemedicine • e-Health • Healthcare redesign • Telemonitoring • Teledermatology • Telecardiology • e-Mental health • Tele-ophthalmology • m-Health • Blended care • Digital health • Implementation

3.1 Fundamentals of Telemedicine

Healthcare systems worldwide are under stress mainly due to the expanding elderly population. The World Health Organization states that the percentage of people over 60-years-old will double to 22% by 2050. This effect is a result of improved sanitation and medical services as well as breakthroughs in medical technologies and pharmaceuticals. Furthermore, low- and middle-income countries often lack adequate healthcare infrastructure and their populations have little access to healthcare services (Mills et al. 2014). Finally, the rise of chronic diseases, such as diabetes, cancer, and dementia, increase demand for long-term healthcare plans (World Health Organization 2015). These problems can only be addressed by restructuring and redesigning our healthcare systems. One of the technologies that is believed to be a big driver and also part of the solution is the Internet in its broadest sense. "Broadest" here means the three primary characteristics of the Internet that in the last decade have changed how many industries work (e.g., travel, finance, retail): (1) its ability to have people efficiently share and access information from and to almost anywhere and anyone, (2) it provides communication (real-time, store, and forward) between actors (human and machine) anywhere in the world, closing the gaps of physical distance and time, and (3) it provides a platform for creating networks and communities. The use of these attributes in the healthcare industry has been referred to as "telemedicine" or "E-health".

The term "telemedicine" has been around since the 1960s and 1970s, when pioneers used telephone and telegraph networks to deliver care to remote locations (Preston et al. 1992). However, by the end of the twentieth century and as the Internet was emerging, its popularity grew and the term telemedicine was heard and read frequently within the healthcare domain. The term covers a spectrum of novel interventions that leverage the capabilities of the Internet. Medical domains dealing with imaging and visual based diagnostics (e.g., radiology, dermatology, pathology) were among the first to start embracing this new technology (Grigsby et al. 1995). The potential for more efficient and cost-effective delivery of healthcare has driven the development of numerous telemedicine services like teleconsultation, telediagnostics, telemonitoring, and telecare in almost all medical fields throughout the world over the next decade with various outcomes in effectiveness and in different implementations and business models (Ekeland et al. 2010; Mistry 2012; Chen et al. 2013). To give some indication of the scope of the field, at the time of writing, MEDLINE had indexed 23,367 articles when searched for "telemedicine" or "e-health."

The terminology used to describe telemedicine services has also exploded the last 10 years. Other associated terms include e-health, telehealth, health 2.0, smart-health, m-health, digital health, blended care, and connected health, which makes it difficult to reach a common understanding of what is being discussed or described. E-health is the term most commonly used and mostly in a broad context, including everything having to do with some electronic/digital function in the domains of wellness, health, and healthcare both in the professional, but even more so in the consumer sphere.

E-health instruments in the consumer sphere range from wearables, self-measurement, self-diagnostics via demotic products such as step counters, smart scales, and anti-depression lighting solutions to a wide range of medical/health apps on mobile devices. "Dr. Google" and websites offering vast libraries of information in these domains exist both with and without validation or medical certification.

In the professional sphere, e-health instruments include, for example, electronic health record (EHR) systems and interoperability systems connecting the EHRs, certified and approved medical devices, prosthetics and robotics, decision support and predictive big data systems, and, finally, what we understand to be telemedicine services:

A care process or the whole of several care processes that meets both of the following two characteristics:

1. *A distance (physical or temporal) is bridged by using both information technology and telecommunications, and.*
2. *There are at least two actors involved in the care process, of which at least one is a registered healthcare professional or under the supervision of a registered healthcare professional.*

Two important notes should be made here. First, using this definition, telemedicine is positioned in the professional domain as a registered healthcare provides has to be involved. A comparison can be made with pharmaceuticals, where self-medication drugs which can be acquired without prescription are counterpart to all consumer sphere e-health instruments freely available to the public and prescription drugs, where a prescription by a healthcare professional is needed, are the counterpart to telemedicine care processes. Just as there are different rule sets in place for over-the-counter and prescription drugs, this comparison immediately outlines an idea on how we could and maybe even should deal with the evaluation, validation and certification, admission, and reimbursement of these telemedicine services. This is elaborated on later in this chapter.

The second argument is that most, if not all, telemedicine services (should) represent a redesign of care processes that already exist, using innovative technologies (the internet and new soft- and hardware). Following this logic, telemedicine is *medicine* (and e-health is *health*); thus, it is to be expected that the prefixes "tele" and "e" in the healthcare domain will disappear when these new services become the industry standard, similar to how nobody talks about e-booking, e-tickets, and e-banking anymore. To get to that industry standard, however, there are some obstacles to overcome in the implementation and upscaling of telemedicine.

3.2   Implementing and Upscaling: The Dutch HMP Model and Use Case

The most commonly heard problem with embedding telemedicine services in regular healthcare systems is that a large proportion of these services remain at a pilot or experimental phase, despite often positive results, and never make it to a larger implementation (Broens 2007). The reasons for this vary and can be found in any of the following categories: technology, acceptance, financing, organization or policy, and legislation. However, the most critical and perennial obstacle to implementation has been the lack of structural financial reimbursement for telemedicine services. Often, it is not a case that the local system of reimbursement cannot handle these redesigned healthcare processes—rather, it is the lack of an appropriated budget.

There are many frameworks and models described in the literature aimed at providing implementation roadmaps for telemedicine services that convey advice on how to avoid or handle these obstacles (e.g., the Health Readiness Instrument for Developing Countries, the Layered Telemedicine Implementation Model, the PACS Maturity Model, the Telemedicine Process Model, and the NHS Maturity model (Broens 2007; Khoja et al. 2007; Haris 2010; Van de Wetering and Batenburg 2009; Wynchank and Van Dyk 2011)). Although these models differ in their approach on some levels, they are united on two accords: (1) they follow the "*start small, think big*" approach and (2) they prioritize their change management strategy.

In The Netherlands, we have developed and successfully applied our own model—the Health Management Practice (HMP) Model—on a large number of telemedicine services using the "start small, think big" approach (Witkamp and van der Heijden 2012). Additionally, the change management strategy was ensured by a dedicated telemedicine provider (KSYOS TeleMedical Centre) commissioned to drive and oversee the implementation. Results of these implementations will be given later in this chapter. The HMP model encompasses a four-phase approach that enables private and public parties to jointly develop, research, and implement new telemedicine services (see Table 3.1).

Table 3.1 Health management practice phases

Phase 1	A specific telemedicine service is developed and is tested internally by the development team for usability and safety for a period of 1–2 months
Phase 2	10–20 future users (health providers and patients) test this telemedicine service for usability and feasibility in regular practice for a period of 3–6 months
Phase 3	50–100 future users (health providers and patients) test for a period of 6–12 months whether the telemedicine service actually contributes to improved efficiency in the healthcare process, a higher production volume, and/or better quality at lower or the same cost.
Phase 4	Many users (between 100 and 1000) in a full implementation of the telemedicine service generate data in real life settings for a period of 1–2 years. These are used to investigate large scale cost efficiency. Results can be used in developing sustainable business cases

The phases are executed in a consecutive manner and are non-overlapping. The completion of all phases for a service takes between 2 and 4 years, however the telemedicine service is already running in real practice after 2 months. More details on HMP can be found in a previous publication (Witkamp and van der Heijden 2012).

The following sections describe how development of the service, evidence of effectives, healthy reimbursement and successful implementation can be achieved in concordance with the HMP phases.

3.2.1 Health Management Development

Telemedicine stakeholders—manufacturers, service providers, end-users (patients, caregivers, healthcare practitioners), policy makers, and health insurers—should all be actively involved in the redesign of the healthcare process to ensure a solid support platform. In phase 1 of the HMP it is important to always start with a clear understanding of the current healthcare pathways, i.e., what technologies are used, in which care process(es), in which health care sector, and what actors (primary and secondary) are involved. The new telemedicine service should not be on top of the old care processes, but should aim to replace parts or the whole process by redesigning the old care process using innovative technologies. Technology combined with redesigned healthcare processes should lead to an integrated telemedicine service, including a description on how to address the following issues: software used, hardware used, infrastructure interoperability, hosting and education that meet (national) requirements of safety, security, certification, connectivity, and user friendliness.

3.2.2 Health Management Research

Independent research should be performed during HMP phase 2, 3 and 4 to evaluate different outcomes, depending on the implementation phase. Ultimately, the aim is to collect effectiveness evidence on the telemedicine service resulting in increased efficiency and better quality of care at equal or lower cost. To determine quality aspects of the telemedicine service, the questions on the elements described in Table 3.2 can be a starting point (Ossenbaard and Duivenbode n.d.). These questions were derived from a think tank of experts organized by the Dutch National Institute for ICT in Healthcare.

The evaluation of telemedicine services has proven difficult through classic randomized controlled trial designs, mostly because such studies tend to be long and drawn out and, therefore, unable to keep up with the fast pace of technology development; that is, the object of the research is like a "moving target" (Ossenbaard and Duivenbode n.d.). Moreover, telemedicine services are often complex interventions with multiple actors and, as such, unsuitable for the RCT models that work so well for pharmaceuticals research (Ossenbaard and Duivenbode n.d.).

Table 3.2 Telemedicine quality elements

Safety	Are the risks or unintended effects of the telemedicine service on the health of the patient known and restricted to an acceptable minimum?
Effectiveness	Is the telemedicine service based on scientific evidence and does it realize the desired effect in terms of process of care or outcomes (cheaper, better, faster)?
Patient centeredness	Does the telemedicine service have a central focus on the needs and preferences of the patient (self-management, ease of use, accessibility, reliability, privacy, etc.)?
Timeliness	Is the telemedicine service available and accessible when required?
Expediency	Does the telemedicine service contribute to reducing overtreatment, under treatment, non-adherence, lack of transparency, or poor care coordination?
Justness	Is the telemedicine service equally useful for everyone, regardless of personal or social characteristics?

New methodologies for evaluation research are being developed specifically to manage these characteristics of telemedicine services, such as the Trials of Intervention Principles (TIP) method (Ossenbaard and Duivenbode n.d.), Multiphase Optimization Strategy Trials (MOST) (Ossenbaard and Duivenbode n.d.), Sequential Multiple Assignment Randomized Trial (SMART) (Ossenbaard and Duivenbode n.d.), Continuous Evaluation of Evolving Behavioral Intervention Technologies (CEEBIT) (Ossenbaard and Duivenbode n.d.), and the Health Technology Assessment-based Model for Assessment of Telemedicine Applications (MAST) (Ossenbaard and Duivenbode n.d.).

The debate on the best methodology is ongoing; however, for those who are implementing telemedicine, the important goal should be to obtain appropriate evidence. There is no one-size-fits-all method and one should choose the method that best fits the enquiry.

3.2.3   Health Management Business Models

Telemedicine stakeholders should all be actively involved in the development of the reimbursement models. When significant effectiveness results on a macro level have been proven in phase 3 of the HMP, the next step is to create a healthy business case to support the full implementation of the telemedicine service. The interested parties together establish a price for the use of the telemedicine service and predefine the performance indicators required for reimbursement. These performance indicators may entail health outcomes as well as logistic outcomes. To assure successful full scale implementation in regular care, active support and marketing from all stakeholders should take place.

The biggest barrier, as mentioned earlier, is the availability of a working budget and for reimbursement. It is up to government, insurers, and relevant parties to work toward the contracting of innovative healthcare services. Indeed, provided that sufficient funds are available, the following six topics may facilitate the safe and expeditious introduction and implementation of telemedicine services and should already be taken into consideration when starting phase 1 of the HMP (Witkamp 2016).

3.2.3.1   Societal Business Case

Providers of telemedicine have demonstrated that their services lead to better, faster care, closer to the patient and at lower cost in phase 1, 2 and 3 of the HMP. Health insurers should not hesitate to compensate promising services, even if the effect in the long-term is likely, but not certain.

3.2.3.2   Business Case Stakeholders

Telemedicine providers should ensure that all stakeholders of the telemedicine service experience benefits. Examples of such benefits are the patient receiving very fast feedback through teleconsultation instead of waiting and travel time, the general practitioner experiencing a learning effect that improves the quality of healthcare they provide, the medical specialist strengthening professional relations with local GPs in the region and having higher job satisfaction, and the hospital benefiting through improved adherence (Witkamp 2016).

3.2.3.3   Low-Hanging Fruit

Parties should scale telemedicine services for simple routine care processes that have already been proven and already have been implemented in exemplar regions in phase 3 of the HMP. These services so far have the largest proven social benefit when scaled up, because routine care processes tend to deal with large numbers of patients resulting in high impact.

3.2.3.4   Current Reimbursement System

Parties should stop identifying existing compensation system as an obstacle to telemedicine implementation. Telemedicine services are a redesign of existing care processes. Thus, within existing laws and regulations, all telemedicine services can and will be reimbursed.

3.2.3.5   High-Quality Care in the Second Line

Parties should reduce benefits for simple routine professional care and increase fees for the care of complex, and serious problems. This allows simple routine care to be redesigned and transferred to primary care under the supervision of medical specialists who, in part, have the ability to free up time to deliver care for which they are trained.

3.2.3.6 Admission

A system is needed where a central body evaluates new telemedicine services and approves them for admission, which, in turn, compels the health insurer to reimburse.

3.2.4 *Health Management Implementation*

Challenges and barriers on the road to a successful telemedicine service implementation can be overcome when a care institution, department within a care institution, or a commercial company acts as a dedicated telemedicine provider, thus offering a single organization that lobbies for telemedicine services, manages the complete telemedicine service implementation, acts as the point of contact for patients, care professionals, and other actors such as government and supervisory bodies. The responsibilities and tasks that a telemedicine provider should incorporate during phase 3 and 4 of the HMP to set up a telemedicine service are:

- Administration, registration, and storage of clinical records.
- Negotiating sustainable reimbursement with healthcare insurers.
- Handle claiming and crediting incorrect claims.
- Imbursement of involved actors (e.g., specialist, general practitioner, telemedicine provider staff).
- Providing clinical liability insurance specifically tailored to telemedicine procedures.
- Providing a telemedicine software platform and keeping it up-to-date in concordance with the latest security standards, legislation, and regulations.
- Providing suitable hardware for telemedicine procedures (e.g., smartphones, diagnostic equipment).
- Acquiring or enforcing the required certifications on quality and safety (e.g., ISO, CE).
- Providing Continued Medical Education-accredited training programs for medical staff.
- Providing project management for telemedicine implementation in a region.
- Providing a helpdesk service for technical and administrative issues.
- Providing yearly reports on performance indicators (e.g., per clinic).
- Providing integration with Electronic Health Records (EHRs) from all involved parties.
- Negotiating and developing communications standards together with EHR providers and other (governmental) actors.

3.3   Best Practices from The Netherlands

In The Netherlands, the largest telemedicine provider is the KSYOS TeleMedical Centre. Founded in 2005 as a healthcare organization, KSYOS contracts with more than 11,000 healthcare professionals—6000 general practitioners, 2500 medical specialists, and 2500 paramedics—and delivers care to over a 1000 patients every day: it is the largest healthcare organization in The Netherlands that solely delivers healthcare by intelligent internet: i.e., telemedicine. KSYOS has implemented various somatic and mental health telemedicine services using the HMP model, e.g., teledermatology in 2005, tele-ophthalmology in 2007, telecardiology and telepulmonology in 2009, and eMentalhealth in 2014.

In the following sections, we discuss the KSYOS general telemedicine processes in patient care and several telemedicine service implementation results of teledermatology, tele-ophthalmology and tele-mental health.

3.3.1   General KSYOS Workflow

Most of the telemedicine processes implemented follow a standardized workflow that is divided into sub-processes, e.g., tele-order, tele-examination, telemonitoring, teleconsultation, and telereferral. Note that not all sub-processes are used in every field and a new patient can start at any of the sub-processes (Fig. 3.1). A healthcare provider (often a GP) orders an examination (e.g., ECG, spirometry, bloodwork, retina photo) through the tele-order system. Examination-specific inclusion criteria can be added. The patient then goes to the location where the examination is performed by a biometrist. This can be at the GP practice, but also in a local shopping mall at an optometrist store or at a medical diagnostic center.

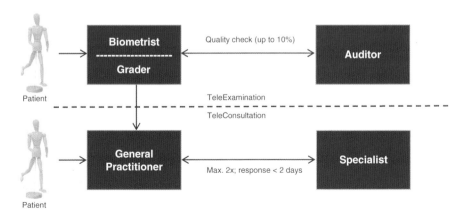

Fig. 3.1 KSYOS workflow for tele-examination and teleconsultation

All biometry is stored and can be accessed online through the secured online KSYOS Electronic Patient Record as PDF, video, or image files accompanied with examination-specific findings. These examinations are assessed by a grader, who can be the same actor as the biometrist but can also be at a different place and time; thus, the patient does not need to be present for the grading. The grader can be a specialist or a paramedic analyst trained specifically for this task. The results (biometry and grading) are presented to the GP who ordered the tele-examination. If an abnormality is found, then the GP can decide to refer the patient physically using a telereferral or to send a teleconsultation request to the regional specialist along with all the data received from the tele-examination, all from within the KSYOS Electronic Patient Record. Additionally, the system selects about 10% of the tele-examinations at random for anonymous auditing, where a specialist reviews the quality of the biometry and grading anonymously. The biometrist and grader thus receive feedback on their work.

3.3.2   Teledermatology

Teledermatology does not utilize a tele-examination process and only uses teleconsultation between the GP and dermatologist. Since 2006, the use of teledermatology has increased every year. By mid-2016, over 3600 general practitioners had performed one or more teleconsultations. Since its introduction in 2005, over 135,000 teledermatology consultations have been performed (Van der Heijden et al. 2011).

Of the 14,897 teledermatology consultations in 2015, 2 evaluation questions posed to the GPs were completed for 10,305 teleconsultations (Van der Heijden et al. 2011). The first question (Q1), "Would you have referred this patient if a teledermatology consultation were not available?" was asked before starting the teleconsultation. The second question (Q2) "Are you referring this patient to the dermatologist?" was asked when the teleconsultation was closed by the GP. Comparing the responses (both questions were answered with YES or NO) to these two questions showed for each teleconsultation if a physical referral was prevented (a prevented referral was counted when the answer to Q1 was YES and to Q2 was NO). The responses showed that 69% of teledermatology consultations were performed to prevent a physical referral (Q1 = YES, N = 7150) and, in this group, ultimately, 70% of the referrals to the specialist were prevented (N = 5021). In addition, 31% of the teleconsultations was performed to obtain specialist advice (Q1 = NO, N = 3155). Within this group, 20% were referred to the dermatologist through a fast-track process, which improved the quality of care for these patients (Fig. 3.2). The average response time for the dermatologists was 5.4 working hours. These results are consistent in all evaluations over the last years and hold true for all 135,000 teledermatology consultations (Van der Heijden et al. 2011).

Apart from preventing unnecessary hospital visits, teledermatology has a significant learning effect on the GP due to the immediate answers received. This leads to better care by the GP over time. After five years of active teledermatol-

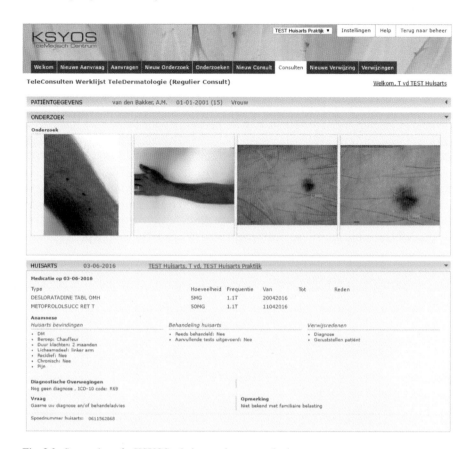

Fig. 3.2   Screenshot of a KSYOS teledermatology consultation

ogy, the GP performs 60% fewer teleconsultations compared with their first year due to the learning effect (Van der Heijden et al. 2011). Moreover, these GPs refer 30% fewer patients to the hospital compared with colleagues who have never done teledermatology, also due to the learning effect. By avoiding immediate referrals, teledermatology has realized a cost saving effect of 18% (Van der Heijden et al. 2011). However, the savings attributed to prevented referrals to secondary care by the learning effect over the years vary between 40% and 60% (Van der Heijden et al. 2011).

3.3.3   Tele-ophthalmology

There are several tele-ophthalmology examination processes. The telefundus screening (TFS) process, which refers to the screening of type 2 diabetes patients for diabetic retinopathy. The other tele-ophthalmology examination processes are focused on other eye diseases such as cataract, macular degeneration, and glaucoma. The optometrist performs eye examinations on own indication or after an order by a GP. The eye examination includes medical history, refraction, tonometry, and fundus photography. The GP can send tele-examination results to a regional ophthalmologist for teleconsultation (Fig. 3.3). Around 50,000 TFS are performed annually through the KSYOS TeleMedical Centre, which, to date, has performed 204,037 screenings (Van der Heijden et al. 2011). These patients have their retina photographed at local shopping centers in optometrist stores, at GP practices, or medical diagnostic centers instead of going to an ophthalmologist at a regional hospital. Twelve percent of TFS are converted into a tele-ophthalmology consultation with a regional ophthalmologist due to a positive grading for retinopathy. After teleconsultation, only 40% of patients are actually referred to the hospital (Van der Heijden et al. 2011). Because of tele-ophthalmology, only 4% (instead of 100%) of type 2 diabetes patients visit an ophthalmologist (Van der Heijden et al. 2011).

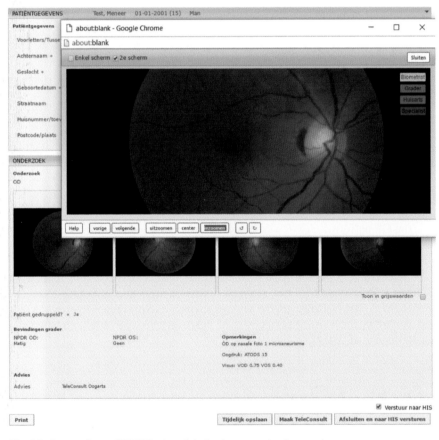

Fig. 3.3 Images from a KSYOS tele-ophthalmology examination

3.3.4 Telecardiology

Telecardiology consists of two types of tele-examinations (telecardiology rest ECG, or TCER, and telecardiology event ECG, or TCEE). Both examinations can be converted to a telecardiology consultation (TCC) with the regional cardiologist. Depending on the clinical context, a GP can give patients a TCER on the spot or the GP can record the cardiac rhythm continuously for 24, 48, or 72 h (even up to 7 or 14 days in a TCEE). Unlike conventional event diagnostics, the advantage of continuous recording is that asymptomatic clinically relevant arrhythmias are indeed registered (for example, paroxysmal atrial fibrillation). Since 2009, there have been 56,803 TCERs performed and, since 2013, 12,137 TCEEs have been performed. Respectively, 65% and 7% of TCERs and TCEEs were converted to a telecardiology consultation (Van der Heijden et al. 2011). Looking at efficiency improvement indicators, in 46% of all TCER consultations and 86% of all TCEE consultations, the GP intended to refer the patient physically to the cardiologist if teleconsultations were not available (Van der Heijden et al. 2011). In these groups, 59% and 49%, respectively, of these referrals were prevented following a teleconsultation. The groups were teleconsultation was used to obtain advice (TCER: 54%, TCEE: 14%) there was a physical referral in 20 and 30% of the cases, respectively. This led to quality improvement as these patients now received advice from the cardiologist and were physically referred on the request of the cardiologist. The average response time by cardiologists was 5.4 working hours (Van der Heijden et al. 2011).

3.3.5 TeleMental Health

This telemedicine service consists of four components: (1) a psychometric tele-examination delivered to the patient as an online questionnaire. The answers are put through an algorithm to analyze the severity of the mental health complaint and to provide advice as to what echelon of care the patient should receive; (2) a blended-care telemonitoring tool, offering 30 programs to treat mild cases of mental disorders (e.g., depression, burn out, stress, insomnia) through online courses utilizing videos, animations, and exercises while also providing online contact with the healthcare provider; (3) teleconsultation services for GPs to gain advice on treatment and medication from, e.g., child psychologists, psychiatrists, and addiction physicians; and (4) a tele-referral system to secondary mental healthcare facilities.

Since its implementation in early 2015, around 1300 GPs have used this service, over 8500 patients have completed the online psychometric tele-examination, and over 17,500 patients have followed an online blended-care program (mostly the burn-out, stress, panic, and mindfulness programs) (KSYOS Research 2016). In both services, the patient is an active actor in the telemedicine process and has logged into a telemedicine system at least once. On average, patients logged into the system nine times per blended care treatment, scored their treatment through a blended care program with an average of 7.7 out of 10 points, and 61% of patients reported a decrease in or even complete disappearance of their symptoms. The health providers using the blended-care programs in their treatment reported that in 20% of cases they needed fewer physical consultations compared with standard treatment and in 26% of the cases they used the same number of physical consultations but felt they provided a higher quality of care (KSYOS Research 2016). In 8% of cases, physicians reported using more physical consultations, whereas the other 46% of cases were reported as "I don't have this knowledge" (KSYOS Research 2016).

3.4   Concluding Remarks

We are faced with a big challenge to make our healthcare systems ready for the surge of patients and demands in the coming years. Redesigning our healthcare processes using new and innovative technologies can help us prepare for that. We should be aware also that when doing so, it is best to aim for those processes that have a routine and simple character, but high turnaround rate, the so-called "low-hanging fruit."

Based on the outcomes of the Dutch telemedicine services introduced by KSYOS, focusing on redesigning these sorts of processes can yield positive results in efficiency, quality, and cost. They have already treated 450,000 patients through their tele-order, tele-examination, teleconsultation, and telemonitoring services in the last 10 years. As far as we know, this is the largest implementation of fully reimbursed telemedicine services in a regular healthcare system in the world. Results show a 70–96% reduction in hospital visits in dermatology and ophthalmology, which translates into an immediate cost reduction of 18%. The response time of 4–5 working hours and the learning effect also have a significant impact on the quality of care delivered. Telemonitoring programs in mental health have demonstrated that the patient as an active actor can result in motivation and ownership of their own health. These results pave the way to similar positive psychology-based blended-care programs in somatic care, especially for lifestyle adjustment in patients suffering from diabetes, chronic obstructive pulmonary diseases, and cardiovascular diseases.

Telemedicine will make it possible for hospitals to concentrate on high-quality specialized care. In many peripheral centers in residential areas, e.g., general practitioner centers, pharmacies, optician stores, physiotherapy centers, and others, more routine care services will be delivered close to the patient by paramedics, caregivers, and the patients themselves under the direction and supervision of the general practitioner and medical specialist at a distance—and at a fraction of the price. This process is not only irreversible in healthcare, but also necessary to continue to meet the changing and increasing demand. Telemedicine services (and e-health instruments in a broader sense) are promising and proven telemedicine services are widely embraced by healthcare providers and patients. The only barrier to scaling up these services is the availability of a budget within regular compensation systems. That obstacle must be removed as soon as possible.

References

Broens THF. Determinants of successful telemedicine implementations: a literature study. J Telemed Telecare. 2007;13(6):303.

Chen S, Cheng A, Mehta K. A review of telemedicine business models. Telemed J E Health. 2013;19(4):287–97.

Ekeland AG, Bowes A, Flottorp S. Effectiveness of telemedicine: a systematic review of reviews. Int J Med Inform. 2010;79(11):736–71.

Grigsby J, Kaehny MM, Sandberg EJ, Schlenker RE, Shaughnessy PW. Effects and effectiveness of telemedicine. Health Care Financ Rev. 1995;17(1):115–31.

Haris F. IT Infrastructure Maturity Model (ITI-MM): a roadmap to agile IT infrastructure. Enschede, Netherlands: University of Twente; 2010.

Khoja S, Scott RE, Casebeer AL, Mohsin M, Ishaq A, Gilani S. E-health readiness assessment tools for healthcare institutions in developing countries. Telemed e-Health. 2007;13(4):425–32.

KSYOS Research. Anonymized database of all telemedicine processes. 2016.

Mills A, et al. Health care systems in low- and middle-income countries. N Engl J Med. 2014;370:552–7.

Mistry H. Systematic review of studies of the cost-effectiveness of telemedicine and telecare. Changes in the economic evidence over twenty years. J Telemed Telecare. 2012;18(1):1–6. Epub 2011 Nov 18

Ossenbaard H., Duivenbode J. Position paper: evaluatie ehealth-technologie in de context van beleid. In press.

Preston J, Brown FW, Hartley B. Using telemedicine to improve health care in distant areas. Hosp Community Psychiatry. 1992;43(1):25–32.

Van de Wetering R, Batenburg R. A PACS maturity model: a systematic meta-analytic review on maturation and evolvability of PACS in the hospital enterprise. Int J Med Inf. 2009;78(2):127–40.

Van der Heijden JP, de Keizer NF, Bos JD, et al. Teledermatology applied following patient selection by general practitioners in daily practice improves efficiency and quality of care at lower cost. Br J Dermatol. 2011 Nov;165(5):1058–65.

Witkamp L, Zonder budget geen ICT-revolutie in de zorg. Medisch contact. 2016.

Witkamp L, van der Heijden JP. Health management practice as a method to introduce teledermatology: experiences from The Netherlands, Telemedicine in dermatology. Berlin, Heidelberg: Springer; 2012.

World Health Organization. World health statistics 2015. 2015; ISBN 978 92 4 156488 5.

Wynchank S. and Van Dyk L., editors. A decision support tool for telemedicine project management. Prove your Hypothesis: telemedicine and eHealth in South Africa, 13–15 Sept 2011. 2011.

Chapter 4
Patient-Centric Strategies in Digital Health

Larry F. Chu, Ashish G. Shah, Dara Rouholiman, Sara Riggare, and Jamison G. Gamble

Abstract It is important to consider that the goal of digital health is to improve the experience of the patient as they traverse the health care system and to ultimately improve their health outcomes. In today's fully connected and digitally integrated world, patients, not providers are the rising stars in digital health innovation. Working from their own experiences and expertise, patients are leading the way in design innovation of novel digital health technologies. As patients become more and more connected, providers must keep up with their patients by utilizing the same technology as their patients. By doing so, providers create a foundation for participatory medicine, leveling power hierarchies and making patients feel comfortable and welcome throughout the process of their care. This chapter explores patient centric strategies in digital health and outlines the foundation of the Everyone Included™ initiative.

Keywords Precision medicine • Physician-patient relations • Patient-centered care • Patient outcome assessment • Diffusion of innovation • Connected doctor • Everyone included • Participatory medicine • Shared decision making • Digital health

L.F. Chu, M.D., M.S. (✉) • A.G. Shah, M.D., M.P.H. • D. Rouholiman, B.S.
J.G. Gamble, M.P.H.
Stanford School of Medicine, 300 Pasteur Drive, Grant Building S268C,
Stanford, CA 94305, USA
e-mail: lchu@stanford.edu

S. Riggare, M.Sc.
Karolinska Institutet, Stockholm, Sweden

© Springer International Publishing AG 2018
H. Rivas, K. Wac (eds.), *Digital Health*, Health Informatics,
https://doi.org/10.1007/978-3-319-61446-5_4

4.1   "Nothing About Us Without Us": The Value of Patients in Digital Health Design

The success of digital health tools and solutions depends on patient participation and engagement. By failing to recognize the value of patient engagement, a number of digital health tools have seen low sale rates, loss of product traction, and a low rates of product adoption by intended users. By directly engaging patients and incorporating them into the design process of digital health tools, valuable insight can be gained by developers. Taking the time to understand the needs of digital health tool end users, better digital health tools can be developed that more precisely address the needs of intended users.

The concept of "nothing about us without us" was first brought to light by disability rights activists in the late 1990s who believed that policy involving the disabled community should be co-created with input from the very community it was designed to impact (Delbanco et al. 2001). Recently, the expression "nothing about us without us" has been adopted by patient communities seeking broader involvement with the health care system (Paul 2016; Schiavo 2014). This concept has moved into almost every corner of health care, from shared decision making in health care to medical conferences (Chu et al. 2016). "Nothing about us without us" also applies to the design of digital health tools which are intended to improve both patient experience and health outcomes.

The creation of novel digital health tools can be thought of in three pathways of patient involvement (Fig. 4.1). In the first pathway, a digital health tool is designed, implemented and validated without any patient involvement. The patient provides input once the device has been released into the market. In the second pathway, patient thoughts, opinions and needs are assessed during the design phase of the digital health tool through focus groups. In this pathway, the digital health tool is developed based on the current needs of the population it is trying to impact. In the third pathway, the patient is brought in as a member of the team and co-creates the digital health tool. By utilizing the third pathway, patient expertise and knowledge surrounding their specific needs can be incorporated into the design process leading

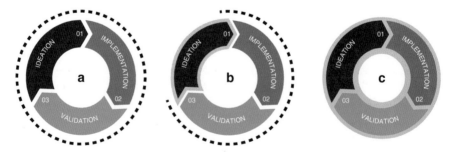

Fig. 4.1 Three pathways of patient-centric digital health innovation. (**a**) The patient is not involved in any phase of design. (**b**) Patient thoughts, opinions and needs are assessed during the ideation phase. (**c**) The patient co-creates as a member of the design team

to more innovative and creative solutions. Many patients are now taking this process into their own hands, creating digital health tools to meet the specific needs of their particular community.

Digital health is thought to spark innovation in health care by providing better tools and solutions which empowers the end-users, patients and providers. Development of any new innovative solution and tool goes through the iterative design process. Iterative design is a methodology based on a cyclic process of ideation, implementation, and validation.

Iterative design begins the innovation process with ideation, working with your community to uncover problems and design solutions to address them. The process continues by implementing the solution in an organization or a targeted population. Validation comes in the innovation process after implementation to test the efficacy of the solution and measure the strengths and shortcomings of the solution.

By turning issues inside out, and bringing all stakeholders to the table at the beginning, we have created a targeted, innovation-focused approach that embraces and expands the contributions of all, that brings elite entrepreneurs and researchers together with empowered patients to create solutions that solve problems, rather than generating solutions in a search of problems. The infinite loop of refinement helps to generate digital health solutions that are effective and efficient and in which all stakeholders are invested. From designing a wearable device to designing a mobile application, including patients in the design process of digital health tools can be manifested in various ways.

4.2 How Patients Are Leading the Way in Digital Health

After passing out on a train platform and receiving a diagnosis of hypertrophic cardiomyopathy, Hugo Campos's life was forever changed. Campos was considered at high risk for sudden cardiac arrest and was fitted with an implantable cardioverter-defibrillator (ICD). As his condition slowly took over his life, he realized that he needed to learn as much as he could about his condition so that he could have educated conversations with his care team. What he really wanted was access to the data that was being collected by his ICD to help guide his interactions and better empower his decisions.

The story of Hugo Campos perfectly illustrates the concept of an empowered patient (ePatient) defined as a patient who is engaged and actively participates in their own treatment and health. The term ePatient was first used by Dr. Tom Ferguson to describe individuals who are equipped, enabled, empowered and engaged with their health care (Ferguson 2007). The ePatient journey begins with the search to truly understand themselves and their own health. Hugo Campos is one of the many ePatients who are redefining Health Care and redefining our thinking of how technology can be used to redefine the doctor-patient relationship. Digital health is increasingly being advertised as a means to facilitate patient empowerment, engagement and innovation (Frist 2014; Birnbaum et al. 2015; Steven and Steinhubl 2013).

In 2016, 15% of consumers in the United States utilized wearable technology and 46% of consumers were active digital health adopters, a 27% increase from 2015 (Terry 2016; Piwek et al. 2016). Pathway C, patient-co-created innovation illustrates a radical transformation in the digital health development sector. Movements like The Quantified Self (QS) and #WeAreNotWaiting are examples of such transformation. The Quantified Self movement promotes individual engagement in self-tracking and analyzing of self-data, with the goal of improving individuals understanding of their bodies and needs to make more informed decisions. The frustration of the type 1 diabetes community stemming from a seeming lack of urgency by the health care industry to utilize digital health tools in monitoring and treating their condition led to the #WeAreNotWaiting movement. The message of the #WeAreNotWaiting movement as described by ePatient Dana Lewis states "we can't wait years and years for better tools and solutions, so we will do everything we can to make today easier." Dana Lewis, who has had type 1 diabetes for over 15 years, started using open-source code to get access to her continuous glucose monitor (CGM) data and make louder alarms for herself. She then utilized other open-source code and commercially available hardware to create a do-it-yourself "artificial pancreas", which was not commercially available for several years after that. In 2015, Lewis launched #OpenAPS, an Open Source Artificial Pancreas System movement for improving access and availability of a hybrid closed loop artificial pancreas system for people with type 1 diabetes (Lewis and Leibrand 2016). Existing digital health tools often fail to address some of the most important and immediate needs of patients and doctors.

Michael Seres experienced this first hand after undergoing only the eleventh small bowel transplant in the United Kingdom. As he recovered, he was required to wear an ostomy bag allowing his bowel to heal. The bag, which is used to collect waste from the intestine, must be changed and monitored manually, a significant burden to patients with a stoma. While still recovering in the hospital, Seres used a Nintendo Wii™ sensor, a battery, and a motherboard to build his very own sensor that would alarm to warn him when his bag was filling up. Today, Michael Seres has turned his sensor into a viable product with FDA approval to improve the lives of ostomy patients such as himself.

Sara Riggare, a Swedish engineer, experienced her first symptoms of Juvenile Onset Parkinson's disease when she was 13 years old. Today, Riggare is pushing the inclusion of patients on all levels of health care and research while pursuing a doctorate in health informatics at Karolinska Institutet in Stockholm. Riggare's research is centered around what she calls "digital selfcare", which includes the way she uses self-tracking to manage her disease and communicate with her physician but also making use of the knowledge that can be found online (Riggare and Unruh. 2015, Riggare et al. 2017).

Campos, Lewis, Seres, and Riggare all have one important thing in common, they don't accept the status quo, they engage, learn, and create what they need to improve their health.

There is a power shift happening in health care which Eric Topol, a cardiologist, geneticist and digital health researcher calls the "Democratization of Medicine", a grassroots movement where patients are developing solutions to their own health problems instead of waiting for the slow moving scientific and medical community (Topol 2015). Patients understand their needs, their own bodies, and have a vested interest in their own health care. Digital health technologies must give patients direct access to personal data that can contribute to their understanding of their health and facilitate preventive care.

4.3   Participatory Medicine: A Successful Collaboration of Patients and Providers Through Digital Health

At the heart of patient-provider communication is the concept of participatory medicine or shared decision making (SDM) which is centered around an open dialogue between patients and providers, where patient's thoughts, opinions and personal expertise are taken into consideration when making clinical decisions. As of 2011, the concept of SDM was supported by 86 randomized clinical trials which suggest SDM increases patient involvement in their health care, increases knowledge gained by patients, increases patient's confidence in decisions and suggests that when SDM is utilized patients often opt for more conservative treatment options (Stacey et al. 2011). Participatory medicine is naturally supported and promoted through digital health technologies such as electronic health (eHealth) and more specifically mobile health technologies (mHealth) which promote ease of communication and sharing of information between providers and patients via portable diagnostic devices. mHealth technologies can be classified into five categories: smartphone-connected devices, smartphone health applications (apps), handheld imaging devices, wearable and wireless devices and miniature sensor technologies (Bhavani et al. 2016).

mHealth technologies are the vital link between the digital patient and the digital clinician and provide a foundation for participatory medicine. From the patient perspective, mHealth technologies facilitate patient self-measures which generate patient specific data and promote behavior modification and patient engagement and participation. Data collected by mHealth technologies from engaged patients can then be transmitted in real-time to providers or stored in the cloud to generate a big-picture of health parameters or to identify individual health concerns. Examples of such technologies include the Withings™ Blood Pressure Monitor, the Sanofi iBGStar® Blood Glucose Monitor, and the AliveCor® Mobile ECG. Data collected by these devices can be stored on the patient's smartphone for later review by a clinician or can be transmitted in real time directly to a clinician for immediate review or to be stored in the patient's electronic health record (EHR). Use of these devices promotes participatory medicine by allowing the patient to collect their own personal healthcare data and share it with the clinician and have also been shown to improve behavioral health outcomes in motivated patients.

While the majority of mHealth devices are aimed at general health outcomes, a number have been designed to address specific health concerns or specific patient populations. An example of such a device is the Ostom-i™ alert sensor developed by 11 Health and Technologies Limited. The Ostom-i™ alert sensor is a smartphone linked device which attaches to an Ostomy bag and alerts the user to the fullness of the bag. Data collected by the Ostom-i™ alert sensor is uploaded onto the user's smartphone which can then be sent directly to providers for their reference. These devices directly engage patients and act as a tool to promote and facilitate patient engagement with their own health care. Furthermore, digital health technologies provide patients with data and knowledge surrounding their specific condition or general health which allows them to act as an informed participant while interacting with care providers.

The future of participatory medicine facilitated by digital health technology will need to incorporate patient input and participation with providers across multiple disciplines. Future technologies such as the "GoalKeeper" system are already being formulated to meet these needs (Amir et al. 2014). The proposed function of the GoalKeeper system is to facilitate communication and implementation of care plans between providers and parents of pediatric patients with complex conditions. The GoalKeeper system will allow parents of children with complex conditions to participate in the design of care plans and relies on status updates provided by parents. This system will directly engage parents of pediatric patients and allow them to directly participate in the care of their child. The GoalKeeper system will use artificial intelligence (AI) to decide how changes in one providers care plan will affect the care plan of other providers. The AI decides which providers will be affected by changes in care plans and choses when and to whom these changes will be reported to. While the GoalKeeper system will only used for parents of children with complex conditions, the technology has potential to be used across multiple patient populations to directly engage patients and allow them to participate in collection of health care data as well as to participate in decision making.

4.4 Social Media and Online Communities of Patients and Providers

Social media and its role in the dissemination of ideas and information has impacted not only the health care system, but a myriad of other industries. Today, ePatients use Twitter, Facebook, YouTube and countless other social media networks rather than the peer-reviewed journals and academic conferences to learn and disseminate new ideas and information. Social media is defined as a computer-mediated tool that enables users to disseminate, collect and share information, ideas, pictures, and videos instantly in virtual communities (Thompson 2015). It provides an inclusive podium where both clinicians and patients benefit from each other's expertise and perspective by disseminating, collecting, and reacting to information that can instantaneously reach and affect millions of people worldwide.

Despite the fact that clinicians remain the top information source in health care, about twenty-five percent of adults in the United States turn to their peers with similar health condition for information and advice (Fox 2011; Landro 2016). A study among people with Parkinson's disease in Sweden showed that even in a generally older community (median age = 68 years) as many as 36% found their knowledge about Parkinson's online (Riggare et al. 2017). Social media gives patients and providers access not only to information and data, but to one another as well. In other words, social media provides a communication platform which broadens our social networks. Today, there are 137 recurring weekly tweet chats, 17,862 chat participants and 66,560 chat tweets pertaining to health care (Audun Utengen n.d.). The dispersion of medical information and advice is no longer limited to the traditional boundaries of doctors' offices and hospitals but has now expanded to incorporate the ePatient community.

Social Media fosters engagement between clinicians and patients in real time. Today, Hugo Campos still does not have access to the data collected by the device implanted in his chest; however, he can use a single lead ECG attached to his smartphone to share his electrocardiogram with his social network in near real-time. This is exactly what he did when he began to feel a fluttering sensation in his chest. Minutes after sharing his ECG results on Twitter, the cardiologists in his social network helped him understand his ECG reading within the context of the symptoms that he was experiencing. This illustrates the power of social media, instant access to information and data needed to make an informed decision. Social media has empowered patients by leveling the traditional information hierarchy, placing patients and physicians on level ground and connecting providers directly to patients in real time.

4.5   The Connected Doctor

In today's world of hyper connectivity, the field of medicine must stay on the cutting edge of the communication revolution. How is a connected doctor defined in our dynamic world of communication technology? At its foundation, a connected doctor may simply be defined as one who utilizes EHRs to write notes and enter data. EHRs were first introduced to the medical community in the 1960s and 1970s and became commonplace around the start of the new millennium (Atherton 2011). In 2011, 57% of physicians reported utilizing EHRs, a 39% increase from 2001 (Analisys Group 2014). As communication technology grows, so to must the connected doctor. Today, simple use of an EHR is not enough to define a connected doctor. Instead, the connected doctor is defined within three parameters: (1) What they are connected to (EHR, online portals, mobile health applications), (2) Who they are connected to (patients, the online community, hospitals, peers, consultants) and (3) How they are connected (internet, smartphones, messaging, mobile health platforms).

While the connected doctor may be thought of as an inevitable happening bringing about great improvements in shared decision making and the ePatient community, it may increase physician burnout rates. In 2011, 45.5% of physicians were found to have symptoms of burnout which increased to 54.5% by 2014. These rates of burnout are higher than are seen in other non-medical occupations (Shanafelt et al. 2015). During this period of increased physician burnout, the use of EHRs increased significantly leading to more time spent on the EHR by physicians (2 h of EHR reporting for every 1 h spent with a patient) (Villares 2016). Physicians are then expected to complete an additional one to two hours of patient-related clerical or EHR work. Furthermore, it has been suggested that physicians are dissatisfied with EHRs which in turn promotes physician burnout (Shanafelt 2016).

While EHRs facilitate improved documentation, order entry, patient safety and improve the billing and reimbursement process, they do not facilitate communication between patients and providers but rather between physicians and the hospital administrative system. Physicians primarily connect to their patients via online portal systems where patients can communicate directly with their providers and have direct access to lab results and other metrics. With the recent advent of mHealth devices and mobile health platforms, providers have direct access to a massive quantity of outpatient health data such as blood pressure, temperature, exercise and diet. Providers may join online patient communities and provide disease-specific or general health related information to an entire community of patients. Provider-provider communication is facilitated by secure, encrypted messaging allowing for easy consults or second opinions. While peer-to-peer interactions are incredibly important for provider communication and decision making the use of artificial intelligence (AI) is becoming a stronger presence in clinical decision support. As the field of precision medicine continues to grow, AI will begin to play a larger role in health outcome predictions allowing providers to treat patients in a preventative manner.

Imagine now the future of the connected doctor. Before a doctor sits down with their patient in person, AI will browse the patients EHR extracting information on allergies, medications, previous hospitalizations and other pertinent health information. The AI system will then incorporate the most current health data such as vital signs and information from health-related questionnaires directly into the EHR for the day's visit. As the doctor has been communicating with the patient via the online portal the reason for the visit is already understood. Once the patient-provider visit begins, information learned during the session is automatically incorporated into the EHR by the AI system instead of the provider. As the provider begins the physical examination, images from connected smart glasses worn by the provider are automatically entered into the EHR and processed by the AI. Medical devices such as the stethoscope are fully connected and integrated into the system and can provide data directly to the providers' handheld smart tablet aiding in their diagnoses. The AI system will evaluate this new information and incorporate it into the EHR with previous data offering a differential diagnosis and providing recommendations for labs and other tests, to be verified by the provider.

As mHealth devices and AI become more prevalent, inpatient medicine will likely change as well. Imagine a patient suffering from congestive heart failure who has been in and out of the hospital due to fluid build-up in the lungs. With an appropriate sensor, a warning can be sent to the medical team alerting them to the fluid buildup. Patients with chronic conditions requiring an indwelling catheter to drain urine often suffer from urinary tract infections. Future sensors may be incorporated into catheter systems with the purpose of detecting bacterial buildup. If bacteria is detected within certain limits, an alert can be sent to the medical team recommending they prescribe a course of antibiotics. Both of these scenarios may prevent extended hospital stays and improve longitudinal health outcomes.

There is no doubt that physicians are becoming increasingly connected. It is important to define the connected doctor as more than just an active use of the EHR. A doctor is truly connected when the EHR provides information back to the physician, when they are constantly connected to their patients through data sharing and a direct line of communication, and when they can send digital information to experts around the world for second opinions. It is also important to recognize that there may be unintended consequences to becoming a fully connected provider. As physicians become more connected, the applications and platforms must be designed to improve work flow and efficiency. With these factors in mind, the future of the connected doctor looks very promising.

4.6   The Everyone Included™ Initiative

In the short time patient-centered care has been recognized as a key element in providing a high level of quality care, there has been a coordinated effort to expand patients' role in their health care. A leading example of this concerted effort has come from the Everyone Included™ initiative. Everyone Included™ is a living framework for health care innovation, implementation and transformation based on principles of mutual respect and inclusivity.

> *"The first step is to identify the ultimate stakeholder–the patient–and then reach out and talk to them. Patients and families are eager to partner. We want to help. We want to be part of the process and we want to be there every step of the way. We want to help set strategic priorities, we want to co-design and co-produce studies, we want our expertise and insight to be valued as the essential part of the team that it is–and we also want our unique offerings to be harnessed to make healthcare better for us and everyone"*
> – Emily Kramer-Golinkoff, ePatient

Digital health like other medical innovations sectors requires validation in the form of empirical research. Everyone Included™ provides a framework for medical research that shatters the silos between researchers, diseases, and stakeholders. Emily's Entourage (EE) is an organization that has been utilizing the Everyone Included™ model to fast track research for new treatments and cures for rare nonsense mutations associated with Cystic Fibrosis. To achieve a breakthrough in time to save Emily Kramer-Golinkoff, a CF patient who founded Emily's Entourage, and others with nonsense mutations of CF, close collaboration between scientists, patients, clinicians, venture capitalists, and many more is required. Emily's Entourage is an example of an organization that brings successful innovation to health care utilizing the principles of Everyone Included™.

Everyone Included™ is the result of collaboration between patients, caregivers, providers, technologists, and researchers which has led to the formation of design and leadership principles intended to drive health care innovation efforts. It formulates a culture in which individuals are trusted and respected for the expertise they

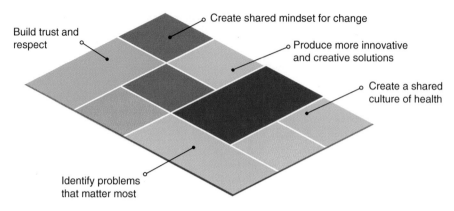

Fig. 4.2 Everyone Included™ value propositions

bring, openness and experimentation is the norm, people have personal ownership of health, individual stories have global impact, and the voice and choice of patients is a part of all stakeholder decisions. The value propositions of Everyone Included™ can be applied towards digital health innovation and include five elements: build trust and respect, create a shared mindset for change, produce more innovative and creative solutions, create a shared culture of health and identify problems that matter most (Fig. 4.2). The creation of digital health solutions requires a collaborative input from all major stakeholders, especially patients. There must be a mutual trust between providers, developers, users and patients to identify the core problems and produce creative solutions.

To accomplish this, the Everyone Included™ initiative has identified six leadership principles which can be implemented into a variety of patient centric design modules. The first leadership principle is "believe in respect, not power hierarchies", this leadership principle aims to break down the walls of traditional power hierarchies which limit creativity and fail to incorporate unique, individual expertise which patients and other stakeholders bring to the table. This is not to imply that hierarchies should be eliminated completely, but rather the power that comes along with hierarchies should be equalized amongst all participants. Second, "leadership can be flexible", this means that leaders respect and incorporate opinions and input from a variety of within team sources while simultaneously remaining true to the vision of their organization. Furthermore, leaders should consider themselves as the center point of a wheel instead of the top of a pyramid. Third, "diverse teams lead to more creative solutions", by creating a team of diverse individuals with different backgrounds and areas of expertise, we believe that more innovative and creative solutions can be reached than if a traditional pyramidal power hierarchy is utilized. Fourth, "diversity requires considerate leadership", a considerate leader within a diverse team keeps the collective "we" in mind while simultaneously recognizing the value, expertise and creativity that diverse teams bring to the table. A considerate leader will also mitigate misconceptions that arise around power and respect, motivating individuals to contribute to their fullest potential by distributing power equally and displaying mutual respect for all team members. Fifth, "create a culture of empathy and consideration", misconceptions and misperceptions inherently accompany diverse teams, however, a considerate leader will create an environment which values taking the time to understand the perspectives and opinions that each team member brings to the table. A considerate leader will foster an environment which addresses the physical and emotional well-being of each team member within a diverse team. The sixth and final leadership principle of Everyone Included™ is "recognize the value of conflict, but reduce its risk". Task conflict is a natural part of team work and if managed properly can lead to more creative solutions by taking alternate viewpoints into consideration.

With careful consideration of the Everyone Included™ initiative, digital health design should follow the third pathway (pathway C) model of ideation, implementation and validation, partnering with ePatients throughout all three steps. The three design steps are further defined as: Ideation; begin the innovation process by working with your community of health care stakeholders, designers, technologists and researchers to uncover problems matter most in your domain or problem area. Focus on designing for problems that matter most through co-design with relevant health care stakeholders using the Everyone Included™ co-creation and leadership principles. Rapidly iterate to optimize your design plans with a diverse team.

Implementation; the best design plan can fail without proper implementation strategies. Work with your team to optimize your plans for implementing change within your organization to avoid pitfalls using Everyone Included™ to anticipate and plan for challenges. Validation; the most important part of any innovation is the measurement of success that tests the effectiveness of the solution.

4.7 Conclusion

By placing an emphasis on patient centrism in digital health, power is put back into the hands of patients and traditional power hierarchies are lowered allowing patients to feel like a participant in their personal health care experience. Through patient involvement in the design of digital health tools, to facilitating shared decision making, collaboration with patients can spark creativity, innovation and the creation of novel digital health tools which more precisely address the issues patients are experiencing. By utilizing Everyone Included™ as a framework for patient inclusion, providers, designers and researchers alike can elevate patient voices to ensure that patients are heard as a valuable and equal member of the health care team.

References

Amir O, Grosz BJ, Gajos KZ, et al (2014) AI support of teamwork for coordinated care of children with complex conditions. 2014 AAAI Fall Symp Ser Arlington, Virginia,13–15 Nov. 2014;2–5.

Analisys Group. Big data in health care. Natl Law Rev. 2014:1–3.

Atherton J. Virtual mentor: history of medicine: development of the electronic health record. Am Med Assoc J Ethics. 2011;13:186–9.

Audun Utengen M Symplur Signals, a healthcare social media analytics platform.

Bhavnani SP, Narula J, Sengupta PP. Mobile technology and the digitization of healthcare. Eur Heart J. 2016;37:1428–38. doi:10.1093/eurheartj/ehv770.

Birnbaum F, Lewis D, Rosen RK, Ranney ML. Patient engagement and the design of digital health. Acad Emerg Med. 2015;22:754–6. doi:10.1111/acem.12692.

Chu LF, Utengen A, Kadry B, et al. "Nothing about us without us"—patient partnership in medical conferences. BMJ. 2016;354:6–11. doi:10.1136/bmj.i3883.

Delbanco T, Berwick DM, Boufford JI, et al. Healthcare in a land called peoplepower: Nothing about me without me. Health Expect. 2001;4:144–50. doi:10.1046/j.1369-6513.2001.00145.x.

Ferguson T, e-Patient Scholars Working Group (2007) E-patients: how they can help us heal healthcare. Patient Advocacy Heal Care Qual 1–126.

Fox S (2011) The social life of health information. Pew Internet Am Life Proj 2011;1–33. doi: http://www.who.int/topics/tuberculosis/en/.

Frist WH. Connected health and the rise of the patient-consumer. Health Aff. 2014;33:191–3. doi:10.1377/hlthaff.2013.1464.

Landro L (2016) Technology and Health Care: The View From HHS - WSJ. Accessed 22 Feb 2017. In: Sept. 25. https://www.wsj.com/articles/technology-and-health-care-the-view-from-hhs-1474855381

Lewis D, Leibrand S. Real-world use of open source artificial pancreas systems. J Diabetes Sci Technol. 2016;1932296816665635 doi:10.1177/1932296816665635.

Paul T. "Nothing about us without us": toward patient- and family-centered care. AMA J Ethics. 2016;18:3–5.

Piwek L, Ellis DA, Andrews S, Joinson A. The rise of consumer health wearables: promises and barriers. PLoS Med. 2016;13:1–9. doi:10.1371/journal.pmed.1001953.

Riggare S, Unruh KT. Patients organise and train doctors to provide better care. BMJ. 2015;6318:h6318. doi:10.1136/bmj.h6318.

Riggare S, Höglund PJ, Hvitfeldt Forsberg H, et al. Patients are doing it for themselves: a survey on disease-specific knowledge acquisition among people with Parkinson's disease in Sweden. Health Informatics J. 2017;146045821770424 doi:10.1177/1460458217704248.

Schiavo R. Nothing about us without us. https://www.emmisolutions.com/blog/2014/10/27/nothing-about-us-without-us. Accessed 24 Mar 2014.

Shanafelt TD, Hasan O, Dyrbye LN, et al. Changes in burnout and satisfaction with work-life balance in physicians and the general US working population between 2011 and 2014. Mayo Clin Proc. 2015;90:1600–13. doi:10.1016/j.mayocp.2015.08.023.

Shanafelt TD, Dyrbye LN, Sinsky C, et al. Relationship between clerical burden and characteristics of the electronic environment with physician burnout and professional satisfaction. Mayo Clin Proc. 2016;91:836–48. doi:10.1016/j.mayocp.2016.05.007.

Stacey D, Légaré F, Col NF, et al. Decision aids for people facing health treatment or screening decisions (review) decision aids for people facing health treatment or screening decisions. Cochrane Libr. 2011; doi:10.1002/14651858.CD001431.pub4.Copyright.

Steven R, Steinhubl M. Can mobile health technologies transform health care? JAMA. 2013;92037:1–2. doi:10.1001/jama.2013.281078.Conflict.

Terry K (2016) Consumer use of digital health tools rising rapidly. In: December 19 http://www.medscape.com/viewarticle/873468. Accessed 21 Feb 2017.

Thompson MA. Using social media to learn and communicate: it is not about the tweet. Am Soc Clin Oncol Educ Book. 2015:206–11. doi:10.14694/EdBook_AM.2015.35.206.

Topol E. The patient will see you now: the future of medicine is in your hands. New York: Basic Books; 2015.

Villares JMM. Allocation of physician time in ambulatory practice: a time and motion study in 4 specialties. Acta Pediatr Esp. 2016;74:203. doi:10.7326/M16-0961.

Chapter 5
Informatics and Mass Data Analysis in Digital Health

Nick van Terheyden

Abstract This chapter reviews the current status of data in the context of digital health and exploring the huge increase in data acquisition in medicine with accompanying move from paper to the Electronic Health Record. The roll out of Electronic Health Records has been filled with challenges and detracting from the physician patient relationship taking the focus away from patients to the technology. But this move to digital information is the gateway to the appliance of science at the point of care but this is dependent on capture of structured codified data or the ability to convert narrative into structured computer readable information. The section offers examples of the benefits in digitizing the patient record and potential opportunities for automating the application of clinical knowledge at the point of care. The key to providing patients with the care they want and clinicians want to give is using this digitized data to offer actionable intelligence and insights at the point of care that make best use of the latest research data to drive the most appropriate treatment Additionally the digitization with new analytics tools applied with automated agents and artificial intelligence will increase the development of disease understanding and opening the door to truly personalized medical care and treatment.

Keywords Big data • Medical informatics • Disease detection • Digital health • Electronic records • Medical records • Health records • HITECH Act

5.1 Introduction

While the rest of the world moved rapidly to the digital age, healthcare has remained a laggard struggling to move from paper to digital records. While this adaptation has been slow to be applied to healthcare, the general consensus is that Electronic

N. van Terheyden, MD
Gaithersburg, MD, USA
e-mail: Drnic1@gmail.com

© Springer International Publishing AG 2018   55
H. Rivas, K. Wac (eds.), *Digital Health*, Health Informatics,
https://doi.org/10.1007/978-3-319-61446-5_5

Byte	: one grain of rice
Kilobyte	: cup of rice
Megabyte	: 8 bags of rice
Gigabyte	: 3 Semi trucks
Terabyte	: 2 Container Ships
Petabyte	: Blankets Manhattan
Exabyte	: Blankets west coast states
Zettabyte	: Fills the Pacific Ocean
Yottabyte	: A EARTH SIZE RICE BALL!

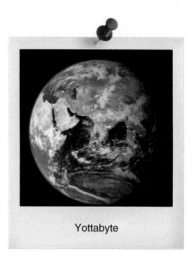

Yottabyte

Fig. 5.1 Visualizing Big Data. Slideshare—What is Big Data. David Wellman

Health Records (EHR[1]) provide a better solution to the capture, use and sharing of clinical data between clinicians and the care team and increasingly the patient and their family.

The generation of data in our world is running at an exponential pace that is accelerating and as The Economist detailed: The Data Deluge (The Economist 2017) the quantity of information is soaring.

> *Everywhere you look, the quantity of information in the world is soaring. According to one estimate, mankind created 150 exabytes (billion gigabytes) of data in 2005. This year, it will create 1200 exabytes. Merely keeping up with this flood, and storing the bits that might be useful, is difficult enough. Analyzing it, to spot patterns and extract useful information, is harder still.*

It is hard to explain what that means but David Wellman of Myriad Genetics (2017) compared 1 byte of data to grains of rice (Fig. 5.1):

1 Byte of data = 1 grain of Rice

1 Kilo Byte (kB) = 1 cup of rice.
1 Mega Byte (Mb) = 8 bags of rice.
1 Giga Byte (Gb) = 3 container lorries.
1 Terra Byte (Tb) = 2 container ships.
1 Peta Byte (Pb) = Cover Manhattan Island.
1 Exa Byte (Eb) = Covers the United Kingdom three times over.
1 Zeta Byte (Zb) = Fills the Pacific Ocean.

---

[1] In this chapter I will use the term Electronic Medical Health (EHR) to denote both and Electronic Medical Records (EMR) and EHR's. Technically an EMR is a narrower version of a health record containing only the medical information.

Medicine is no different and in fact is second only to astronomy in the rate of acquisition and creation of data. Not only have the major-medical advances increased exponentially, but our capacity to absorb and process this information as humans remains steadfastly limited. Our medical education system remains resolutely stuck in traditional methods suited to an age when knowledge was limited and our understanding of the human body and causes of disease were incomplete. In many cases we failed too understand the underlying science behind a disease and the treatments were at best ineffective and at worst harmful.

> Medicine used to be simple, ineffective and relatively safe. Now it is complex, effective and potentially dangerous
> Sir Cyril Chantler (Chantler 1999)

As you will read elsewhere in this book not only is the healthcare system changing, but we must change the medical education system to adapt to this new environment that is data rich. The new generation of doctors are digital natives expecting and using the readily accessible knowledge in their day to day activities and will expect and need to do the same as clinical professionals in the new age of Digital Health.

For the current clinical professionals who have traditionally relied on the unaided mind to recall the knowledge imbued through the study of medicine and updated over time by access to journals and research can no longer keep a pace with the moves updates and changes let alone recall the information appropriately and reliably for each case and patient they are treating. The human mind is notoriously unreliable at recall and, as the size of the knowledge domain expands, so to rises the human inability of recall. We are now expecting our clinicians to process somewhere of the order of six billion pieces of data in a 15 min encounter.

In this chapter we review the digitization of the medical record, the positive and negative impact this has had on day to day clinical practice and the impact this will have on the future of medicine—both the practice as well as research and discovery.

5.2   Medical Errors and the EHR

On November 29, 1999 The Institute of Medicine (IOM) published the seminal report "To Err Is Human" which highlighted the jaw dropping statistic that "at least 44,000 people, and perhaps as many as 98,000 people, die in hospitals each year as a result of medical errors that could have been prevented." Medical Errors were now a major cause of death ranking above cancers, road traffic accidents and AIDS. The smoking gun was the inability of the current documentation system and medical notes to provide the necessary information required for the healthcare system to have even a chance of preventing these errors.

They follow up in March 2001 with a follow up report "Crossing the Quality Chasm: A New Health System for the 21st Century" which took direct aim at the technology infrastructure of the healthcare system and the siloed approach to medicine and the sharing of data. For many of that time seeing a patient was something of a shot in the dark when it came to information. If the patient had any clinical notes, stored in a traditional manila folder, their appearance concurrent with you seeing them was unpredictable and oftentimes clinical staff were relegated to asking the patient for details of their past diagnoses and treatments—information that suffered the same human reliability recall issues that clinicians faced. Featured in this report were the high rates of medication errors a major problem with incorrect dosing, preventable allergic reactions and overt mistakes—all problems that digital systems were highly suited to monitoring and preventing. Their guidance was to eliminate the hand written note containing clinical data and the need to move to an automated digital systems.

Since there we have seen a steady flow of similar reports highlighting the high rate of medical errors, the cost in human life and economic terms of these errors and the ongoing failure to effectively digitize and computerize the medical record. There have been multiple ongoing efforts to digitize the healthcare records in the United States including one of the early programs to create the Veterans Administration Medical Records System "VistA"—which stands for the Veterans Information Systems and Technology Architecture. This started life as a gigantic hack that predated the IoM report and while it had its problems it has continued to receive high ratings from the clinical users. Ultimately it fell foul of the rapid change of technology and politics and is being replaced by a commercial EHR.[2]

Around the world many other countries have moved en masse to digitize their medical records. Some of the smaller countries like Denmark which has a centralized computer database to which >98% of primary care physicians, all hospital physicians and all pharmacists now have access as do the patients. Other countries include New Zealand, Sweden and Germany are all far down the path to digitization. The progress of medical record digitization around the world is documented elsewhere (The Commonwealth Fund 2017).

The Health Information Technology for Economic and Clinical Health (HITECH) Act, enacted as part of the American Recovery and Reinvestment Act of 2009, was signed into law on February 17, 2009, to promote the adoption and meaningful use of health information technology. This $30 Billion dollar investment has moved the USA into the Digital Age for medical records with over 80% of physicians using some for of EHR and over 3/4 of hospitals adopting some basic form of an EHR. For all that investment and focus there have been significant challenges many centered around the continued siloed nature of the information, despite it being digitized and the failure to integrate the many systems and sources of data effectively. But the

---

[2]You can read more about the history of the VistA system here http://www.politico.com/agenda/story/2017/03/vista-computer-history-va-conspiracy-000367

biggest push back to the technology has come from the clinical professionals who find the technology distracting their focus away from the patient to the screen. This was captured in the Journal of American Medical Association "The Cost of Technology" (Toll 2012).

The drawing was unmistakable. It showed the artist—a 7-year-old girl—on the examining table. Her older sister was seated nearby in a chair, as was her mother, cradling her baby sister. The doctor sat staring at the computer, his back to the patient—and everyone else.

The criticism has been valid in many cases and some of the blame is a result of taking an existing processes and systems and attempting to automate it rather than rethinking from scratch. The EHR currently still has the look and feel of a paper record—even using many of the "paper" terms such as folders and tabs that came from the paper medical record. A better approach would have been to rethink the format and storage of clinical data as John D. Halamka, M.D., M.S., the Chief Information Officer of Beth Israel Deaconess Medical Center has advocated. He has suggested a Facebook or WikiPedia like medical record that could be a living "breathing document," updated my multiple contributors. While that comes with some authentication and validity challenges it represents a novel and alternative way of thinking about patients clinical data and how to store, share and use this data more effectively and is likely to be part of future developments.

But despite the negative impact of the EHR roll out even the most resistant clinicians would not accept going back to the world of paper. No one wants to return to the era of paper based medical record that were not available without he patient, that could only be accessed by one person who had to have physical access to the record. No one wants to return to the era of clinical records that contained indecipherable hieroglyphics that could not be decoded with certainty. No one wants to return to the immense volumes of paper that accompanied many of the chronically sick patients who accumulated paper notes, test results and reports at an alarming rate measured in inches of folders. No one wants to return to the paper based record that was incomplete, and un-searchable that could contain the necessary information but was impossible to tell if it did or to find it. No one wants to return to an era of paper that was incapable of tracking the content and securing it and determining who had accessed the information.

5.3   The EHR Is Here to Stay

Fundamental to the advances in healthcare is the foundation of accessible knowledge and the ability to access and apply this for the benefit of the patient. Tied to this is the desire to apply this knowledge to the appropriate context of the patient giving them right treatment at the right time. To achieve this under the tsunami of data and knowledge in medicine that is changing and learning at an exponential rate.

Table 5.1 Landmark clinical trials and current rate of use for selected procedures

Clinical procedure	Landmark trial	Current rate of use
Flu vaccination	1968 (7)	55% (8)
Thrombolytic therapy	1971 (9)	20% (10)
Pneumococcal vaccination	1977 (11)	35.6% (8)
Diabetic eye exam	1981 (4)	38.4% (6)
Beta blockers after MI	1982 (12)	61.9% (6)
Mammography	1982 (13)	70.4% (6)
Cholesterol screening	1984 (14)	65% (15)
Fecal occult blood test	1986 (16)	17% (17)
Diabetic foot care	1983 (18)	20% (19)

Yearbook of medical informatics: managing clinical knowledge for health care improvement 2000

Medicine has continued to make incredible progress in the diagnosis and treatment of disease but the pace with which these insights and innovations reach day to day clinical practice has remained stubbornly slow (Table 5.1). Studies suggest that it takes an average of 17 years for research evidence to reach clinical practice (it took 25 years for Beta blockers treatment for heart patients) (Balas and Boren 2000).

It takes an estimated average of 17 years for only 14% of new scientific discoveries to enter day-to-day clinical practice Practice-Based Research (2017).

Patients want access to the latest treatments, and physicians want to deliver the best possible care but under the data deluge this is an insurmountable task for any human and can only be done with support by technology. The EHR captures the patient data in digital form—not all of it structured or coded but sufficient to provide input to automated clinical systems that reconcile the clinical data with the latest advances in medical diagnosis and treatments. The record remains incomplete with EHR records distributed in different incompatible systems and many elements remain locked away in free form narrative that continues to challenge natural language processing engines. We have and continue to make progress in computerized understanding of the clinical narrative but it is inconsistent and incomplete. In the interim, having some of the record digitized as discreet data already offers opportunity for automated insights, alerts and augmented clinical care that helps the clinical team offer the best options based on the latest data and most recent clinical research.

Simple improvements with automation allow patients to be identified and targeted for preventative screening or a treatment. For a busy family practitioner seeing more than 40 patients in a clinical session, sometimes limited to a few minutes, there is little time available for identifying preventative intervention opportunities. They are pressured to review existing data, distill the latest patient provided information and capturing this and the findings of a clinical examination into the EHR, which leaves little time to identify additional clinical intervention opportunities for immunization, review of cardiovascular risk including life style interventions and guidance or preventative screening. But with digitized clinical information the never tired, never forgetful, never overwhelmed EHR can be programmed to identify patients:

- The 70 year old who has not had their Influenza immunization.
- The 52 year old who has not been seen recently and has not yet had a screening Colonoscopy.
- The Diabetic patient who has not had their screening eye exam done in the last 2 years.

As the process for capture of information and our ability to understand the free form narrative so too will the functionality and support that is derived from the EHR increase. That ability can also be used and to date has been in some specific cases to analyze the clinical research data with new tools. Artificial Intelligence (AI) tools have been developed that can analyze large volumes of structured and unstructured data found in clinical research papers and then offers a knowledge base that can be queried and will generate and evaluate clinical and diagnostic hypothesis. This will open up a new era of medical diagnosis:

- Bringing Evidence to the Point of Care
- Consumption of medical records, results etc. offering differential diagnosis and probability analysis with links to underlying literature sources
- Draws on the specifics of a patient case and vast volumes of clinical data and medical
- Highly granular results tailored to a particular patient's conditions, demographics, history
- True personalization of medicine based on large cohort historical data analysis

For established treatments and protocols we can now provide care and treatments with consistency using established knowledge for the benefit of the patient, for example:

- Medication dosage: guidelines, clinical research findings for specific patient.
- Adverse drug reactions: computational model + research database.
- Treatment options: contextualized to patient.
- Standard of care: aligning treatment to standards.
- Trending guidelines: recently published, pre-official.
- Post-operative discharge and follow up.
- Entry of symptoms or symptomatic trends can trigger alerts for follow up.
- Ongoing refinement based on dynamic interaction and learning.

Ultimately, this automation will start to offer a medical avatar embodied with the collective knowledge and wisdom of the human race and available for instant access to be applied to each and every patient for treatment and management of chronic conditions.

The digitization of healthcare will open new doors to diagnosis and treatment and revolutionize the way we approach clinical research. We have already seen this in practice with an update to the seminal and much referenced Framingham Heart Study that was initiated in 1948 that recruited and studied 15,000 participants over three generations. The gathering of this data limited by a manual process and following up with the participants every 2 years (History of the Framingham Heart

Study 2017). The results from this study form the basis of our models for diagnosing and treating heart disease focusing on blood pressure, cholesterol and obesity. The study identified the life style changes we recommend to patients to reduce their weight, stop smoking, decrease stress and increase physical activity and exercise. The discovery and subsequent mediation of these risk factors is largely credited with a 75% decline in mortality rates due to heart-related disease in the last half century.

But the new game in town is the recruiting a million smartphone users to create the largest heart study of its kind (Health eHeart 2017). Researchers at the University of California, San Francisco (UCSF) are recruiting a million participants to join a decade long heart health study in what amounts to a large scale digital version of the Framingham study but on steroids. The sheer scale of the participants, the frequency of data collection and the scale of the different data elements being collected will generate enormous amounts of data offering a more granular picture of individuals and their health and collecting it at a fraction of the cost of traditional manual methods. This is just the start of an incredible journey into the world of digital health data that will generate new insights and opens the door to filling the huge gaps in patient data that take place between the infrequent and brief visits they have to physician offices and hospitals. You can read more about the capture and use of that data in the chapter "Quantified Self."

Once these EHR systems are integrated and include all the data generated by the patients, as well as the exploding domain of genomic and proteomic data, the emerging cadre of smart algorithms and artificial intelligence tools can sift through the EHR looking for patterns and helping us understand, treat, and ultimately prevent disease. As we expand our knowledge and understanding of disease we can focus on the prevention rather than the cure for diseases. Identifying them before they occur and mitigating or even preventing the outbreak of conditions. Not only is this great care but it is also very cost effective as the majority of the cost in our healthcare system is linked to expensive treatments that attempt to cure late stage disease.

Gone will be the waste that currently takes places as we test treatments on patients to determine if they are suitable to their individual condition. We will be able to identify the precise treatment for a single individual who's unique genetic make up, their individual biome and living circumstances affect their responsiveness to drugs and therapies. Based on the large data sets we will match them with other individuals who had the same characteristics and share the same genetic and micro biome make up and have already identified the cause and treatment for the condition. No more returning to the doctors office after a week to review the treatment choices and change therapy based on trial and error—the availability of the complete digitized medical record offers customized precision medical therapies that will work first time, saving time, health and money as we move rapidly to personalized medical care.

Our understating of disease will expand as we start to make the connections between previously unknown causative factors. A recent paper published in Australia offered an alternative approach to the treatment of asthma focused on diet that would change the gut microbiome and reduce or even remove the need for drugs to treat asthma (The Canberra Times 2017) You can read more about driving healthy habits and keeping patients committed to positive lifestyle changes in the chapter Serious Gaming.

For those of you concerned about the future and the replacement of humans by technology the study done by the Mayo Clinic in 2006 (Bendapudi et al. 2006) identified the most important characteristics patients feel a good doctor must possess. The Ideal clinician is:

- Confident
- Empathetic
- Humane
- Personal
- Forthright
- Respectful
- Thorough

These facets are entirely human and will be hard for technology to replace. The role of clinicians and healthcare staff will change and be augmented by the technology easing the burden of data gathering and memorization. The right information and knowledge will be available to review with patients allowing the focus to be the clinician/patient personal interaction.

It should be abundantly clear that the adoption and importantly full interoperability of a fully digitized health record will be fundamental to our future of medicine. The addition of multiple other data streams including patient generated data, genomics, proteomics and diagnostic imaging data will only make the need even more acute for the EHR to store, secure, backup and allow the use of our digital medical record. This data is coming from an increasing number of sources and is coming at an increasing rate that will challenge the current capabilities of our EHR. As clinicians or patients we need to have this data digitized and accessible so we can tap into the incredible trajectory of medicine that will access and use this data to offer treatments that are better and more economical.

References

Balas EA, Boren SA. Yearbook of medical informatics: managing clinical knowledge for health care improvement. 2000. http://www.ihi.org/resources/Pages/Publications/Managingclinicalknowledgeforhealthcareimprovement.aspx. Accessed 26 May 2017.

Bendapudi NM, Berry LL, Frey KA, Parish JT, Rayburn WL. Patients' perspectives on ideal physician behaviors. Mayo Clin Proc. 2006;81(3):338–44. doi:10.4065/81.3.338.

Chantler C. The role and education of doctors in the delivery of health care*. Lancet. 1999;353(9159):1178–81.

David Wellman of Myriad Genetics: What is Big Data. http://www.slideshare.net/dwellman/what-is-big-data-24401517. Accessed 26 May 2017.

Health eHeart—million smartphone users recruited to heart study. 2017. https://www.health-eheartstudy.org. Accessed 26 May 2017.

History of the Framingham Heart Study. 2017. https://www.framinghamheartstudy.org/about-fhs/history.php. Accessed 26 May 2017.

Practice-Based Research—"Blue Highways" on the NIH Roadmap https://www.ncbi.nlm.nih.gov/pubmed/17244837. Accessed 26 May 2017.

The Canberra Times. Radical asthma treatment unveiled in Canberra. http://www.canberratimes.com.au/act-news/were-at-the-tip-of-a-new-paradigm-radical-asthma-treatment-unveiled-in-canberra-20170326-gv735a.html. Accessed 26 May 2017.

The Commonwealth Fund, What is the status of electronic health records? http://international.commonwealthfund.org/features/ehrs/. Accessed 26 May 2017.

The Economist: the data deluge. http://www.economist.com/node/15579717. Accessed 26 May 2017.

Toll E. The cost of technology. JAMA. 2012;307(23):2497–8. doi:10.1001/jama.2012.4946.

Chapter 6
"Healthcare on a Wrist": Increasing Compliance Through Checklists on Wearables in Obesity (Self-)Management Programs

Thomas Boillat, Homero Rivas, and Katarzyna Wac

Abstract Increasingly, healthcare can get on our wrists. Unhealthy lifestyle habits (e.g., sedentary behavior, nutrient-poor diets) result in higher levels of chronic diseases (e.g., CVD, obesity) and, paradoxically, the first step in disease management requires radical lifestyle changes, away from the unhealthy ones. These changes are difficult for patients and require day-to-day planning and adherence to new behaviors (increased physical activity, special diet programs) for best health outcomes in a long-term. We envision an important role of personalized, miniaturized Information Technologies (IT), specifically smart watches—supporting the patient's self-management efforts in any daily life context, acting as a reminder for specific activities and documenting the patient's progress via checklist-based approach. We delineate the requirements and design choices for the WATCH-list—an example of self-management service for obesity patients' compliance to diet programs. We discuss the chronic illness self-management and role of IT in increasing the patient's self-efficacy of activities contributing to health, in turn increasing the patient's compliance to these activities and therefore facilitating better health outcomes in a long term.

T. Boillat
Stanford University, Stanford, CA, USA

University of Lausanne, Lausanne, Switzerland
e-mail: tboillat@stanford.edu

H. Rivas
Stanford University, Stanford, CA, USA
e-mail: hrivas@stanford.edu

K. Wac (✉)
Stanford University, Stanford, CA, USA

University of Copenhagen, Copenhagen, Denmark

University of Geneva, Geneva, Switzerland
e-mail: wac@stanford.edu

© Springer International Publishing AG 2018
H. Rivas, K. Wac (eds.), *Digital Health*, Health Informatics,
https://doi.org/10.1007/978-3-319-61446-5_6

Keywords Consumer health informatics and personal health records • Mobile health • Tracking and self-management systems • Ubiquitous computing and sensors • Physiologic modeling and disease processes • User-centered design methods (includes prototyping)

6.1   Towards an IT-Enabled Chronic Care

The paradox of health and life expectancy in the twenty-first century is that while advancements in technology and medicine enable us to live longer, our modern lifestyle habits (e.g., sedentary behavior, nutrient-poor diets) increase the probability of becoming chronically ill and experiencing long-term limitations, until death (Lee 2003; Oh et al. 2005). In Europe almost 86% of deaths in 2015 were due to a chronic illness like ischaemic heart disease, cardiovascular disease (CVD), hypertensive heart disease, Chronic Obtrusive Pulmonary Disease (COPD), diabetes or cancer, and the number is increasing (WHO 2005). Moreover, 78% of overall medical care is spent by people with one or more chronic conditions, and 60% of it—by people with multiple chronic conditions (comorbidity).

Yet, the current, legacy health systems are designed more for acute *cures* rather than a longitudinal chronic *care*. Chronic diseases are long-term conditions that cannot be easily managed via a single (set of) measurement(s) assessing the patient's health state and single (set of) treatment(s). Paradoxically, the first step in disease management requires lifestyle changes away from the modern lifestyle habits, which brought the patient to the state of illness at first. These changes are difficult for patients and require day-to-day planning and adherence to new behaviors (more physical activity, special diet programs) for best health outcomes in a long-term. Overall, chronic diseases require continuous assessment of the patient's health state and ideally, early interventions, preventing further worsening of this state and the disease exacerbations.

There are number of attempts towards redesign of current health systems to improve chronic care management. The most prominent proposal is the Innovative Care for Chronic Conditions (ICCC) framework by the World Health Organization (WHO) (WHO 2002), based on Wagner's Chronic Care Model (CCM, Fig. 6.1) (Wagner et al. 2001).

This framework focuses on necessary changes in: (1) the patient and his community (micro-level) domain—increasing the patient's knowledge, confidence, and self-management skills and awareness of the importance of regular self-monitoring; (2) the healthcare organization and care team (meso-level) domain—increasing preparedness of teams for patient care; and (3) the policy and financial (macro-level) domain—developing sustainable business models for better chronic care management. The complexity of the framework lies in the fact that all these domains are highly interdependent and the proposed set of changes are hampered by lack of strong evidences for their efficiency and effectiveness (Porzsolt and Stengel 2006).

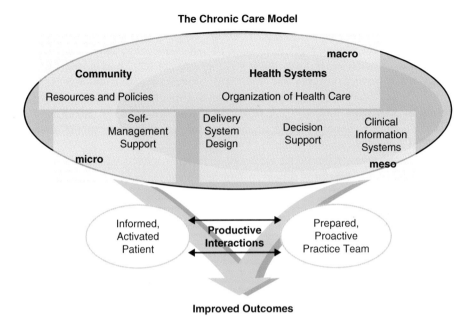

Fig. 6.1 The chronic care model

The ICCC emphasizes the role of regular patient self-monitoring and observation of the course of disease, and there exists some research demonstrating the importance and benefits of self-management in chronic care. For example, Linden et al. (Linden et al. 1996) surveyed that CVD patients self-measurement can help to manage and even significantly decrease their blood pressure, heart rate, and cholesterol. Richardson et al. (Richardson et al. 1990) shows that patient-self care increase survival among cancer patients. Lorig et al. (Lorig et al. 1999) conducted clinical trials with patients suffering from heart disease, lung disease, stroke, or arthritis and proved that a disease self-management program can improve health status while reducing patient hospitalization, Norris et al. (Norris et al. 2001) acquired similar results in case of diabetics' patients, while Verberk et al. (Verberk et al. 2007) with patients suffering from hypertension. Rice et al. (Rice et al. 2010) proved that self-management for COPD patients reduces their hospitalization rate, while Vieira et al. (Vieira et al. 2010) showed that self-monitored home-based rehabilitation might improve quality of life for the COPD patients.

Recently we observe an increasing miniaturization and availability of computing, storage, and communication resources for IT systems (Hansmann et al. 2003), as well as the availability of improved sensors for human vital signs and environmental conditions measurements. These developments enable the development of telemedicine systems providing services for ambulatory monitoring of a patient's condition and, if required, for an ambulatory intervention (Istepanian et al. 2004). These services enable the acquisition of data for monitoring of the patients' condition outside the healthcare center; in many cases these services are designated for home use. The data acquired could then be used by patients for self-management, as well as by healthcare teams to make an informed decision upon a patient's state. To date, there exists a number of manufactured and marketed systems that provide ambulatory monitoring services, however, they are not employed in the chronic disease management process (Wac et al. 2010) because they have not been exhaustively evaluated for use in regular clinical practice. Also, the impacts of these monitoring devices seem limited (Case et al. 2015; Rosenberger et al. 2016) as it is unclear how they should be designed and what functionalities they should offer to maximize diet program compliance.

In this chapter we focus on the methodological approach towards use of ambulatory monitoring services that support patient self-management in chronic care, and especially in the obesity management care. As obesity management requires management of strict diet and other lifestyle activities, where we see a role of IT, acting as a reminder for specific activities and documenting the patient's progress via checklist-based approach. More specifically, we investigate the capacity of smart watches in order to guide diet programs and thus increase their efficiency.

6.2   Challenges Linked to Obesity and Diet Control

Obesity is the first non-infectious pandemic; in the USA, 70% of people are overweight, 30% are obese, and 20 million people are morbidly obese. Obesity management includes, amongst the others, adherence to physical activity and nutritional programs, both becoming either a sole lifestyle-based treatment or as a preparation for the surgery. In case of the latter, existing studies report that patients who are capable of losing 10% of their weight prior to surgery can decrease complications during the surgical intervention, while keeping a strict diet after the procedure also has a direct negative impact on complications (BMI Stanford Hospital and Clinics 2015). Diabetes, high blood pressure, sleep apnea, reflux disease, and many other medical problems can virtually disappear in obesity patients with significant weight loss (BMI Stanford Hospital and Clinics 2015). Evidence reveal that periodic consultations increase diet program compliance by providing more guidance, helping maintain diet programs.

On the other hand, early detection of variations can prevent derivation from initial target, and allow physicians and nutritionists to adapt diet programs for better results. Thus, the combination of high frequency plus high consistency of dietary self-monitoring improves long-term success in weight management (Peterson et al. 2014). On the other hand, recent research shows that self-management of physical activity and diet can also lead to behavioral weight loss programs (Turner-McGrievy et al. 2013). In this view, technology-supported behavioral change interventions will be a part of twenty-first-century health care (Spring et al. 2013). Electronic devices such as smartphones provide applications that allow patients to more efficiently keep track of their diet, compared to traditional paper-based journals (Turner-McGrievy et al. 2013).

Today, weight loss programs are most of the time distributed as paper copies of information that patients are supposed to remember and apply. Very often, following a strict diet requires patients to make a set of significant daily lifestyle changes and remembering detailed timing. More personalized, patient-centric guidance is needed; specifically to monitor patients' compliance to their diet programs. Thus, it is critical for these patients to have the means to follow these diets, but existing paper-based recommendations aiming to support them is difficult to handle and can only passively remind them to, amongst the others, take their six different meals and supplements.

6.3 Traditional Diet Program in Bariatric Patient Care

Diet programs for obesity patients are usually split into two time periods: before and after bariatric surgery. The former aims to decrease patient weight prior surgery to reduce the risk of complication and to limit stomach activity. The latter intends to smoothly prepare the stomach and the digestive system to receive solid foods after surgery (e.g., gastric bypass, sleeve gastrectomy). Diet programs before surgery typically consist of high protein liquid shakes, food supplements such as vitamins or iron and physical activities. Patients are recommended to drink between four and six shakes in a day and take food supplements in between to maximize the supplements' effect. Other recommendations (e.g., drinking water, physical activity) are usually communicated to increase diet programs compliance.

On the other hand, diet programs after surgery are more diverse and also longer. They traditionally start with high protein (HP) shakes, similar to the pre-surgery diet for approximately 1 month. They are then followed by 1 week of pureed phase including eggs, nonfat yoghurts, pureed refried beans or poached salmon.

Thus, diet programs usually include specific food menus, drinks, supplements and/or drugs and physical activities (Fig. 6.2). Until reaching a sustainable solid food diet after surgery, patients go through three to five different diet programs

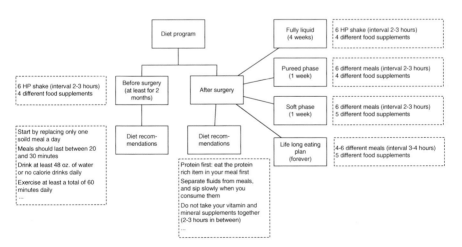

Fig. 6.2 Model of a typical diet program in bariatric care

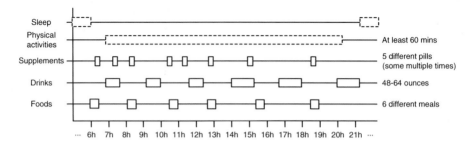

Fig. 6.3 Daily activities included in a typical diet program prescribed in bariatric care

enabling them to lose weight and prepare their body for new lifestyle choices. As a result, per a diet program, a patient nowadays is supposed to remember up to 20 activities, each of which requiring to be performed at a specific time throughout the day (Fig. 6.3).

6.4   IT-Enabled Support for Diet Programs in Bariatric Patient Care

Paper documentation is the most common medium that hospitals and clinics give to bariatric patients for describing elements of a diet program. Very often the diet program includes a paper checklist that is meant to guide patients on a daily basis. It contains the different activities, sequentially placed, that patients have to do—from food to food supplements and drugs. In addition to this checklist, more detailed information is given on the bariatric and digestive systems to help patients better understand the underlying reasons behind the different diets. This aims to increase the patients' literacy, potentially increasing their motivation.

In few cases, hospitals or clinics recommend mobile applications for smartphones such as "myfitnesspal" or "loseit."[1] Compared to the paper documentation, diet programs on digital artifacts such as mobile applications are easy to carry, to access and information is also easy to find. There is no need to search information across multiple dozen of pages, i.e., application search functions enable it.

As alternatives to official mobile applications, there exists third parties ones that either already contains standardized diet programs or that allow patients to re-enter their own programs. However, these mobile applications are often not recommended by hospitals or clinics because it is unclear how information is treated and used.

While recent smartphones offers activity tracking capacity, there exists many different types of wearables that aim to monitor physical activities and motivate

---

[1] https://www.myfitnesspal.com and http://loseit.com

their users with some gamification techniques (e.g., earn medals, batches). These metrics and techniques are usually very generic and their impacts on weight loss are effective only for patients' with specific personality characteristics, as the weight loss may be a long term goal, with daunting daily lifestyle changes contributing to it (Chung et al. 2017). A recent study reveals that wearables were less efficient than traditional self-monitoring methods (Jakicic et al. 2016), over a 24-month period. More specifically, the 470 participants (respectively one group of 234 and another of 237) were asked to follow a program including a low-calorie food diet and physical activities. Both groups attended group counseling sessions as well as interventions via phone calls and text messages. While one group self-monitored its progress via a website, the other received wearables. The research reveals that participants using wearables lost on average 2.4 kg less than the other group.

Another type of wearables that is getting much attention is smartwatches. They are considered as the extension of smartphones, with a privileged access to people's attention. Compared to smartphones that often require efforts to access them, smartwatches are able to display (short) information much faster (Narayanaswami and Raghunath 2000). They are often the first intermediary between users and their mobile devices (Pradhan and Sujatmiko 2014). In order to provide users relevant information, smartwatches leverage their sensors (e.g., GPS) to send contextualized notifications. Research shows that smartwatches can be used as a mediator between nurses and patients (Ali and Li 2016). Through this device, nurses can monitor activities of patients as well as communicate with them. Unlike mobile devices, smartwatches are always on patients' arm and notifications are an efficient way in order to send messages to patients. While smart watches seem to be well-defined by academics, in reality watch manufacturers rather use it as a marketing tool. Thus, there exists many different types of smart watches. On the one hand, traditional computer companies have embraced the watch market with fully digital watches that differ from traditional watches by their colorful touchscreens.

On the other, traditional watch manufacturers are adding electronic pieces in their mechanical movements. In this view, there are mainly three different mechanisms to display the data collected through embedded sensors. Firstly, to insert the data on the "cadran," either analogically or digitally (Table 6.1, left column). Secondly, to superpose a digital screen on top of the traditional "cadran" (Table 6.1, right column). Lastly, to place in additional module in the "wristlet." In this latter option, only the module is connected to a smartphone, the watch itself is not.

Thus, smartwatches have different capacity that depends on the characteristics (Tables 6.1 and 6.2). The latter impact the smartwatches' functionalities as well as the dependency to a smartphone. For instance, given it has no screen, to access the data collected by the Withings Activité Steel (Table 6.2), one needs a smartphone. Oppositely, the Samsung Gear S3 can receive a SIM card (Table 6.1) that enables the smartwatch to receive calls, messages and communicate with the Internet without a smartphone.

Table 6.1 Characteristics of two selected smartwatches

Brand and name	Apple watch 2	Samsung gear S3
Example model		
Price	$399	$349 and $399 with 4G LTE
Size	42.5 × 36.4 × 11.4 mm	46 × 12.9 mm
Screen (ifcolor, iftactile)	1.65 in., OLED 2	1.3 in., super AMOLED
Weight	34.2 g	63 g
Memory	8 Gb	4 Gb
User interactions capabilities	Multi-level touchscreen, digital crown, button Personalized screen Speaker	Touchscreen, steel bezel, buttons Personalized screen Speaker
Activity trackers embedded	Heart rate sensor, accelerometer, gyroscope, GPS, GLONASS	Heart rate sensor, accelerometer, gyroscope, barometer, GPS
Activity tracker functionalities	Steps, exercises (e.g., running, swimming), standing, heart rate	Steps, exercises (e.g., running), standing, heart rate
Other sensors embedded (for wearer's context)	Ambient light sensor	Ambient light sensor
Short-range connectivity	Wi-Fi (802.11b/g/n 2.4 GHz), Bluetooth 4.0	Wi-Fi (802.11b/g/n 2.4 GHz), Bluetooth 4.2, NFC
Long-range connectivity	N/A	4G LTE, 3G UMTS
Waterproof	50 m	1.5 m
Battery life	18 h	72 h
Phone (in)dependency	Medium	Low
Compatibility	iOS	Samsung android, android with small limitations, iOS with big limitations
Programmability	Low, impossible to have background logging without user interacting with the watch	High, possible to have background logging without user interacting with the watch

Table 6.2 Characteristics of two selected mixed-smartwatches

Brand and name	Withings Activité steel	Kairos HYBRID SSW158
Example model		
Price	$129.95	$2,400
Size	36.4 × 11.5 mm	46 × 17.1 mm
Screen (ifcolor, iftactile)	No digital screen	1.8 in. TOLED
Weight	37 g	155 g
Memory	N/A	N/A
User interactions	Only via smartphone	Touchscreen, Speaker
Activity trackers embedded	Accelerometer	Gyroscope, accelerometer, GPS
Activity tracker functionalities	Steps, exercises (swimming, running), sleep	Steps
Other sensors embedded (for wearer's context)	Day and Night motion sensor	N/A
Short-range connectivity	Bluetooth 4.0	Bluetooth 4.0
Long-range connectivity	N/A	N/A
Waterproof	50 m	30 m
Battery life	8 months	2 days
Phone (in)dependency	High	Medium
Compatibility	Android, iOS	Android, iOS, Windows phone
Programmability	N/A	N/A?

6.5 Personalized Diet Programs on Wearables: WATCH-List Service

In this section delineate the requirements and design choices for the WATCH-list—an example self-management service for obesity patients' compliance to diet programs deployed on a smart watch. It is supporting the patient's efforts in any daily life context, acting as a reminder for specific activities and documenting the patient's progress via checklist-based approach.

6.5.1 Checklists as Application Structure

An application structure that fits particularly well for codifying and documenting knowledge on small screen is checklist. Checklists are cognitive tools that are used in many fields (e.g., aviation, nuclear) for their effectiveness to comply with a given activity set (including the order of activities) and their capacity to reduce human errors (Hales and Pronovost 2006). They have the abilities to democratize knowledge by means of sequential steps, while they reduce workload, improve quality, communication, and collaboration (Winters et al. 2009). Checklists are used to support short memory and guide workers in their routines. In surgery for instance, they have demonstrated their capacity to remind surgeons verify some elements, which help decrease complication and mortality rates in operating rooms (Haynes et al. 2009).

6.5.2 WATCH-List Functional Requirements

Codification of the diet program by means of interactive and contextualized checklists: It implies that the smartwatch application displays the activities that a patient has to perform (e.g., drink 4 Oz of HP shake, take 2 pills of Vitamin B12) based on the patient's diet program and time of the day.

Centralization of diet programs: The smartwatch application is not only an interface between the device and a patient, but also between patients and their care (surgical) teams. Because the diet program is centralized (e.g., in a cloud infrastructure) it is also accessible by surgical teams who can keep track of patients' activities.

Documentation of patients' activities: The smartwatch application allows patients to interact with the diet program and thus keep track of the activities that are performed and the remaining ones.

Track patients' activities: The smartwatch should embed sensors such as accelerometer, GPS or heart rate to provide information about patients' activities and medical health state.

Context-aware notifications: They indicate patients what they have to eat, drink or what supplements they have to take at the right time.

Remote interface: It allows a care team (e.g., nutritionists, surgeons, psychologists) to create and modify individual diet programs. The modifications are then on the patients' smartwatch user interface.

6.5.3 WATCH-List Non-functional Requirements

Multimodal user interactions: The smartwatch checklist application should offer different physical affordances (e.g., touchscreen and buttons) for accessing its functionalities. Patients' morphology can potentially prevent them to use a smartwatch touchscreen or digital crown.

Work in a standalone mode: The smartwatch should not require an additional device such as a smartphone in order to work. It is not realistic to impose patients to carry a smartphone all day long only for the purpose of a diet application on a smartwatch. It implies that the smartwatch must be able to receive a SIM Card in order to access Internet and receive updates or personal notifications from the surgical team.

Battery-life of 1 day: Battery duration is a recurrent topic with smartwatches and can impact their usefulness in many different domains. In our case, the watch should last at least 18 h, while it can be charged overnight.

Digital screen bigger than 1 in.: The smartwatch application requires a digital screen not smaller than 1 in. to display the different checklists and other information.

Vibration and visual notifications: Notifications are a powerful mechanism to inform patients about what they have to do. The smartwatch must be able to display these in a visual as well as silent manner (i.e., vibration).

Security and privacy: Information related to patients and their diets must be stored, exchanged and treated securely. It implies to secure data not only on the watch but also on the centralized infrastructure where diet programs and patient data is stored.

Fully personalized and contextualized: Patients must be able to individually customize the application according to their preferences (e.g., font-size, font color, background color).

6.5.4 Personalized Diet Programs on Smartwatches

Using smartwatches as technology for supporting and executing diet programs offers new opportunities to faster the time for clinics to intervene when irregularities occur with patients. Because diet programs and their completion are stored centrally, clinics can access their progression and quickly detect abnormalities in diet programs. More specifically, when documenting the different activities via a smartwatch (e.g., first meal has been taken, vitamin D too), the application stores the different actions and replicates them into the centralized diet program system. Then, various types of analysis can be performed to detect behavioral patterns with patients and also across patients. In this context, an emerging concept that is increasingly used to analyze the relationships between actions and their impacts is process mining. The latter provides a set of tools that support multiple ways to discover, monitor, and improve processes based on event logs (van der Aalst 2011). It thereby enables a link to be established between process models and "reality". It means to compute the difference between the activities that a patient is supposed to do in order to follow his or her diet (bottom part of Fig. 6.4) and his or her actual execution (top part of Fig. 6.4). Additionally, patients can also document their emotions to inform the clinic on the difficulties to follow the diet program. In return, when possible, nutritionists can adapt the diet program to make it more pleasant for patients.

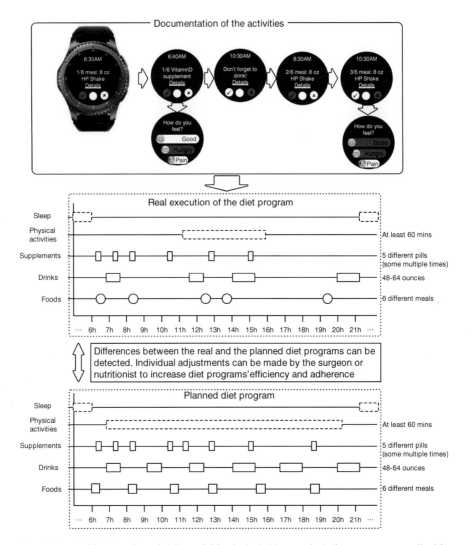

Fig. 6.4 Real life execution of daily activities included in a typical diet program prescribed in bariatric care

6.6   Towards Chronic Self-Management by IT Design

The IT solutions, including smartwatches as in the above WATCH-list service case—will have an increasingly important role in self-management of patient's health. From the psychological perspective, the patient's efforts and performance in self-management strongly correlate with the patient's *self-efficacy*, i.e., their beliefs that they can manage to achieve the desired (health) outcomes (Bandura 1977). In this section we discuss the role of IT solutions like WATCH-list in increasing the

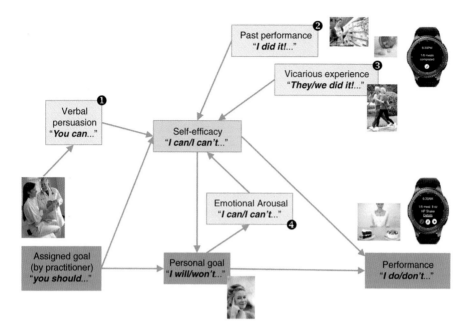

Fig. 6.5 Model of the patient's performance with respect to health activities and the role of IT in it

patients' self-efficacy of activities contributing to health (e.g., physical activity, diet programs).

Self-efficacy of health is a complex psychological concept that varies over time for the same person, according to his or her current health state and treatment plan. It is highly correlated with the patient's self-management efforts and hence its health outcomes (Sarkar et al. 2006; Bethancourt et al. 2014; Strecher et al. 1986; Ross and Mirowsky 2010; Lorig et al. 2000). In Fig. 6.5 we draw the dependencies between these activities and the patient's state.

A doctor assigns to a patient responsibility of a set of activities and performance goals ("you should") (e.g., follow a diet program), based on which the patient derives his or her own action plan, embedded in his or her daily life activities ("I will/ I will not"). This action plan influences then the actual performance of the patient ("I do/I don't"). Additionally the performance is influenced by the patient's self-efficacy of the activities contributing to these goals ("I can/I cannot").

There are four different sources of self-efficacy as distinguished in the literature (Sarkar et al. 2006). Namely, the self-efficacy is influenced by (1) the verbal persuasion of the expert (a doctor), pointing out that the patient "can" do specific activities. (2) Secondly, own past experience ("I did it!") influences the self-efficacy positively, in case of fulfilled goals, and it influences it negatively, in case of unfulfilled goals. (3) Performance of others, which the patient has observed or participated in ("They/we did it"), also influences patient's self-efficacy. (4) Finally, own emotional arousal ("I can!/I can't!") related to a given activity, may influence the self-efficacy, especially at the moment of performance.

The literature suggests that the poorly performing patients experiencing unhealthy outcomes may be in a 'vicious circle', where the subsequent past experienced failures and poor performance (related to the self-efficacy sources: (2) and (3)), may result in a relapse of their self-efficacy (Bethancourt et al. 2014; Strecher et al. 1986; Ross and Mirowsky 2010; Lorig et al. 2000). As we shown in the example WATCH-list service above, the smartwatch and checklist embedded in the patients' daily life can help accounting and documenting the performance of the patient, and facilitate to fuel patients' self-efficacy via "past performance" evidence (e.g., "1/6 meals completed" as in Fig. 6.5). In this context, the above-mentioned personalization of performance goals that are feasible and actionable for a patient is important.

WATCH-list like solutions shall aim at documenting the past successful experiences of the patients, increasing their self-efficacy and potentially fuelling the sustainable lifestyle changes and long terms health outcomes. We continue the research in a direction of the service design elements for IT-based services, enabling the self-management of a patient's health by assuring the self-efficacy of health according to different patients' state and needs, thus improving their health outcomes (Wac et al. 2015; Wac and Rivas 2015).

6.7 Discussion

Wearable technologies, such as smartwatches, offer new opportunities to support chronic care and enables patients' self-management. Compared to traditional chronic care management that requires patients to regularly travel to a clinic, wearables provide more flexibility and actively include patients in the process. However, one of the reasons that the existing ambulatory monitoring services are not used for patient self-management in chronic care is lack of randomized controlled trials of sufficient power[2] that provide supporting evidence for their effectiveness and efficiency. To date, few studies investigate the capacity of wearables to support patients in weight loss programs (e.g., (Jakicic et al. 2016)). Moreover, with respect to use of these services themselves, there is lack of methodological support to embrace these systems, i.e., lack of sufficient knowledge among patients and teams about how to make proper use of the service to collect the reproducible data of a clinical value and how to make a use of this data being collected outside the healthcare center.

While in most research wearables are used to collect data linked patients' activities (e.g., steps, sleep) as well as to motivate patients via the concept of gamification (Chung et al. 2017), we argue that this technology offers alternative capacity. Via the WATCH-list concept, we describe the design of a smartwatch application that aim to implement personalized diet programs and guide patients in their execution

---

[2] number of patients enrolled in a study, that enables to reliably detect the size of the effect of the study intervention

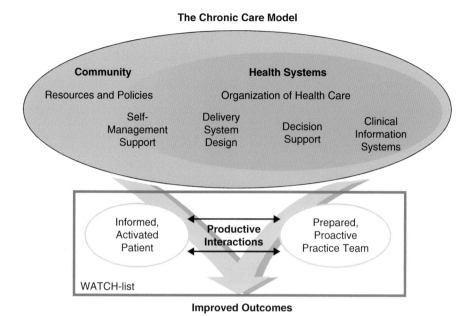

Fig. 6.6 The role of IT-enabled services like WATCH-list in operationalizing the chronic care model

by means of contextualized notifications. Because data on diet programs' completion is centralized, WATCH-list also serves as an early-warning system for clinics that can proactively contact patients when abnormalities occur. Thus, it reduces the intervention time and eventually increases diet programs' compliance.

This benefits of WATCH-list on chronic care are more tangible in the context of the Chronic Care Model (Wagner et al. 2001) (Fig. 6.6). While traditional activity tracking systems only enable self-monitoring of patients' activities (the left circle), we argue that WATCH-list has the ability to link patients and clinics via the documentation of the activities. Thus, it creates productive interactions that increase the level of awareness of both patients and clinics towards increasing the adherence and the efficiency of diet programs.

References

Ali H, Li H. Designing a smart watch interface for a notification and communication system for nursing homes. In: Human aspects of IT for the aged population. Design for Aging. Springer International Publishing. 2016, pp. 401–11.

Bandura A. Self-efficacy: toward a unifying theory of behavioral change. Psychol Rev. 1977;84(2):191.

Bethancourt HJ, Rosenberg DE, Beatty T, Arterburn DE. Barriers to and facilitators of physical activity program use among older adults. Clin Med Res. 2014;12(1–2):10–20.

BMI Stanford Hospital and Clinics. Eating after bariatric surgery: a medical nutrition therapy handbook. Bariatric and Metabolic Interdisciplinary Clinic, Stanford Hospital and Clinics. 2015.

Case MA, Burwick HA, Volpp KG, Patel MS. Accuracy of smartphone applications and wearable devices for tracking physical activity data. JAMA. 2015;313(6):625–6.

Chung AE, Skinner AC, Hasty SE, Perrin EM. Tweeting to health: a novel mHealth intervention using Fitbits and twitter to Foster healthy lifestyles. Clin Pediatr (Phila). 2017;56(1):26–32.

Hales BM, Pronovost PJ. The checklist—a tool for error management and performance improvement. J Crit Care. 2006;21(3):231–5.

Hansmann U, Merk L, Nicklous MS, Stober T. Pervasive computing: the mobile world. 2nd ed. Germany: Springer; 2003.

Haynes AB, et al. A surgical safety checklist to reduce morbidity and mortality in a global population. N Engl J Med. 2009;360(5):491–9.

Istepanian RSH, Jovanov E, Zhang YT. M-health: beyond seamless mobility for global wireless healthcare connectivity-editorial paper. IEEE Trans Inf Technol Biomed. 2004;8(4):405–12.

Jakicic JM, et al. Effect of wearable technology combined with a lifestyle intervention on long-term weight loss: the IDEA randomized clinical trial. JAMA. 2016;316(11):1161–71.

Lee R. The demographic transition: three centuries of fundamental change. J Econ Perspect. 2003;17(4):167–90.

Linden W, Stossel C, Maurice J. Psychosocial interventions for patients with coronary artery disease: a meta-analysis. Arch Intern Med. 1996;156(7):745–52.

Lorig KR, et al. Evidence suggesting that a chronic disease self-management program can improve health status while reducing hospitalization: a randomized trial. Med Care. 1999;37(1):5–14.

Lorig KR, Sobel DS, Ritter PL, Laurent D, Hobbs M. Effect of a self-management program on patients with chronic disease. Eff Clin Pract. 2000;4(6):256–62.

Narayanaswami C, Raghunath MT. Application design for a smart watch with a high resolution display. In: The Fourth International Symposium on wearable computers. IEEE Press. 2000, pp. 7–14.

Norris SL, Engelgau MM, Narayan KV. Effectiveness of self-management training in type 2 diabetes. Diabetes Care. 2001;24(3):561–87.

Oh H, Rizo C, Enkin M, Jadad A. What is eHealth (3): a systematic review of published definitions. J Med Internet Res. 2005;7(1)

Peterson ND, Middleton KR, Nackers LM, Medina KE, Milsom VA, Perri MG. Dietary self-monitoring and long-term success with weight management. Obesity. 2014;22(9):1962–7.

Porzsolt F, Stengel D. In: Porzsolt F, Kaplan R, editors. Optimizing health: improving the value of healthcare delivery. New York, NY: Springer; 2006.

Pradhan D, Sujatmiko N. Can smartwatch help users save time by making processes efficient and easier. Master's thesis. Finland: University of Oslo; 2014:18.

Rice KL, et al. Disease management program for chronic obstructive Pulmonary disease: a randomized controlled Trial. Am J Respir Crit Care Med. 2010;182(7):890–6.

Richardson JL, Shelton DR, Krailo M, Levine AM. The effect of compliance with treatment on survival among patients with hematologic malignancies. J Clin Oncol. 1990;8(2):356–64.

Rosenberger ME, Buman MP, Haskell WL, McConnell MV, Carstensen LL. Twenty-four hours of sleep, sedentary behavior, and physical activity with nine wearable devices. Med Sci Sports Exerc. 2016;48(3):457–65.

Ross CE, Mirowsky J. Why education is the key to socioeconomic differentials in health, Handbook of medical sociology. 6th ed. Nashville: Vanderbilt University Press; 2010.

Sarkar U, Fisher L, Schillinger D. Is self-efficacy associated with diabetes self-management across race/ethnicity and health literacy? Diabetes Care. 2006;29(4):823–9.

Spring B, Gotsis M, Paiva A, Spruijt-Metz D. Healthy apps: mobile devices for continuous monitoring and intervention. IEEE Pulse. 2013;4(6):34–40.

Strecher VJ, McEvoy DeVellis B, Becker MH, Rosenstock IM. The role of self-efficacy in achieving health behavior change. Health Educ Q. 1986;13(1):73–92.

Turner-McGrievy GM, Beets MW, Moore JB, Kaczynski AT, Barr-Anderson DJ, Tate DF. Comparison of traditional versus mobile app self-monitoring of physical activity and dietary intake among overweight adults participating in an mHealth weight loss program. J Am Med Inform Assoc. 2013;20(3):513–8.

van der Aalst WMP. Process mining: discovery, conformance and enhancement of business processes. New York: Springer; 2011.

Verberk WJ, et al. Self-measurement of blood pressure at home reduces the need for antihypertensive drugs. Hypertension. 2007;50(6):1019–25.

Vieira DS, Maltais F, Bourbeau J. Home-based pulmonary rehabilitation in chronic obstructive pulmonary disease patients. Curr Opin Pulm Med. 2010;16(2):134–43.

Wac K, Rivas H. Emerging mHealth innovations for patient self-management support. In: International Conference on E-health networking, application & services (HealthCom), Boston, USA, 2015, pp. 574–7.

Wac K, Dey AK, Vasilakos AV. Body area networks for ambulatory psychophysiological monitoring: a survey of off-the-shelf sensor systems. In: Proceedings of the Fifth International conference on body area networks, Greece, 2010, pp. 181–7.

Wac K, Fiordelli M, Gustarini M, Rivas H. Quality of life technologies: experiences from the field and key challenges. IEEE Internet Comput. 2015;19(4):28–35.

Wagner EH, Austin BT, Davis C, Hindmarsh M, Schaefer J, Bonomi A. Improving chronic illness care: translating evidence into action. Health Aff (Millwood). 2001;20(6):64–78.

WHO. The innovative care for chronic conditions framework (ICCC). Geneva, Switzerland: WHO; 2002.

WHO. Chronic illness statistics for 2005. Geneva, Switzerland: WHO; 2005.

Winters BD, Gurses AP, Lehmann H, Sexton JB, Rampersad CJ, Pronovost PJ. Clinical review: checklists—translating evidence into practice. J Crit Care. 2009;13(6):210.

Chapter 7
From Quantified Self to Quality of Life

Katarzyna Wac

Abstract *"Know Thyself"* is a motto leading the Quantified Self (QS) movement, which at first originated as a "hobby project" driven by self-discovery, and is now being leveraged in wellness and healthcare. QS practitioners rely on the wealth of digital data originating from wearables, applications, and self-reports that enable them to assess diverse domains of their daily life. That includes their physical state (e.g., mobility, steps), psychological state (e.g., mood), social interactions (e.g., a number of Facebook "likes") and environmental context they are in (e.g., pollution). The World Health Organization (WHO) recognizes these four QS domains as contributing to individual's Quality of Life (QoL), with health spanning across all the four domains. The collected QS data enables an individual's state and behavioral patterns to be assessed through these different QoL domains, based on which individualized feedback can be provided, in turn enabling to improve the individual's state and QoL. The evidence of causality between QS and QoL is still being established, as only data from limited cases and domains exist so far. In this chapter, we discuss the state of this evidence via a semi-systematic review of the exemplary QS practices documented in 609 QS practitioners' talks and a review of the 438 latest available personal wearable technologies enabling QS. We discuss the challenges and opportunities for the QS to become an integral part of the future of healthcare and QoL-driven solutions. Some of the opportunities include using QS technologies as different types of affordances supporting the goal-oriented actions by the individual, in turn improving their QoL.

Keywords Human-computer interaction • Mobile health • Tracking and self-management systems • Ubiquitous computing and sensors • Physiologic modeling and disease processes

K. Wac
Department of Computer Science, University of Copenhagen, Copenhagen, Denmark

Quality of Life Technologies Lab, University of Geneva, Geneva, Switzerland
e-mail: katarzyna.wac@unige.ch

© Springer International Publishing AG 2018   83
H. Rivas, K. Wac (eds.), *Digital Health*, Health Informatics,
https://doi.org/10.1007/978-3-319-61446-5_7

7.1   Introduction

Quantified Self (QS) is a relatively young trend, where individuals focus on tracking own state and behavioral patterns with the help of old-fashioned paper-and-pencil methods, or, on a growing scale – with a support of personalized devices (wearables and smartphones) for continuous, ideally unobtrusive tracking. The QS movement is lead by the motto *"Know Thyself"* and has been enabled by the high spread and adoption of the Internet and its services, as well as ubiquitous availability of personal devices like smartphones with embedded sensors, enabling implicit and explicit tracking services. For example, in the United States in 2015, 89% of the population used the Internet, and 72% owned a smartphone, and these numbers are increasing yearly (Poushtr 2016). Self-tracking is a real trend in the US. It is estimated that 60% of the US population in 2013 tracked some aspect of their life (e.g., weight, exercise, mood), 33% of adults tracked health indicators or symptoms (e.g., blood pressure, blood sugar, headaches, or sleep patterns), and 12% tracked a health indicator on behalf of someone they cared for (Fox 2013). Added together, seven out of ten US adults said they tracked at least one health indicator. It was shown that 50% of these trackers record their notes in some organized way, such as on paper (29%) or using technology (21%), i.e., 8% of trackers use a medical device (e.g., a glucose meter), 7% use an app or another tool on their mobile phone or device, 5% use a spreadsheet, 1% use a website or another online tool. It was also shown that 46% of self-trackers admitted that tracking changed their overall approach to maintaining their health or the health of someone for whom they provided care. For 40% of them tracking led them to get a first-hand medical consultation or motivated them to get a second opinion, and for 34% of them it affected a decision about how to treat an illness or condition. As Fox (2013) has shown, self-trackers are more likely be living with chronic conditions themselves or be caring for a loved one, who is living with such a condition; and overall, they are more likely to report that tracking had an impact on their health.

These self-trackers are essentially QS practitioners. They rely on the wealth of digital data originating from QS technologies embracing wearables, applications, and self-reports that enable them to track different aspects of their physical or psychological health, social interactions and environmental conditions they are in. These four aspects constitute the individuals' Quality of Life (QoL), defined by World Health Organization (WHO 1995) as *"individuals' perception of their position in life in the context of the culture and value systems in which they live and in relation to their goals, expectations, standards and concerns"*; health spans across all the four domains. The collected QS data enables an individual's state and behavioral patterns assessment in the different QoL domains, based on which individualized feedback can be provided, in turn enabling to improve the individual's state and hence enabling to improve their QoL. The evidence for correlations/causalities between QS and QoL is still being established, as only data for limited cases and domains exist so far. Along our research we have already mapped a selection of large collaborative research projects in different QoL domains (Wac et al. 2015). We have concluded that most of the projects are in the domains of a person's physical health (majority), and some in social interactions, and environmental resources. The least number of projects are related to the psychological health aspects; although this domain is quickly catching up. In this chapter we further discuss the evidence for the QS/QoL correlations/causalities by mapping a selection of QS approaches in different QoL domains and analyzing this evidence. Specifically, we systematically assess 609 QS-community endorsed practices (answering question "*what do* people track") and the 438 latest personal wearable technologies enabling QS (answering question "*what can* people track"). Given the QS practices and wearables database we by no means claim to have a complete set of data, as the selected data sources may be incomplete, as well as the field is evolving, and some recent advances may not be documented yet. Furthermore, in this chapter, we also discuss a broad range of challenges (e.g., lack of evidence, privacy and security aspects) and opportunities (unobtrusiveness, longitudinal data collection) for the QS approach to become an integral part of the future healthcare and QoL-driven solutions, including the opportunity for the QS technologies as different types of affordances supporting the goal-oriented actions by the individual, in turn improving his/her QoL.

7.2   Quantified Self (QS)

Quantified Self (QS), referred to as, amongst the others, "self-tracking", "life-logging", "personal analytics" or "personal informatics", is a term encompassing a form of self-monitoring/self-tracking of individual's daily life activities and analyzing patterns and trends in, e.g., physical activity, nutrition, weight, mood, productivity data, usually to enable the individual's engagement with and reflection upon these patterns and trends, and potentially leading to behavior change strategies build upon this data (Choe 2014). The QS-enabled engagement is data-driven and very personal, as opposite to engagement with generic lifestyle recommendations like "move more" "eat more greens" without an indication of what exactly means "more", and where does the individual stand on this goal. More specifically, the QS tracking focuses on quantification of the daily life of individuals and ways of improving different aspects of their activities, like getting more physical activity, losing weight, eating better or getting better quality sleep; as supported by the quantitative data captured by the individuals. The QS encompasses the objective (e.g., steps), as well as subjective (e.g., mood or pain assessments) data being collected by the individual (Swan 2013).

The QS concept has been coined in the US by Gary Wolf and Kevin Kelly (the WIRED magazine[1] journalists) in 2008 building the Quantified Self community since then (Wolf and Kelly 2014). In 2012 the QS community involved 7000 self-trackers organized in 50 meeting groups around the world (so-called "meet-ups"), while today it involves over 125,000 self-trackers along 100+ meet-ups. In fact, the QS concept has been known for longer, Samuel Pepys was the first self-tracker in 1660–1669, he kept a daily written diary with personal, professional and public

---

[1] https://www.wired.com.

activities and events and own reflections (Pepys 1660). Self-tracking has become easier and more accessible with the advent of personal mobile technologies – either enabling easier capturing of data in electronic form (e.g., like notes on a smartphone, within an app) or capturing the events and data automatically and unobtrusively via an app or a wearable device. The mobile apps and wearables constitute the QS technologies that enable self-trackers to easier capture the data, aggregate and organize it, analyze it (e.g., statistically), interpret and display it in a meaningful ways. That in turns enables the self-tracker to define actions to take, in turn changing the resulting data being collected. The QS movement has grown significantly, also influencing the research in healthcare, by inspiring health and state tracking solutions delivered on mobile platforms, and being referred to as mhealth (K Wac 2012). Diverse scientific journals and magazines cover the QS movement theme from healthcare perspective, like Biotechnology by Nature (Elenko et al. 2015) and Translational Medicine by Science (Steinhubl et al. 2015). The QS practice is sometimes seen as "narcissistic" and "self-centered", but the behavior is argued as being the result of the self-tracker being curious about own life and state and trying to improve own behaviors, in turn improving own QoL. The fact is, that many of the QS self-tracking projects fade with time, i.e., once the target behavior has been changed and is maintained by an individual (Eysenbach 2005).

According to (Lupton 2016), there are five different practices of QS: private, pushed, communal, imposed and exploited. The *private* QS practice implies an intrinsic motivation for data being collected for own use and self-improvement, optimization of life along the slogan: "self-knowledge through numbers". An example of "private" QS results research includes our research on Heart Rate (HR) patterns over three months (Katarzyna Wac 2014) or 12 years of longitudinal study and self-experimentation with weight control by (Roberts 2012). The *pushed* QS practice implies that there is an incentive for engaging individuals in data collection, where the data serves other actors or agencies, e.g., healthcare practitioners, insurance companies, and so on. The *communal* QS practice implies that data collected by an individual is being shared with a community on a social media for, e.g., competition, social comparison or encouragement purposes. The imposed QS practice implies that individuals are obliged to collect some QS data and share with other actors or agencies, e.g., due to workplace compliance (e.g., truck drivers) or when participating in drug addiction program. The exploited QS practice implies that data collected by an individual is being exploited commercially for another purpose (e.g., advertising) or sold in bulk for a better understanding of the target population. In this chapter we focus mostly on the *private* QS practice, enabling the individual to self-track to improve their behaviors and resulting QoL.

7.3   Context and Methods

In this section, we discuss the state of the art in Quantified Self (QS) domain via a semi-systematic assessment of (1) the exemplary QS practices and (2) the latest available personal wearable technologies enabling the self-tracking in QS practice.

By no means we claim this discussion to be exhaustive, as the selected data sources may be incomplete, as well as the field is evolving, and some recent advances may not be documented.

7.3.1   Quantified Self Talks

At each of the QS community meet-up, there are a series of self-tracking projects being presented voluntary by the community members. Each QS talk is structured along three questions, imitating a scientific approach to a topic, i.e., "What did you do", "How did you do that" and "What have you learned". Answering the first question enables to elaborate on the self-tracker's "research" context and question(s), as well as assumptions taken (if any). Answering the second question leads to elaboration on research methods employed, while answering the third – on the results and findings, especially brought back to the self-tracker personal experience and context. Usually, based on the self-experimentation, a self-tracker point outs some causality between tracked variables, or at least a correlation, that enables them to make more informed decisions in their daily life and improve the tracked aspects. The meet-up talks of the exemplary QS practices' from around the world are being selected by the QS community managers (Wolf & Kelly) and are being posted on the official QS Vimeo channel.[2]

Previously, Choe et al. (2014) analyzed 53 talks posted along 2008–2013 from the QS website and then 30 talks posted from 2013–2014. Choe et al. (2015) focused on analyzing the talks by their visualization content and insights, i.e., *how* people track what they track and how they visualize the data. They found that the top variables that self-trackers experimented with were: physical activity, food consumption, weight, mood, work productivity and cognitive performance. Additionally, 56% of the self-trackers monitored the designated data with a wearable, 40% with an excel spreadsheet and 21% with custom software app or "pen and paper" method (multiple overlapping answers were possible per a self-tracker). In this chapter, we focus on further analysis of the QS talks for *what* do people track.

At the time of this research there were in total 1006 talks available online for 2008–2016. However, some talks were (a) duplicated (i.e., same speak, same talk, different venue), (b) "meet-up" introductory talks, or other (c) event-based talks ("Quantified Self Public Health Symposium 2015"), (d) panel discussions, (e) philosophical talks, or discussed (f) a specific broader aspects of self-tracking (e.g., ethics, privacy, scientific approaches), or (g) a self-tracking concept at large (i.e., without an individual's self-tracking project behind), or (h) a framework for data fusion and/or data analytics or a product/service enabling self-tracking. These talks were omitted from our analysis; we have included only talks presenting a personal self-tracker story. For each of the talks, the self-tracker has improved some of the aspects of the analyzed behaviors, or learned something new, as presented in the talk

---

[2] http://vimeo.com/qslabs.

(Answering the question "what did you learn"?); however the analysis of these results is beyond the scope of this book chapter. Overall, we have identified 609 talks being then analyzed for the purpose of our research to answer the question on "what *do* people track"?

7.3.2   Quantified Self Technologies: Wearables (and Apps)

Self-tracking is on a growing scale enabled by the ubiquitous availability of personal computing and communication devices and services—including personal wearable devices and mobile applications and services. We have analyzed the state of these QS technologies by analyzing a database of wearables available from Vandrico Inc.[3] (being lead by Deloitte), which is free and claims to be an up-to-date source of information about the latest technologies. At the time of this research there were a total 438 wearables available online for 2001–2016 and beyond (i.e., some wearables were marked as "to be released soon"). Each wearable has already a meta-data identifying its sensors, e.g., accelerometer, its goal, i.e., what phenomena are to be tracked (e.g., physical activity, sleep) and where is the wearable to be placed (e.g., wrist). Many of the wearables are also paired with their web-based services for advanced analytics and visualization. In our analysis we do not discuss the wearable or the web-based components separately; we are just focusing on "*what can* people track" with a specific device.

7.3.3   Methods: Data Acquisition and Tagging

To analyze the information about the self-tracking projects presented along with the 609 QS talks and the self-tracking possibilities of 438 wearables, each talk, and each wearable has been assigned a tag or set of tags representing the behavioral topic/aspect being tracked.

The tags to code the talks were either (a) derived from the talk/wearable description itself (e.g., 'nutrition', physical 'activity') or (b) assigned following the similarity of the topic with the domain represented by a tag, e.g., 'gluten-free diet' tracking has been coded as 'nutrition', 'steps' or 'running' coded as 'activity'. This way, for example, the 'activity' tag corresponds to talks/wearables tracking different types of daily life (physical) activities, of different duration, location, intensity, and include the calories burned, movements tracking of different parts of the body, and motion tracking. Moreover, the 'weight' tag embraces topics related to weight loss and fat loss and muscle management. 'Brain activity' corresponds to any EEG-based brain activity tracking or influencing it via neuro-feedback or influencing own focus, attention, intelligence or alertness with nutrition, caffeine, alcohol, intake of oils or medica-

---

[3] http://www.vandrico.com.

ments. The 'communication' tag embraces wearables that are hands-free, remote, and go beyond the SIM-enabled phone. The 'interaction' tag corresponds to any new interaction techniques, either gesture-based or based on novel interfaces including 3D sound and vision, haptic, microphone, and screens. A 'relationship' tag is used for the topics related to social interaction and communication – to distinguish them from the above-ones specifically relating to novel communication and interaction modalities.

There were in total 160 unique tags identified for the QS talks, and 58 tags for the wearables, and as some of these were overlapping, 192 unique tags have been leveraged in the further data analysis.

After each QS talk/wearable has been coded with the tag(s), clouds of tags were created. A cloud of tags is a visualization of a frequency of a given tag in a given set of words as a weighted list. The absolute frequency of a tag corresponds to a font size—the more frequently the tag has appeared, the larger the font size. In the figures, a color of the tags does not have any meaning. Tag clouds were created with the Wordle[4] web application. The results are as follows.

7.4   Quantified Self Talks

The 609 analyzed talks have been given mostly in years 2012–2015 (i.e., there are around 100–120 talks/year). Most of the talks (90%) have one tag describing the self-tracking project discussed; at most a talk would have five tags. Figure 7.1 presents the distribution of topics discussed in the talks encoded as tags.

As one can conclude from the figure, physical activity (97 talks) and nutrition (72) are the most likely to be tracked by the individuals, followed by weight (47), sleep (47), productivity (31) and emotions (28). Concerning the emotions, self-trackers focus on both positive (e.g., happiness, content, gratitude, 14 talks)

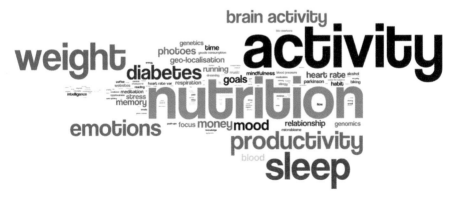

Fig. 7.1 Quantified Self Talks: behavior self-tracking projects focus

---

[4] http://www.wordle.net/.

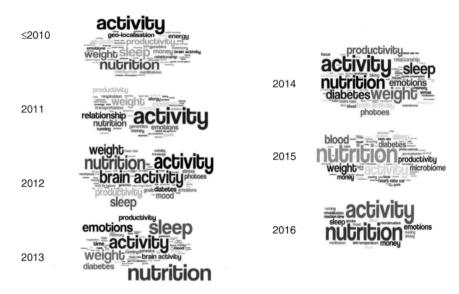

Fig. 7.2 Quantified Self Talks: self-tracking projects' distribution focus in time

and negative ones (stress, anger, grief, 14 talks). The least tracked, i.e., only by one individual, are, for example: flossing teeth, exposure to light, odd events, lying or flying.

Figure 7.2 presents the distribution of topics discussed in the talks encoded as tags and arranged over the years, in which the talk has been given (assuming being approximate to the year, the self-tracking project took place).

From Fig. 7.2 we conclude that 'activity' was always a prevalent topic to be tracked, along all the years with 'nutrition', 'sleep' and 'weight' gaining importance in time. 'Brain activity' (22 projects) was popular in 2012 with the advent of wearable, portable and affordable EEG-based brain trackers (e.g., Emotiv). Genetics (8), genomics (8), blood (12) and microbiome (5) analysis become popular along the years, since commercial companies started to provide affordable and easy to use tests to consumers at large.

7.5 Quantified Self Technologies

The QS self-tracking is on a growing scale enabled by ubiquitous availability of specific technologies embraced within the personal computing and communication devices and services. These devices and services collect multiple types of high-resolution data (e.g., location, physical activity) longitudinally and unobtrusively, provide some type of service visualizing this data to its user and are minimally obtrusive and wearable (even fashionable in some cases).

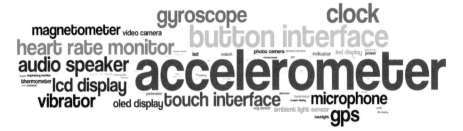

Fig. 7.3 Quantified Self Technologies: embedded sensors/interaction elements

7.5.1 Raw Sensor Data Acquisition

The 438 analyzed QS devices were released primarily in 2014 (155 devices), 2013 (73) and 2015 (57), while some are under development and will be released in 2017 (labeled as 'upcoming announcement' in the database, 71 devices) others will be released later (i.e., labeled as 'undisclosed release date', 82 devices). Figure 7.3 presents the raw sensors or interaction elements embedded in the analyzed wearable.

The raw sensor embedded in a wearable is mostly an accelerometer (209), gyroscope (83), some type of button-based interface (116), touch interface (73), kinesthetic interface (vibrator, 71) or LCD-based display (70), digital clock (100), heart rate monitor (82), GPS (78), including microphone (64) and audio speaker (78).

7.5.2 Behaviors Tracked/Enabled

Based on the raw sensor data or an interaction element, higher-level behaviors or behavioral aspects can be enabled or tracked, as presented in Fig. 7.4.

Wearables can track physical activity (207), sleep (47), geo-localization (20), phone notifications (57) and phone controls (44), as well as enable behaviors or novel form of interactions (e.g., gesture) with connected objects (29) and/or communications (17). There are other wearables that can track other behaviors or phenomena including eating, foot pressure, urinary infections and dreaming.

7.5.3 Positioning on the Body

Concerning the placing of the QS technology/wearable on the body, the most frequent positioning is the wrist (204), followed by the head (78), torso (22), chest (15) and ear (12) or arm (12). 26 out of 438 wearables can be put anywhere on a body to track the designated data. Figure 7.5 presents the wearables positioning distribution.

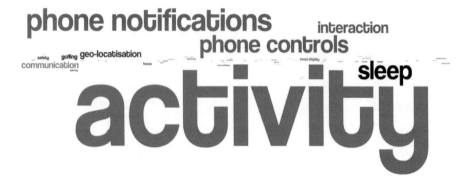

Fig. 7.4 Quantified Self Technologies: behaviors tracked/enabled

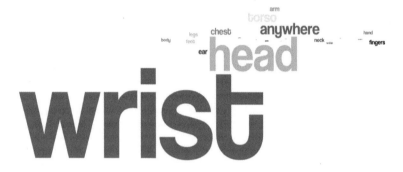

Fig. 7.5 Quantified Self Technologies: positioning on the body

7.5.4 Raw Data Sensor and Behaviors and Positioning on the Body

It is interesting to analyze the technological progress over time with respect to the types of sensors being integrated into the QS technologies, types of behaviors tracked or enabled by these sensors and their positioning on the body. Figure 7.6 presents a time-line of the conceptual development of wearables since 2010 for three variables of wear-able technology: raw sensors, tracked/ enabled behavior and positioning on the body.

From Fig. 7.6 we observe that early development (i.e., around 2010–2102) implies that QS "sensors" are just buttons and (simple) displays, while accelerom-eters appeared in 2013 and became an integral part of a wearable. Following that, (physical) activity was always an integral tracked behavioral variable, with phone notifications and controls appearing along the way, especially powered by advance-ments in short range communication like Bluetooth, enabling data exchange between a wearable and a phone. The most common positioning is the wrist. However, some recent advancements in miniaturization have enabled them to be placed on the head, torso, or become "anywhere"-based wearables.

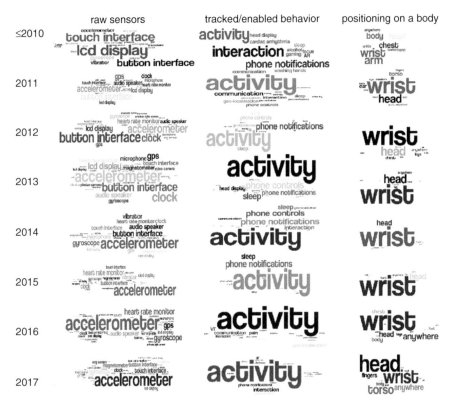

Fig. 7.6 Quantified Self Technologies: timeline for the diversity of sensors and behaviors and positioning on the body

7.5.5 Behaviors and Positioning on the Body

Figure 7.7 presents our research findings from the perspective of the human body—and wearables positioning on the body. Namely, it visualizes what behaviors a wearable can provide data for or what behaviors it can enable depending on where the wearable is placed on the body.

The physical activity type of behavior is a prevalent behavior being tracked from toe to head; anywhere on the body. Human hands become an interface for phone controls and phone notifications. Novel wearables in the area of interaction and communication are interfaced through hands or some part of the head. Especially the head has become a natural positioning for wearables enabling augmented/virtual reality (AR/VR). These developments are propelled by the emerging developments in personal electronic devices, having ever-increasing capacity of batteries and computing and communications capabilities, while being miniaturized to become unobtrusive part of everyday objects.

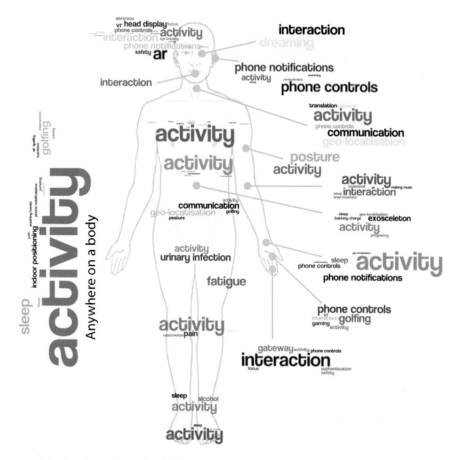

Fig. 7.7 Quantified Self Technologies: positioning on the body and behaviors

7.6 Quality of Life (QoL)

The World Health Organization (WHO) in 1995 has defined QoL as an "*individuals' perception of their position in life in the context of the culture and value systems in which they live and in relation to their goals, expectations, standards and concerns*" (WHO 1995). Along with that, the WHO has also defined the assessment scale - WHOQOL, which assesses the individual's QoL across four domains, i.e., physical and psychological health, social relationships and environmental, and 24 sub-domains (Fig. 7.8). The sub-domains include a variety of subjective and objective aspects being collectively exhaustive and mutually non-exclusive, i.e., there exist overlaps and correlations between these aspects, like, e.g., influence of noise (i.e., environment) on the sleep and rest (i.e., physical health). Health is an aspect of the

QoL Domain	Facets incorporated within QoL domains	CODE
Physical Health	Activities of daily living	phy-adl
	Dependence on medicinal substances, medical aids	phy-meds
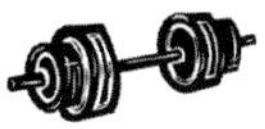	Energy and fatigue	phy-energy
	Mobility	phy-mobility
	Pain and discomfort	phy-pain
	Sleep and rest	phy-sleep
	Work capacity	phy-work
Psychological Health	Bodily image and appearance	psy-bodyimage
	Negative feelings	psy-negativefeel
	Positive feelings	psy-positivefeel
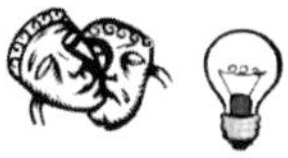	Self-esteem	psy-selfesteem
	Spirituality/religion/personal beliefs	psy-beliefs
	Thinking, learning, memory and concentration	psy-thinking
Social relation.	Personal relationships	soc-relationships
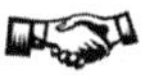	Social support	soc-support
	Sexual activity	soc-sex
Environment	Financial resources	env-finances
	Freedom, physical safety and security	env-freedom
	Health and social care: accessibility and quality	env-healthcare
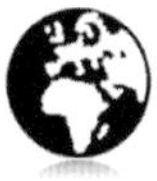	Home environment	env-home
	Opportunities for acquiring new information and skills	env-info
	Participation in/opportunities for recreation/leisure	env-leisure
	Physical environ. (pollution / noise / traffic / climate)	env-environ
	Transport	env-transport

Fig. 7.8 Quality of life domains and codes for the QS talks and technologies

individual's life that spans across all the different QoL domains. The column titled "code" in Fig. 7.8 corresponds to a WHOQOL-based coding of findings in our research as presented in the further sections of this chapter.

Since the WHO proposal, there have been many specialized QoL scales developed to evaluate a person's QoL. For example, there are scales for a given physical and psychological health condition (e.g., cancer), a given population (e.g., elderly), ethnicity (e.g., a Hispanic) or professional role (e.g., a nurse). There are even separate scales being developed for the QoL of animals. Additionally, current QoL research focuses on disabilities and older populations, specifically enabling them to have larger mobility (Schulz 2012; Kanade 2012).

In our research, we employ the WHOQOL as the most generic and applicable model across health states, populations, ethnicities, and professional roles of an individual. Additionally, in this chapter, we focus on an analysis of a potential role of QuantifiedSelf in improving QoL of any healthy, able-body individual.

7.7 From Quantified Self (QS) to Quality of Life (QoL): Where Is the Evidence?

Having presented our research material on Quantified Self (talks and technologies), as well as the approach to Quality of Life (QoL), in this section we qualitatively analyze the link between the two. The overarching question we attempt to answer is "if" and "how" the QS practice of self-tracking contributes to the QoL of the QS practitioners, i.e., self-trackers. The QS practice implies a behavior tracking (behavior assessment)—which may pave the way for behavior change, i.e., individual engages in self-experimentation (e.g., change of diet habits) that itself may be tracked by the QS technologies (e.g., nutrition logger, glucose level measurements), and which resulting behavioral effects may also be tracked by the QS technologies (e.g., better sleep). The QS technologies can serve as a behavior assessment tools in any point of the behavior change; supporting the behavior change with quantitative data. We explicitly do not employ any specific behavior change model drawn from psychology to fit our research into; as our research is rather exploratory and aims at understanding the current state of the art in the QS domain and its potential for the QoL improvement, rather than testing specific theories.

From the theoretical standpoint, (Petit and Cambon 2016) hypothesize that the practice of QS may have positive influence on his/her health by (1) transforming the individual's relation to own body and health and (2) by empowering the individual to leverage their self-tracking efforts to better control their health and health-related decisions. For both hypotheses, a common denominator is that individuals practicing QS make better health decisions, which in turn leads them to have a better health state and quality of life. There are some example studies supporting at least partially these hypotheses for specific populations focusing on self-management of movement/physical activity and gait-related disorders (Shull et al. 2014) or self-management of type 2 diabetes (Goyal et al. 2016). What is important to notice in the context of our research is that, the QS community is self-selected and attracts highly motivated individuals to improve their own health state and quality of life. The above-posed hypotheses are likely to be confirmed for the highly motivated individuals (although there is no clear evidence documented within the literature yet).

What is not yet evident is the efficacy of using QS-inspired, self-tracking and mobile health technologies to transform the relationships with their own health, including health decision-making and behavior change in patient populations. So far the technology with the most evidence for behavior change is the SMS-based interventions in smoking cessation (Free et al. 2013a; Free et al. 2013b). The use of QS tools and methods as a support for disease prevention or management via behavior changes, both regarding their role (transformation of relationship vs. empowerment), as well as their efficacy, must be researched further, especially in clinical populations. We cannot put forward yet a hypothesis that the QoL of patients' practicing QS would improve with time. Therefore, in the following paragraphs, we focus on general discussion considering the individuals practicing QS voluntarily, and we discuss their potential improvement of QoL, as enabled by the QS tools and methods.

As we can conclude from the previous section, the QS tracking focuses on the daily life of individuals and ways of improving different aspects of their activities, like getting more physical activity through a day, losing weight, eating better or having a better quality sleep. Ideally, QS enables the individuals to create and keep healthier habits, and in case they are suffering from a disease requiring medical opinion and treatment—track pain or other symptoms, which then could be discussed with a healthcare practitioner at their next visit. Overall, the QS methods and tools presented in the previous section can potentially contribute to an improvement of different aspects of individual's physical and psychological health, social relationships or environmental conditions; and as these are the main dimensions of the individuals' QoL. This way the QS practice can potentially contribute to the individual's QoL.

7.7.1   Methods

This section maps the state of the art in the QS domain (i.e., the exemplary 609 QS practices and the 438 latest available personal wearable technologies), on the space of QoL domains, as defined by the WHO (employing the codes from the 'code' column in Fig. 7.8). We answer questions like "What *do* people track, which may contribute to their QoL"? (based on the QS talks), and "What *can* people track, which may contribute to their QoL"? (based on the QS wearables space).

7.7.2   Results

To get a picture on the state of the art in the QS domain and its potential contribution to the QoL, for all the QS talks and QS technologies considered in our research, we have coded their main tag regarding the corresponding QoL domain. In practice, that means that the results from Fig. 7.1 and Fig. 7.4 have been coded into the WHO QoL domains, as presented in the Figs. 7.9 and 7.10. Therefore, Fig. 7.9 encodes the behaviors being tracked by the QS practitioners or behaviors being able to be collected via wearables—as contributing to specific WHO QoL sub-domains in the physical or psychological health, social relationships of environmental domains.

The top WHO QoL sub-domains, in which QS practitioners self-track, include activities of daily life (physical activity, nutrition, etc., 315 talks), medications (65), sleep (52) and work (33) in the physical health domain, thinking (116), body image embracing weight (54), positive feelings (including mood, happiness, content, gratitude, 47 talks) and negative feelings (stress, anger, grief, 14) within the psychological health domain. Within the social relationships domain, QS practitioners self-track relationships (14), and within the environmental domain—status of their finances (20).

Fig. 7.9 Quantified Self Talks: self-tracking projects focus coded along the WHO QoL domains

Fig. 7.10 Quantified Self Technologies: behaviors tracked/enabled coded along the WHO QoL domains

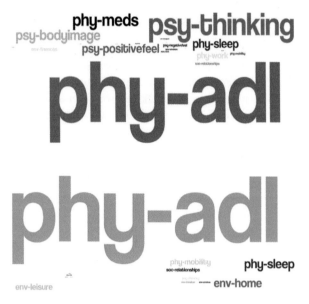

The top WHO QoL sub-domains, enabled to be self-tracked by the currently available technologies include activities of daily life (mainly physical activity, 341 wearables), sleep (48), mobility (30) and medications (5) in the physical health domain, and thinking (13) within the psychological health domain. Within the social relationships domain, QS technologies enable new forms of human communications usually via a novel interface, e.g., kinesthetic, EEG (18), and within the environmental domain—status of their home environment (including home control, 45), get some leisure activities (32), practice their freedom via security and authentication/authorization enabling wearables (10) or check the status of their environment (pollution, noise, temperature, etc., 9 technologies).

Figure 7.11 enables us to compare the QS self-tracking space ("what people do track"?) with QS potential self-tracking space enabled by the QS technologies ("what can people track"?), as mapped along the WHO QoL sub-domains in the physical or psychological health, social relationships of environmental domains.

As it can be concluded from Fig. 7.11, concerning the physical aspects of what QS self-trackers would like to track, and which technologies are not yet available, we can see that nutrition and productivity tracking can still be improved. For the psychological tracking, weight (although impossible to be measured via a wearable), as well as negative emotions and in the future—complex states of beliefs and self-esteem would be important for assessment, although neither being tracked now, nor being able to be tracked. For the social relationships, the relationship status, as well as sex-related aspects would be of interest to be tracked automatically via technologies. Social support is very important for mental health (Rueger et al. 2016; Wedgeworth et al. 2016), although neither being tracked now, nor being able to be

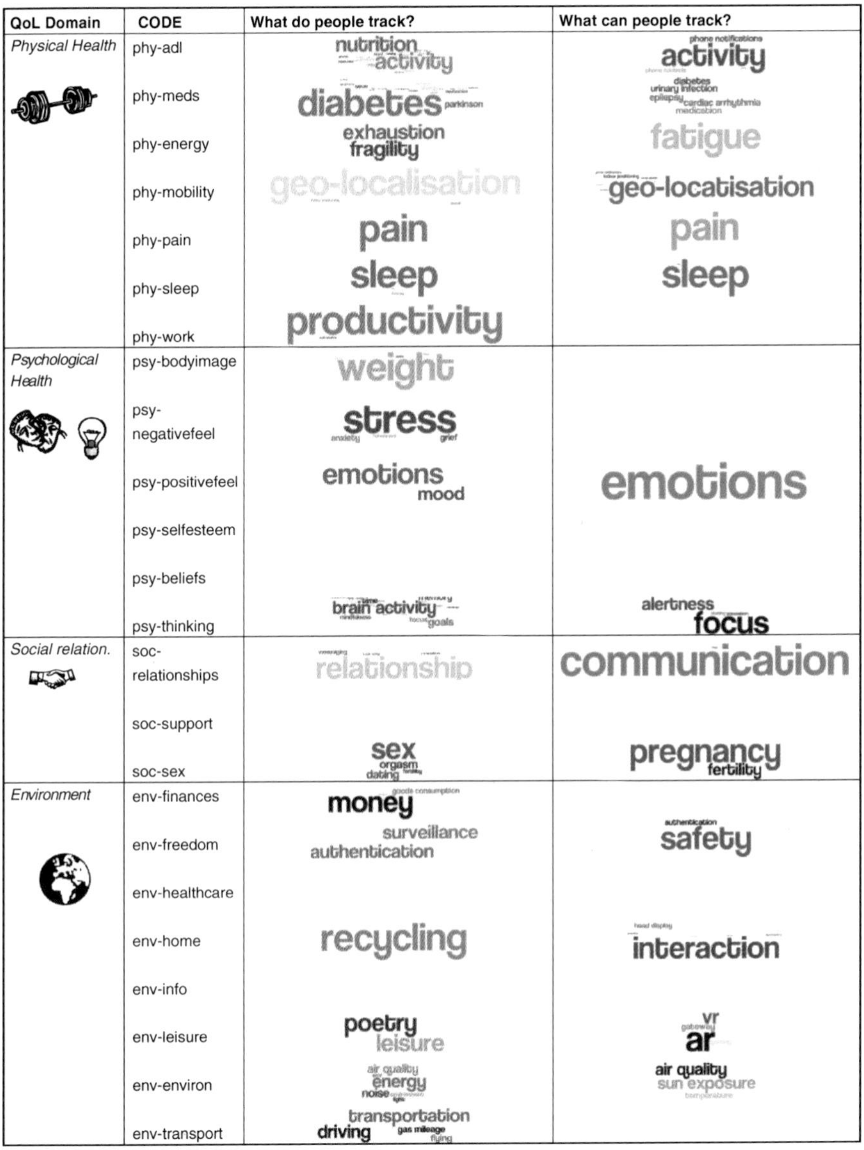

QoL Domain	CODE	What do people track?	What can people track?
Physical Health	phy-adl	nutrition activity	activity phone notifications
	phy-meds	diabetes parkinson	diabetes urinary infection epilepsy cardiac arrhythmia medication
	phy-energy	exhaustion fragility	fatigue
	phy-mobility	geo-localisation	geo-localisation
	phy-pain	pain	pain
	phy-sleep	sleep	sleep
	phy-work	productivity	
Psychological Health	psy-bodyimage	weight	
	psy-negativefeel	stress anxiety grief	
	psy-positivefeel	emotions mood	emotions
	psy-selfesteem		
	psy-beliefs		
	psy-thinking	brain activity memory focus goals	alertness focus
Social relation.	soc-relationships	relationship	communication
	soc-support		
	soc-sex	sex orgasm dating	pregnancy fertility
Environment	env-finances	money goods consumption	
	env-freedom	surveillance authentication	safety authentication
	env-healthcare		
	env-home	recycling	interaction head display
	env-info		
	env-leisure	poetry leisure	vr ar
	env-environ	air quality energy noise	air quality sun exposure
	env-transport	transportation driving gas mileage flying	

Fig. 7.11 QoL domains vs. QS talks and technologies

tracked. For the environmental aspects, technologies could evolve to track individuals' finances, leisure activities and transportation means. Access to healthcare, information, and knowledge is neither being tracked now, nor being able to be tracked, yet it may become a need in the future.

7.7.3 Behavioral Routines and QS Technologies as "Affordances"

Feldman and Pentland (2003) analyzed different types of routines, especially in the organizational context, distinguishing the ostensive and performative aspects of routines. The *ostensive* aspect of a routine enables people to guide, account for, and refer to specific performances of a routine (i.e., is the theory of the routine), and the *performative aspect* creates, maintains, and modifies the ostensive aspect of the routine (i.e., is the practice of the routine, e.g., context or other activities informing the theory). (Boillat et al. 2015) extended the theories of (Feldman and Pentland 2003) by researching how mobile applications act as affordances enabling specific goal-oriented actions in individual's routines. An *affordance* of an object or an action or an environment relates to a design space of possibilities (e.g., actions) that it enables. (Boillat et al. 2015) has considered mobile applications as affordances contributing to the ostensive and performative aspects of an individual's routine. In this chapter, we employ and further extend the work of (Boillat et al. 2015) assuming QS technologies (wearables and their corresponding mobile apps) as affordances and we discuss their support for the ostensive and performative aspects of a routine.

In Table 7.1, we employ work of (Feldman and Pentland 2003) and (Boillat et al. 2015) to represent the role QS technologies in relation to the goal-oriented action in performing daily routine behaviors in diverse QoL domains.

As it can be seen from the table, the role of QS technologies in relation to routine behaviors can be 'representing' or 'influencing', both applied to ostensive and performative aspects, as follows.

In the case of the QS technologies 'representing' ostensive aspects of routine behaviors, these technologies—and specifically their user interface with forms, checklists and visual elements—enable to codify the patterns of behaviors given the specific behavior types (e.g., physical activity) and goals (e.g., 10'000 steps a day). The specified behavior types and goals may or may be not driven by the latest state of the evidence in the health and QoL field (Higgins 2016).

In the case of the QS technologies 'representing' performative aspects of routine behaviors, these technologies—and specifically their sensing elements (e.g., accelerometer, Heart Rate)—enables them to document and trace the behavior outcomes—either during execution or through time-based logs (to be viewed after the behavior occurs).

In the case of the QS technologies 'influencing' ostensive aspects of routine behaviors, these technologies—and specifically their user interface with visual elements—enable them to enrich (and thus also influence) the representation of the routines by enabling the access to real-time and historical behavioral data and behavioral routines.

In the case of the QS technologies 'influencing' performative aspects of routine behaviors, these technologies- and specifically their interactive elements (e.g., screen, tactile or auditory feedback)—enables them to guide the individual by

Table 7.1 Roles of QS technologies as affordances in daily routine behaviors

QS Technology affordance role in a routine (Feldman and Pentland 2003)	Affordance categories (based on Boillat et al. 2015) of QS technologies supporting individual routine behaviors	
'Representing' (ostensive aspect)	*Knowledge codification affordance*	
	Codify the patterns of behaviors through the mobile application's storyboard and navigation elements.	– Dashboard with defined goals for behavior – Different behavioral goals categories (physical activity, sleep)
	Codify the behaviors via forms and checklists	– A predefined selection of behavioral goals, e.g., 10,000 steps or 10 floors in a day – By means of graphical interface, users can define their own behavioral goals, e.g., wake up at 7 am. – Behavioral goals are possible to be defined for weekends/ weekdays, work time (9 am-5 pm), morning/ afternoon/ evening etc.
	Codify the behaviors via interactive visual graphics	– Visualization of behavioral goals via interactive visual graphics, e.g., "Happy Hill" goal representing a goal of 10 floors to be achieved each day
'Representing' (performative aspects)	*Document and trace affordance*	
	Document the outcome of a routine behavior during execution	– Up-to-date real-time behavioral data visible (e.g., 5378 steps just now) with indication on how it relates to a predefined behavioral goal(s) (e.g., 10,000 steps)
	Trace the observable behavior of individuals through logs	– Historical behavioral data (with indication on how it relates to a predefined behavioral goals) data available
'Influencing' (ostensive aspects)	*Enrichment affordance*	
	Enrich routines through seamless access to information	– Up-to-date real-time behavioral data, as well as behavior goal(s) data visible anytime
	Enrich the representation of routines	– Visualization of routines via interactive visual graphics e.g., Castle along one day, while "Happy Hill" (10 floors) the next day

(continued)

Table 7.1 (continued)

QS Technology affordance role in a routine (Feldman and Pentland 2003)	Affordance categories (based on Boillat et al. 2015) of QS technologies supporting individual routine behaviors	
'Influencing' (performative aspects)	*Guidance affordance*	
	Guide individuals by constraining the way of behaving and standardizing instances of routines	– Users get visual / acoustic / vibration notification to help them reach their goals. – Reminders enabling to achieve a behavioral goal, e.g., "do not be a sitter" (goal being to stand up every hour)
	Guide executants by validating the behavior performed	– Notifications, if behavioral goals are partially achieved, e.g., 50% of a goal
	Guide individuals in individual ways of behaving by generating context-dependent routine instances	– Detecting when users are outside and encourage them to extend their walk "You need only 500 more steps to reach your next activity level"

constraining or encouraging them to behave a certain way (e.g., feedback upon specific Heart Rate levels when performing physical activity) and validating behaviors just conducted against the pre-defined goals.

The table above represents a general view of the field of QS technologies and their role in relation to the goal-oriented action in performing daily routine behaviors in diverse QoL domains. For each QS technology instantiation analyzed earlier in this chapter, this table could be adapted to its specific behaviors enabled/tracked and its specific sensing and interaction capabilities. Considering a specific QS technological instantiation, e.g., a wearable as an affordance within the context of routine behaviors may open new avenues for design choices for this instantiation—depending on its role concerning to the targeted routine behavior and its ostensive or performative aspect for the routine itself.

7.8 Discussion

In this section, we discuss the challenges and opportunities for QS to become an integral part healthcare and QoL-driven solutions. Additionally, in the scope of the opportunities, we analyze the QS approaches as different types of *affordances* supporting the behavioral routines and goal-oriented actions by the individual, in turn enabling them to improve their QoL.

7.8.1 QS Technologies for QoL Improvements: The Challenges and Opportunities

The Quantified Self field paves the way for self-monitoring and self-knowledge, and, as we show in this chapter—there are a variety of aspects individuals already track (leveraging on a growing scale QS technologies) and can track automatically (via QS technologies), enabled by advances in miniaturized, personalized devices, including smartphone and diverse mobile apps.

The challenges to be tackled before the QS technologies and developments can enable the QoL improvements and provide clear evidence for these improvements are as follows. First of all, what can be concluded from the results, is that what individuals "do track" differs from what QS technologies "enable them to track"—there is especially a shortage of technologies enabling behavior and state tracking in psychological health and social relationships domains. That can stem from the fact that phenomena in these domains are highly subjective, and cannot be easily quantified based on data solely monitored on, e.g., a wrist. The research in affective computing domain addresses this issue leveraging psychophysiological computing (Ciman and Wac 2016; Wac and Tsiourti 2014) and we can expect major developments in years to come.

Within the QS technologies themselves, we shall consider the accuracy and reliability of the devices themselves, for example, how "a step" is defined (Case et al. 2015; Piwek et al. 2016). The accuracy of the devices will become increasingly important when introducing the behavioral interventions for QoL improvements; inaccurate assessment data may lead to inaccurate interventions and in turn even negatively influence one's QoL. There is already research to improve the accuracy of QS technologies and specifically personal wearable devices in a uniform way (Case et al. 2015), and recently the US-based FDA recommendations have been put forward to positively influence the accuracy of these wearables (Cortez et al. 2014). However, to enable the community (including the scientist) to understand and potentially improve the accuracy of the QS technologies, the manufacturers and service providers shall, ideally, publish the results of their accuracy evaluations in a peer-reviewed manner as well as enable an open, standardized, interoperable access to their data streams.

Additionally to the openness of the data, the QS technologies users must know how their data is secured and where it is stored and with whom it is shared (Lobelo et al. 2016). The data security and privacy may be an important aspect of the adoption of these technologies, especially in Europe (Leibenger et al. 2016), where the new the European Union's new General Data Protection Regulation (2016/679 GDPR) will come into effect as a law across the EU after 25th May 2018. Some scientists have already discovered that even the companies, which seemed to be trustworthy by the QS community, are turning their user's data for profit.[5]

---

[5] C. de Looper, "Runkeeper is the latest mobile app to run afoul of privacy advocates", available from http://www.digitaltrends.com/mobile/runkeeper-user-tracking/, May 2016.

Overall, the QS technologies and development do not provide clear evidence for QoL improvements, i.e., no strong evidence is available to date besides small indicative studies in fields of physical health. An obvious problem is, that the self-quantification experiments lack the rigorous controls and double blind of pharmaceutical trials. These results could also be effects of (a) inaccurate devices (as discussed above), (b) placebo effects (Shapiro 1968) (i.e., results acquired solely by a psychological effect of QS activity) or (c) the Hawthorne effect (Adair, and G., J. 1984) (i.e., results acquired due to an "observer" effect of QS activity).

Nevertheless, there are opportunities for the QS technologies and developments to provide clear evidence for QoL improvements, as follows. First of all, the QS technologies field is expanding, as technologies get on a growing scale more and more miniaturized and hence minimally obstructive, more personalized, with more computing and communication power and longer battery lifetime (following Moore's law (Schaller 1997)(Minerva and Crespi 2017)), enabling to conduct longitudinal QS data collection and analytics with masses.

Looking from the perspective of the QoL assessment and improvement, this field it is a very complex field and much research must be done in understanding the causality and correlations between the different QoL domains (physical, psychological, social interactions, environmental) and their contributions to the individual's QoL. That must be done for both: healthy and pathologic populations. Some attempts are already documented in the literature (Bergland et al. 2016; Da Silva and Pereira 2017; McKee et al. 2015). The new research methods enabling to model these correlations and causalities are needed. Towards this end, the QS technologies may pave the way for experimentation within the four QoL domains, especially in $N = 1$ conditions, where the correlations and causalities could be disclosed and modeled for an individual. Such approach has been already introduced in the literature, especially for QS technologies-enabled behavior change and management and treatment options in chronic illness (Schork 2015; Swan 2013; Patel et al. 2015).

Many patients are self-trackers that have found QS-enabled solutions in areas that the traditional health system would never have studied or applied to their specific case. Given that these patients organize themselves on dedicated online social platforms, e.g. PatientsLikeMe.com, many of the individual patient's self-experiments could be aggregated to form hypotheses with respect to, e.g., most effective management and treatment options for given patient and health state (age, gender, socioeconomics, broader context of life, health history), enabling the individuals' QoL improvements. The hypotheses could be then further tested in new populations for their effectiveness. Such an approach would pave the way for highly personalized behavior change interventions leading to QoL improvements.

7.8.2   Limitation of the Work

The limitation of this survey is that it is not exhaustive and may miss important developments regarding QS technologies embedded in wearables, not yet documented due to their novelty. The same applies for the phenomena being tracked—potentially interesting aspects of QS individuals' life may not be documented yet, although widely tracked and contributing the QoL improvements.

The opportunities for future work include more detailed analysis of the Quantified Self community as a whole, potentially getting into meta data of each single QS talk in each single city given worldwide, and understanding what is currently tracked and with which level of depth and if there is a success outcome (e.g., increased awareness or behavior change). As for the QS technologies, recent approaches and innovative ideas may be interesting to track on e.g., kickstarter.com platform—dedicated for upcoming design-based ideas for future products and services. Overall, the completeness of our approach may be challenged and fulfilled with further research in this domain.

7.9   Conclusive Remarks

This chapter has surveyed exemplary QS practices and latest available personal wearable technologies enabling Quantified Self approach and understanding "what do people track", "what can people track" and how the tracked data can contribute to their Quality of Life improvements in physical, psychological, social interactions and environmental health domains. The least developments are within the mental health and social interactions domains. Overall, the evidence for the QS technologies contributing to individual's QoL mostly lacks so far. We discussed challenges to be overcome and the opportunities for the QS to become an integral part of the future healthcare and QoL-driven solutions, including an opportunity for the QS technologies as different types of affordances supporting the goal-oriented actions by the individual, in turn improving their QoL.

Based on the progress witnessed in the domain, as well as the current state of the art, as documented in here and in related articles (Wac et al. 2015), we envision that the QS approach embracing the QS technologies and improving the individual's QoL will be available for general public, and it will be embedded in the fabric of our daily life. It will be automated, accurate, easy to use, affordable, longitudinal and comfortable. Therefore little effort is required for self-tracking and self-improvement of own QoL. We envision that more and more individuals will be willing to and open to the possibility of higher self-awareness, understanding potentials behavioral choices, willing to change themselves for better QoL of themselves and those around them. We will be able to become scientists with ourselves being own subject to research – enabled by QS technologies to extend the mind and the body of oneself – and becoming an "exoself" (Swan 2013). The choice is ours if and how we wish to *"Know Thyself.*

Acknowledgments This research is supported by the Swiss NSF MIQmodel (157003), AAL ANIMATE (6-071) and CoME (7-127) projects, and COST actions (1303, 1304). I appreciate the help of the QoL team members and collaborators with getting the data required for this chapter (especially Alexandre De Masi) and for overall feedback (especially Thomas Boillat).

References

Adair JG. The Hawthorne effect: a reconsideration of the methodological artifact. J Appl Psychol. 1984;69(2):334–45. http://doi.org/10.1037/0021-9010.69.2.334

Bergland A, Meaas I, Debesay J, Brovold T, Jacobsen EL, Antypas K, Bye A. Associations of social networks with quality of life, health and physical functioning. Eur J Phys. 2016;18(2):78–88. http://doi.org/10.3109/21679169.2015.1115554

Boillat, T., Lienhard, K., & Legner, C. (2015). Entering the World of individual routines: the affordances of mobile applications. Proceedings ICIS 2015. http://aisel.aisnet.org/icis2015/proceedings/ISstrategy/14.

Case MA, Burwick HA, Volpp KG, Patel MS. Accuracy of smartphone applications and wearable devices for tracking physical activity data. JAMA. 2015;313(6):625. http://doi.org/10.1001/jama.2014.17841

Choe, E. K. (2014). Designing self-monitoring technology to promote data capture and reflection. Retrieved from https://digital.lib.washington.edu/researchworks/handle/1773/26199

Choe EK, Lee NB, Lee B, Pratt W, Kientz JA, Choe EK, et al. Understanding quantified-selfers' practices in collecting and exploring personal data. In: Proceedings of the 32nd annual ACM conference on Human factors in computing systems - CHI '14. New York: ACM Press; 2014. p. 1143–52. http://doi.org/10.1145/2556288.2557372.

Choe EK, Lee B, Schraefel M. Characterizing visualization insights from quantified selfers' personal data presentations. IEEE Comput Graph Appl. 2015;35(4):28–37. http://doi.org/10.1109/MCG.2015.51

Ciman M, Wac K. Individuals' stress assessment using human-smartphone interaction analysis. IEEE Trans Affect Comput. 2016:1–1. http://doi.org/10.1109/TAFFC.2016.2592504

Cortez NG, Cohen IG, Kesselheim AS. FDA regulation of mobile health technologies. N Engl J Med. 2014;371(4):372–9. http://doi.org/10.1056/NEJMhle1403384

Da Silva JP, Pereira AMS. Perceived spirituality, mindfulness and quality of life in psychiatric patients. J Relig Health. 2017;56(1):130–40. http://doi.org/10.1007/s10943-016-0186-y

Elenko E, Underwood L, Zohar D. Defining digital medicine. Nat Biotechnol. 2015;33(5):456–61. http://doi.org/10.1038/nbt.3222

Eysenbach G. The law of attrition. J Med Internet Res. 2005;7(1):e11. http://doi.org/10.2196/jmir.7.1.e11

Feldman MS, Pentland BT. Reconceptualizing organizational routines as a source of flexibility and change. Adm Sci Q. 2003;48(1):94. http://doi.org/10.2307/3556620

Fox, S. (2013). .The self-tracking data explosion

Free C, Phillips G, Galli L, Watson L, Felix L, Edwards P, et al. The effectiveness of mobile-health technology-based health behaviour change or disease management interventions for health care consumers: a systematic review. PLoS Med. 2013a;10(1):e1001362. http://doi.org/10.1371/journal.pmed.1001362

Free C, Phillips G, Watson L, Galli L, Felix L, Edwards P, et al. The effectiveness of mobile-health technologies to improve health care service delivery processes: a systematic review and meta-analysis. PLoS Med. 2013b;10(1):e1001363. http://doi.org/10.1371/journal.pmed.1001363

Goyal S, Morita P, Lewis GF, Yu C, Seto E, Cafazzo JA. The systematic design of a behavioural mobile health application for the self-management of type 2 diabetes. Can J Diabetes. 2016;40(1):95–104. http://doi.org/10.1016/j.jcjd.2015.06.007

Higgins JP. Smartphone applications for patients' health and fitness. Am J Med. 2016;129(1):11–9. http://doi.org/10.1016/j.amjmed.2015.05.038

Kanade T. Quality of Life Technology. Proc IEEE. 2012;100(8):2394–6. http://doi.org/10.1109/JPROC.2012.2200555

Leibenger D, Möllers F, Petrlic A, Petrlic R, Sorge C. Privacy challenges in the quantified self movement – an EU perspective. Proc Privacy Enhanc Technol. 2016;2016(4):315–34. http://doi.org/10.1515/popets-2016-0042

Lobelo F, Kelli HM, Tejedor SC, McConnell MV, Martin SS, Welk GJ. The wild wild west: A framework to integrate mhealth software applications and wearables to support physical activity assessment, counseling and interventions for cardiovascular disease risk reduction. Prog Cardiovasc Dis. 2016;58(6):584–94. http://doi.org/10.1016/j.pcad.2016.02.007

Lupton D. The diverse domains of quantified selves: self-tracking modes and dataveillance. Econ Soc. 2016;45(April):1–22. http://doi.org/10.1080/03085147.2016.1143726

McKee KJ, Kostela J, Dahlberg L. Five years from now. Res Aging. 2015;37(1):18–40. http://doi.org/10.1177/0164027513520329

Minerva, R., & Crespi, N. (2017). Technological evolution of the ICT sector. SpringerNew York53–87. http://doi.org/10.1007/978-3-319-33995-5_3.

Patel MS, Asch DA, Volpp KG. Wearable devices as facilitators, not drivers, of health behavior change. JAMA. 2015;313(5):459–60. http://doi.org/10.1001/jama.2014.14781

Pepys, S. (1660). Diary of samuel pepys. https://books.google.com/books?hl=en&lr=&id=Y35K AAAAYAAJ&oi=fnd&pg=PA1&ots=0IaL7LkXbd&sig=oNa59Jp7sOq2Cx_IGhcMa7AaZQo #v=onepage&q&f=false.

Petit A, Cambon L. Exploratory study of the implications of research on the use of smart connected devices for prevention: a scoping review. BMC Public Health. 2016;16:552. http://doi.org/10.1186/s12889-016-3225-4

Piwek L, Ellis DA, Andrews S, Joinson A, Yang B, Rhee S, et al. The rise of consumer health wearables: promises and barriers. PLoS Med. 2016;13(2):e1001953. http://doi.org/10.1371/journal.pmed.1001953

Poushtr, J. (2016). Smartphone ownership and internet usage continues to climb in emerging economies.http://www.pewglobal.org/2016/02/22/smartphone-ownership-and-internet-usage--continues-to-climb-in-emerging-economies/#fn-35095-2.

Roberts S. The reception of my self-experimentation. J Bus Res. 2012;65(7):1060–6. http://doi.org/10.1016/j.jbusres.2011.02.014

Rueger SY, Malecki CK, Pyun Y, Aycock C, Coyle S. A Meta-analytic review of the association between perceived social support and depression in childhood and adolescence. Psychol Bullet. 2016;42(10):1017–67. http://doi.org/10.1037/bul0000058

Schaller RR. Moore's law: past, present and future. IEEE Spectr. 1997;34(6):52–9. http://doi.org/10.1109/6.591665

Schork NJ. Personalized medicine: time for one-person trials. Nature. 2015;520(7549):609–11. http://doi.org/10.1038/520609a

Schulz, R. (2012). Quality of life technology handbook. https://books.google.dk/books/about/Quality_of_Life_Technology_Handbook.html?id=nrE7LfUiO5oC&pgis=1.

Shapiro AK. Semantics of the placebo. Psychiatr Q. 1968;42(4):653–95. http://www.ncbi.nlm.nih.gov/pubmed/4891851

Shull PB, Jirattigalachote W, Hunt MA, Cutkosky MR, Delp SL. Quantified self and human movement: a review on the clinical impact of wearable sensing and feedback for gait analysis and intervention. Gait Posture. 2014;40(1):11–9. http://doi.org/10.1016/j.gaitpost.2014.03.189

Steinhubl SR, Muse ED, Topol EJ, Barrett PM, Komatireddy R, Haaser S, et al. The emerging field of mobile health. Sci Transl Med. 2015;7(283):283rv3. http://doi.org/10.1126/scitranslmed.aaa3487

Swan M. The quantified self: fundamental disruption in big data science and biological discovery. Big Data. 2013;1(2):85–99. http://doi.org/10.1089/big.2012.0002

Wac K. Smartphone as a personal, pervasive health informatics services platform: literature review. Yearb Med Inform. 2012;7(1):83–93.

Wac K. Beat-by-beat getting fit : leveraging pervasive self-tracking of heart rate in self-management of health. Stanford: Association for the Advancement of Artificial Intelligence; 2014.

Wac K, Tsiourti C. Ambulatory assessment of affect: survey of sensor systems for monitoring of autonomic nervous systems activation in emotion. IEEE Trans Affect Comput. 2014;5(3):251–72. http://doi.org/10.1109/TAFFC.2014.2332157

Wac K, Fiordelli M, Gustarini M, Rivas H. Quality of life technologies: experiences from the field and key research challenges. IEEE Internet Comput. 2015;99:1. http://doi.org/10.1109/MIC.2015.52

Wedgeworth M, LaRocca MA, Chaplin WF, Scogin F. The role of interpersonal sensitivity, social support, and quality of life in rural older adults. Geriatr Nurs. 2016;38(1):22–6. http://doi.org/10.1016/j.gerinurse.2016.07.001

WHO. The World Health Organization quality of life assessment (WHOQOL): position paper from the World Health Organization. Soc Sci Med, 1995;41(10):1403–1409. http://doi.org/10.1016/0277-9536(95)00112-K.

Wolf G, Kelly K. Quantified self: self knowledge through numbers. 2014. http://quantifiedself.com website, Visited April 207

Chapter 8
3D Printing

Michael Gelinsky

Abstract Three-dimensional printing which was used for prototyping purposes only at the beginning has evolved to a real option for industrial production purposes. Also for a variety of medical applications it is of utmost interest as three-dimensional objects easily can be prepared, based on patient-specific 3D data. Already used are 3D printed models for educational and training purposes as well as for planning of complex surgical intervention. In addition, 3D printing is commonly used now for fabrication of surgical sawing and drilling templates. For manufacturing of patient-specific implants more and more 3D printing technologies are applied, currently mostly utilizing non-degradable biomaterials like metals or ceramics. But also degradable implants already can be generated, as well as tissue constructs—if bio-printing technologies are applied, utilizing living cells. This chapter provides an overview how 3D printing is currently emerging as an important tool for individualized medicine and patient-specific therapies.

Keywords Additive manufacturing • Patient-specific • Implant • Biomaterial • Bioprinting

8.1 Basics of Additive Manufacturing

Additive manufacturing (AM), also referred to as 3D printing, describes a class of manufacturing technologies in which material is added in a layer-by-layer fashion to directly produce a three-dimensional object (Gibson et al. 2014). Prerequisite is a digital dataset that defines the dimensions of the object and, for the manufacturing process itself, additional information about the step-wise assembly process

M. Gelinsky
Centre for Translational Bone, Joint and Soft Tissue Research, University Hospital and Medical Faculty, Technische Universität Dresden, Fetscherstr. 74, 01307 Dresden, Germany
e-mail: michael.gelinsky@tu-dresden.de

H. Rivas, K. Wac (eds.), *Digital Health*, Health Informatics,
https://doi.org/10.1007/978-3-319-61446-5_8

(Fig. 8.1). AM, therefore, can be seen as a further development of technologies like computer numerical controlled (CNC) milling, which are still subtractive methods, but already make use of the principles of computer aided design/computer aided manufacturing (CAD/CAM).

AM was first introduced in the field of prototype development (and, therefore, called "rapid prototyping") in mechanical engineering and design but evolved into a class of production technologies applied to all kinds of industries, including the biomedical field, in the meantime. In medicine, digital data describing the patient's anatomy that can be used for the CAD/CAM process is commonly available as computed tomography (CT) and 3D magnetic resonance imaging (MRI), which have emerged as standard medical imaging techniques.

AM is an umbrella term for a variety of technologies covering a whole range of materials (metals, ceramics, polymers, and living cells suspended in soft hydrogels) as well as dimensions. Nowadays, instruments for the production of parts measuring 1 m^3 are available as well as high-precision "printers" that achieve sub-micron resolution. This diversification makes it difficult to provide a concise introduction to AM with respect to its full range of applications. The advantage of AM is that in most cases, less raw material is needed (which is of great importance if the raw material is expensive as in the case of most medical implants or devices) and no tools specific for the part to be manufactured are needed. As soon as the digital dataset of the object is available, the production process can begin. Another benefit is that with AM, various geometries can be realized (e.g., those with internal, closed cavities), which are not possible using conventional methods. This process is already used, for example, in the aircraft and space industries to manufacture novel parts that are lighter compared with conventional ones and sometimes offer improved mechanical stability.

As this chapter is not focused on AM in general, an exhaustive description of the variety of established technologies cannot be given here; however, an increasing

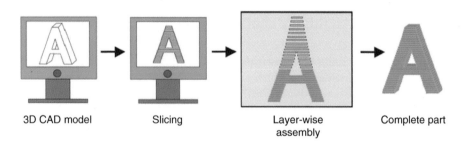

3D CAD model   Slicing   Layer-wise   Complete part
                                        assembly

Fig. 8.1 Principle of additive manufacturing in which a three-dimensional object is created by material addition in a layer-by-layer fashion (scheme provided by the European Space Agency (ESA), www.esa.int)

number of books are available that provide in-depth insight into all aspects of this fast-growing research field and its numerous applications (Gibson et al. 2014; Chua and Leong 2015; Gebhardt and Hötter 2016). As mentioned above, methods and respective 3D printers are available nowadays to manufacture very small to very large objects from all types of materials. Each AM technology has advantages and disadvantages; therefore, a proper selection has to be done depending on the proposed application.

For objects to be utilized in medicine, aspects like material selection, reproducibility, and accuracy of the manufacturing process are of special importance. In addition, if possible, one-step technologies, like selective laser sintering/melting (SLS/SLM), are applied in which layer-by-layer material deposition and formation of the final product are combined in a single process. However, these technologies cannot be utilized to incorporate sensitive pharmaceutical or biological components due to issues such as applicability under sterile or even GMP conditions, which are of greater relevance.

Many studies predict strong growth rates of AM in all medical fields in response to further rapid technological development and price reduction of the respective hardware and software. From this evolution, the utilization of AM in medicine will definitely benefit and probably will become one of the major fields of application in the future.

8.2 Present Landscape of 3D Printing in Healthcare

In principle, 3D printing could be used for producing most of the devices, implants, and even tissue engineering constructs utilized in medical education and clinical practice today. However, as illustrated in the left graph in Fig. 8.2, AM is only cost-effective for small quantities, whereas the cost per unit is significantly lower if identical parts are produced in large amounts by conventional manufacturing technologies. On the other hand, the particular strength of AM is that the complexity of the part does not significantly influence the production costs (Fig. 8.2, right). Therefore, it is unlikely that AM will replace conventional, established technologies for production of large quantities of identical parts, but will be used especially for small quantities (e.g., patient-specific implants or devices; see Sect. 8.4) or for manufacturing very complex structures.

The utilization of 3D printing in medicine was initially driven by medical needs, especially for the therapy of large skull defects. As the shape and size of the human skull differs much more than that of the long bones, each skull defect has its specific location and dimensions; thus, patient-specific implants (PSI) are needed for a proper treatment. With the development of CAD/CAM technology, such implants were manufactured first based on subtractive methods, like CNC milling, and later

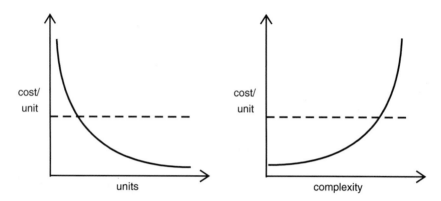

Fig. 8.2 Comparison between conventional manufacturing (*continuous line*) and AM (*dashed line*) concerning the relationship between unit number and cost per unit (*left*) as well as the complexity of the object to be manufactured and cost per unit (*right*). The graphs were adapted from Ch. Sandström (2013)

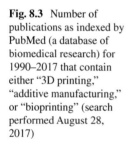

Fig. 8.3 Number of publications as indexed by PubMed (a database of biomedical research) for 1990–2017 that contain either "3D printing," "additive manufacturing," or "bioprinting" (search performed August 28, 2017)

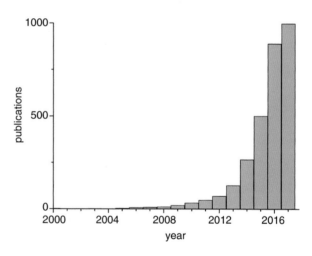

by AM in the 1990s using novel stereolithographic techniques. However, limitations concerning "processable" materials and the high price of the required printers prevented the broad application of 3D printing in medicine for over two decades. However, in the last couple of years and driven by the fast development of AM in general and drop in hardware prices, 3D printing has started to be utilized and further explored in all disciplines of healthcare; indeed, a separate industry based on 3D printing applications in medicine has begun to develop. The tremendous increase in research activity is nicely reflected by the fast-growing number of publications on AM in the biomedical fields as shown in Fig. 8.3.

As usual for new medical applications and technologies, gaining approvals is a time-consuming process that delays their translation into clinical practice. In the case of AM and patient-specific implants and devices, the U.S. Food and Drug Administration (FDA) issued a first draft on "Technical Considerations for Additive Manufactured Devices" (US Food and Drug Administration 2016) in May 2016, which is only the first step of a long-lasting procedure. Nevertheless, in many countries, selected AM-based technologies have already been implemented in clinical applications like manufacturing of PSI made of approved materials like titanium or conventional ceramics.

8.3   3D Printing in Medical Education and Surgical Planning

Probably the fastest growing field in 3D printing applications in medicine is currently that of 3D models for medical education and surgical planning. Both can be described together as the only significant difference is that for medical education, standardized, or at least typical, anatomical models are produced, whereas for surgical planning, patient-specific and, therefore, unique units are fabricated. "Medical education" includes utilization in anatomy courses for first-semester students as well as training devices for complex surgeries, such as cochlear implants, for which models have been developed that can be treated using conventional surgical instruments to simulate all steps of the real intervention. Ethical concerns exist regarding the utilization of formalin-preserved cadavers and exposure of staff and students to toxic gaseous formaldehyde. Therefore, the use of anatomically correct, 3D printed models made of polymers might offer a practical alternative. Recently, McMenamin et al. described the advantages of using 3D printing compared with using preserved cadavers or plastinated specimens for anatomical teaching (McMenamin et al. 2014). It was pointed out that AM allows for the fast and easy manufacture of realistic, multi-colored models of any anatomical object with high accuracy and reproducibility, whereas embalmment as well as plastination processes are very time-consuming. In addition, with 3D printing, as many copies as needed can be produced and the specimen can be scaled down and up, the latter being of interest for very small and/or complex objects. Given that the prices for 3D printers and suitable polymers are falling, printed models will likely present an interesting alternative from a financial point of view.

In contrast, 3D printed models for surgical planning do not replace any established methodology, but rather are a clear add-on to existing procedures. We have to distinguish between the two types of models. In the case of surgical planning, the model specimen is atypical; i.e., it represents the pathological situation of one specific patient, whereas teaching models would be anatomically typical. These models are used like a touchable 3D image to facilitate defining the strategy of a surgical intervention in case of very complex or risky treatments. The other type of model is used already to test the applicability of the surgical intervention by, e.g., probing the width and geometry of blood vessels concerning the optimal size of a catheter or stent. Whereas for anatomical teaching and pre-operative planning the mechanical and haptic properties of the printed models are not of primary interest, this is one of the major issues for AM of models for surgical training or simulation of a specific surgical intervention. Table 8.1 summarizes the requirements of these different approaches for the respective 3D printing technology. Unfortunately, the terminology of the various types of models is not clearly defined yet.

Whereas 3D printed models for surgical planning were used only in very few cases in the past (mostly in neuro- and maxillofacial surgery), this application is rapidly developing and is now being explored in all surgical disciplines. A variety of studies have described the opportunities and advantages of 3D printed models and most authors argue strongly in favor of using the new possibilities of AM in selected, i.e., complicated, complex, and/or risky cases. Such models could consist of only one (unicolored) material, representing only one type of tissue, e.g., bone in orthopedic surgery. Figure 8.4 (left) shows an example of 3D printed models for

Table 8.1 3D printing models for anatomical training and surgical planning/simulation

	Typical or patient-specific	Dimensional accuracy	Haptic/mechanical similarity	Processability with surgical instruments
Anatomical training	Typical	Medium	Not important	Not important
Surgical training	Typical	Medium	Important	Important
Surgical planning	Specific	High	Not important	Not important
Surgical simulation	Specific	High	Important	Important

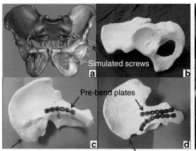
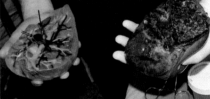

anterior acetabular wall   Posterior acetabular wall

Fig. 8.4 3D printed models for surgical planning. *Left*: models representing parts of a pelvis for planning of internal fixation of acetabular fractures. Note that the 3D models were also used for pre-bending the metal plates prior to their implantation in real surgery. (**a**) A schematic design of the virtual fixation for the fractured acetabula including number, length, and orientation of simulated screws (green). (**b**) 3D model of the fractured part of the acetabula. (**c**) Fixation with a pre-bend plate is simulated on the physical model of the anterior and (**d**) posterior acetabular wall, respectively (image taken from Zeng et al. (2016) with permission). *Right*: model of the right lobe of a liver used in a living donor transplantation compared with the real lobe (photograph taken from Zein et al. (2013) with permission)

planning the reconstruction of complex acetabular fractures. In other cases, multi-material (multicolor) printing is necessary to visualize different structures, like blood vessels, within one organ, tissue, or anatomical region. In Fig. 8.4 (right), a printed liver lobe is shown in which the liver mass is reproduced with a transparent polymer so that the arteries, veins, and bile ducts are printed in different colors to remain visible.

Numerous additional examples for utilization of 3D models for surgical planning could be given here, but it is obvious that this new option is of special relevance for rare, complex, and especially risky surgeries in which specialists from several disciplines are involved (Gillaspie et al. 2016). Real 3D models not only facilitate discussion between the surgeons, but also help inform the patient by showing what is intended to be done and the possible risks of the intervention.

In principle, for AM of models used for medical education and surgical planning, all types of technologies and materials can be utilized; however, polymers are the most frequently used material. As mentioned earlier, models used for surgical training or simulation should be composed of materials that mimic the properties of natural tissues as closely as possible and that can be manipulated with standard surgical instruments. For some tissues, like bone, printable materials are already available that fulfill this requirement very well; for other tissues, such materials are still under investigation. In a recent publication by Chae and co-workers (2015), an overview is given about AM technologies, commercially available printers, and the software needed for translation of the DICOM dataset (coming from medical 3D imaging like CT or MRI) to a CAD file format (like .stl), suitable for the 3D printing process.

For the implementation of 3D printed models for surgical planning in clinical practice, two general options are available: digital data processing and (or) printing can either be outsourced to a commercial service or established in-house. Some big hospitals, e.g., in the U.S. the Mayo and Cleveland Clinics, already have their own 3D printing facilities, which are usually attached to the radiology departments. As a function of size, complexity, and detail of the model, the full process, including data processing and manufacturing, requires between a few hours and 1–3 days. With increasing printing speeds, this period will decrease further.

8.4 Patient-Specific Implants (PSI) and Devices

The logical next step after printing anatomical and surgical models is to fabricate patient-specific implants and devices by AM, i.e., parts that are inserted in the living human body. Astonishingly, this step was done first as an advancement of already established technologies like CNC milling and based on the principles of CAD/CAM. As mentioned earlier, the first important application was PSI for skull defects as those can hardly be treated with conventional, standardized implants. At first, such PSI were only manufactured as replacements of bone tissue or joints (consisting of bone and articular cartilage), using mechanically stable biomaterials like titanium, aluminum oxide, or zirconium oxide. Later, degradable polymers like polycaprolactone (PCL) and polylactide (PLA), non-degradable polymers like

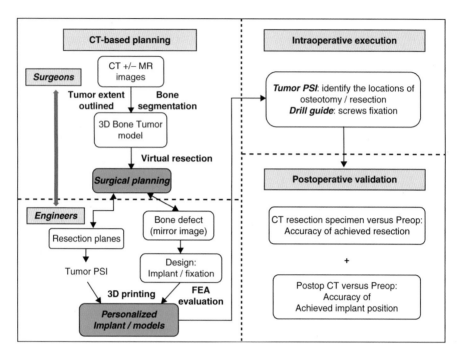

Fig. 8.5 Workflow of PSI manufacturing for a patient, suffering from bone cancer, based on CT data (scheme taken from K. C. Wong et al. (2015) with permission). *FEA* finite element analysis, *PSI* patient-specific instrument

PEEK, and additional bioceramics (e.g., hydroxyapatite) were introduced for this application. In the meanwhile, a multitude of biomaterials and technologies is used for the AM of PSI. Quality standards of the raw materials used for the 3D printing processes of course must be as high as those for the conventional manufacture of medical devices.

In principle, the workflow for PSI manufacturing is similar to that used for the printing of surgical models; however, in case of implanted parts, a thorough preoperative validation has to be performed. In case of load-bearing implants, besides the accuracy of the part concerning its size, the mechanical properties also have to be taken into account. Ideally, this includes a finite element analysis and modeling. In Fig. 8.5, the typical workflow of PSI planning, manufacturing, validation, and utilization is depicted, taken from a real clinical case in which a customized metal implant for a cancer patient suffering from a pelvic tumor was applied (Wong et al. 2015). Selected images from this study are shown in Fig. 8.6 to demonstrate the most important steps of the process.

If a PSI is used for treatment of an existing defect (e.g., a skull defect), then the implant has to fit perfectly to the geometry of the lesion. In the case of utilization of a customized implant that replaces tissue (e.g., a tumor) to be resected during the same surgery, both the location and dimensions of the resected area as well as the implant have to match the preoperative plan. To ensure accordance, in many cases,

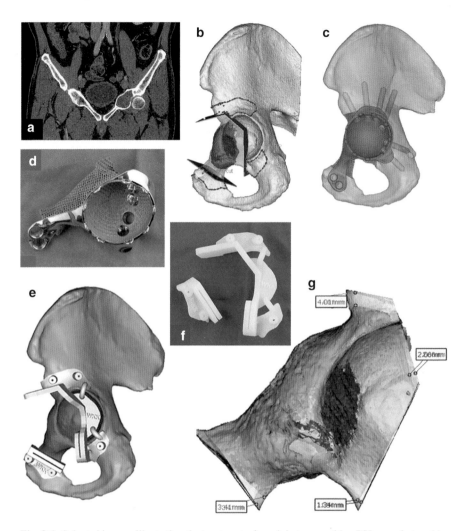

Fig. 8.6 Selected images illustrating the treatment of a pelvic tumor with a PSI manufactured by 3D printing (images taken from K. C. Wong et al. (2015) with permission). (**a**) CT scan of a patient with a chondrosarcoma affecting the left acetabulum (*red arrow*). (**b**) Virtual definition of the resection planes. (**c**) Virtual positioning and planning of the implant including screws to be used for fixation. (**d**) PSI manufactured by selective laser melting of Ti6Al4V (shown after surface finishing). (**e**) Virtual design of patient-specific saw guides to help meet the resection planes during surgery as defined in (**b**). (**f**) Saw guides made of polyamide and fabricated by selective laser melting. (**g**) Comparison of the CT image of the resected tumor specimen (shown in *blue*) with the dataset of the surgical planning (*yellow* and *red*); deviations are indicated in millimeters

saws and/or drill guides have to be used, which again are fabricated by 3D printing (Fig. 8.6e, f). In a very thorough study performed by Wong and co-workers, compliance between the digital model, the resection margins, and implant position were analyzed after surgery and deviations of 1–4 mm were measured (Fig. 8.6g), although these did not affect good clinical outcomes (Wong et al. 2015). The utilization of templates like saw and drill guides in surgery was very recently reviewed by Chen et al. in an own publication (Chen et al. 2016).

The additive manufacturing of PSI, surgical instruments, and tools like tracheal tubes by means of different 3D printing technologies and biomaterials is currently being investigated intensively in all surgical disciplines. In a study published recently by Martelli and co-workers, the utilization of 3D printing in surgery was systematically reviewed by collecting the main advantages and disadvantages mentioned in 158 original papers (Martelli et al. 2016). The main advantages of 3D printing were found to be the facilitation of preoperative planning, better accuracy of the patient-specific part and reduced surgical time. The disadvantages were mainly deviations between the virtual model and the real 3D object, the long time needed for the whole process, and additional costs.

As already discussed in Sect. 8.2 and shown in Fig. 8.2, AM is only cost-effective for small lot sizes or the fabrication of very complex objects. Thus, it will not replace the conventional technologies used for the mass production of standardized implants or medical devices, but it does offer great advantages for manufacturing PSI from which (by definition) only a single copy has to be fabricated. It is obvious that this leads to problems concerning the regulatory approval of such implants or devices as the normal procedures, like standardization of the production process and quality control, cannot be performed for unique parts for which only one copy exists. As mentioned earlier, discussions regarding the respective legal aspects have just begun (recently described and discussed by Morrison and co-workers (2015)) and it will be a long and complicated process to define suitable new regulatory principles for AM and PSI.

It is self-evident that if implantable devices can be fabricated by 3D printing, then devices like prostheses, orthoses, or individual polymer casts for fracture stabilization also can be made using AM technologies. This new field of research, which is rapidly developing like all 3D printing-related applications, was reviewed recently by Lunsford et al. (2016) who summarized and assessed 20 original papers published on this topic.

The logical next step after the establishment of 3D printing for fabricating PSI and medical devices and replacing or supporting human tissues would be to utilize AM for tissue regeneration. For this, the term "3D bioprinting" has been coined and its respective developments will be discussed in the following section.

8.5   3D Bioprinting

Tissue engineering (TE) describes the formation of living tissue outside of a living organism, i.e., in a tissue culture lab (*in vitro*). In most cases, a 3D scaffold is seeded with cells and then further cultivated until cell and tissue differentiation occur. If a clinical application is intended, then the scaffold should consist of a biodegradable material to act as an artificial extracellular matrix only for a limited period of time, but then give space for the regenerating new tissue. 3D printed biomaterials can be used as scaffolds for TE, which offers the opportunity to create artificial tissues of predesigned shape and size. However, conventional cell seeding has several limitations; in particular, only one cell type or mixture of cells can be seeded onto one construct.

In contrast, 3D bioprinting allows for the inclusion of multiple cell types with high spatial resolution as the cells are mixed with the respective biomaterial prior to printing. During the AM process, therefore, biomaterial(s) and cells are positioned together, which enables the fabrication of complex tissue models. As a side effect, very high seeding efficiency is guaranteed as the cells are immobilized in the scaffold material during manufacture. Two main classes of technique can be distinguished: (1) spherical cell/biomaterial droplets or cell aggregates are used as building blocks (Gudapati et al. 2016), or (2) cells are suspended in a hydrogel and extruded continuously in a strand-like fashion (Ozbolat and Hospodiuk 2016). Mostly inkjet printing technologies are used for the first type of application, whereas extrusion-based bioprinting (also called 3D plotting, direct writing, or robotic dispension) is achieved by pneumatic or mechanical extrusion. Both groups of technologies have advantages and disadvantages. The main disadvantage of the droplet-based method is that hardly macroscopic objects can be fabricated as they would be needed for clinical applications. In addition, the utilization of cell spheres as building blocks requires extremely high cell numbers, which remains difficult to achieve. For extrusion-based bioprinting, suitable soft hydrogels are applicable for 3D scaffold fabrication as well as protecting the cells during the printing process and allowing further cell growth afterwards (Malda et al. 2013). As cells cannot be kept alive in concentrated or highly crosslinked gels, in most cases a second, stiffer material is used to provide mechanical stability. This supporting material can be a thermoplastic polymer like PCL (Schuurman et al. 2011) or an additional, highly concentrated hydrogel (Melchels et al. 2016). In an alternative, simpler approach recently published by Schütz and co-workers, a low concentrated alginate hydrogel, known to be suitable for bioprinting but too soft for scaffolding purposes, was blended with methylcellulose to achieve a higher viscosity during the printing process. After scaffold fabrication, the cell-loaded construct was crosslinked with calcium ions to stabilize the alginate part of the blend. As the methylcellulose is not affected by calcium crosslinking, it gets dissolved over time, providing suitable conditions for the cultivation of embedded human mesenchymal stroma cells (hMSC) for up to 21 days (Schütz et al. 2017). It also could be demonstrated that hMSC still can be differentiated toward the adipogenic lineage after bioprinting with this biopolymer hydrogel blend. In Fig. 8.7, a 2 cm × 2 cm scaffold consisting of 30 layers of the abovementioned hydrogel blend and suspended hMSCs (cell line hTERT-MSC) is shown, printed without additional supporting material: note the completely open macropores in z-direction.

3D bioprinting is currently developing as a distinct research field (Chua and Yeong 2015), having strong interactions with AM, TE, microfluidics, and organ-on-a-chip technologies. Concerning possible clinical applications of bioprinted tissue

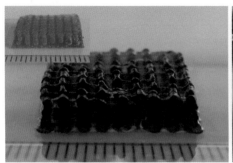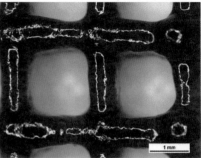

Fig. 8.7 3D bioprinted construct (2 cm × 2 cm, 30 layers) consisting of an alginate/methylcellulose blend with embedded hMSCs. *Left*: image shows scaffold 1 day after printing; living cells were stained with MTT (*insert*: cell-free control). *Right*: view on the same scaffold from above, clearly showing the open macropores in the z-direction and a well preserved strand shape. Scaffolds were printed as described by Schütz et al. (2017), but using the cell line hTERT-MSC instead of primary cells

models, we have to take into account that only very few classical TE applications have been translated to real therapies so far, even though partly established in the lab more than two decades ago. The high regulatory hurdles are due to the utilization of living human cells and, therefore, similar in TE and bioprinting. Nevertheless, practical applications of bioprinted human tissue equivalents are reasonable and possible, mostly in the pharmaceutical industry for the testing of new drugs (Pati et al. 2016). The development of vascularized and fully functional tissue/organ models is currently under intensive investigation, but it is still unclear when bioprinting will be introduced into clinical practice.

8.6   Future Predictions of 3D Printing

As 3D printing has evolved to a very innovative and fast-growing field of research, it is difficult to predict its future direction. Currently, we see intensive investigation by researchers from all over the world as well as rapid progress concerning hardware and software development by companies and the commercialization of numerous applications. This includes implementations of AM in medicine as described above. Already, companies in industrialized countries are producing PSI and models for preoperative planning based on CT or MRI data from specific patients. As the development of more personalized therapies continues to trend globally, 3D printing will definitely play a stronger role; however, the velocity and degree of translation will be restricted by financial as well as regulatory issues.

References

Chae MP, Rozen WM, McMenamin PG, Findlay MW, Spychal RT, Hunter-Smith DJ. Emerging applications of bedside 3D printing in plastic surgery. Front Surg. 2015;2:ID25. (14 pages)

Chen X, Xu L, Wang W, Li X, Sun Y, Politis C. Computer-aided design and manufacturing of surgical templates and their clinical applications: a review. Expert Rev Med Devices. 2016;13:853–364.

Chua CK, Leong KF. 3D printing and additive manufacturing. Principles and applications. 4th ed. Singapore: World Scientific Publishing; 2015.

Chua CK, Yeong WY. Bioprinting, principles and applications. Singapore: World Scientific Publishing; 2015.

Gebhardt A, Hötter J-S. Additive manufacturing: 3D printing for prototyping and manufacturing. Munich: Hanser; 2016.

Gibson I, Rosen D, Stucker B. 3D printing, rapid prototyping, and direct digital manufacturing. 2nd ed. New York, NY: Springer; 2014.

Gillaspie EA, Matsumoto JS, Morris NE, Downey RJ, Shen KR, Allen MS, Blackmon SH. From 3-dimensional printing to 5-dimensional printing: enhancing thoracic surgical planning and resection of complex tumors. Ann Thorac Surg. 2016;101:1958–62.

Gudapati H, Dey M, Ozbolat I. A comprehensive review on droplet-based bioprinting: past, present and future. Biomaterials. 2016;102:20–42.

Lunsford C, Grindle G, Salatin B, Dicianno BE. Innovations with 3-dimensional printing in physical medicine and rehabilitation: a review of the literature. Phys Med Rehabil. 2016;8:1201–12.

Malda J, Visser J, Melchels FP, Jüngst T, Hennink WE, Dhert WJ, Groll J, Hutmacher DW. 25th anniversary article: engineering hydrogels for biofabrication. Adv Mater. 2013;25:5011–28.

Martelli N, Serrano C, van den Brink H, Pineau J, Prognon P, Borget I, El Batti S. Advantages and disadvantages of 3-dimensional printing in surgery: a systematic review. Surgery. 2016;159:1485–500.

McMenamin PG, Quayle MR, McHenry CR, Adams JW. The production of anatomical teaching resources using three-dimensional (3D) printing technology. Anat Sci Educ. 2014;7:479–86.

Melchels FP, Blokzijl MM, Levato R, Peiffer QC, de Ruijter M, Hennink WE, Vermonden T, Malda J. Hydrogel-based reinforcement of 3D bioprinted constructs. Biofabrication. 2016;8:035004. (9 pages)

Morrison RJ, Kashlan KN, Flanangan CL, Wright JK, Green GE, Hollister SJ, Weatherwax KJ. Regulatory considerations in the design and manufacturing of implantable 3D-printed medical devices. Clin Transl Sci. 2015;8:594–600.

Ozbolat IT, Hospodiuk M. Current advances and future perspectives in extrusion-based bioprinting. Biomaterials. 2016;76:321–43.

Pati F, Gantelius J, Svahn HA. 3D bioprinting of tissue/organ models. Angew Chem Int Ed Engl. 2016;55:4650–65.

Ch. Sandström. 3D Printing – why it isn't (only) a hype. 2013. Accessed on Sept 1, 2016. http://disruptiveinnovation.se/?cat=81.

Schütz K, Placht A-M, Paul B, Brüggemeier S, Gelinsky M, Lode A. 3D plotting of a cell-laden alginate/methylcellulose blend: towards biofabrication of tissue engineering constructs with clinically relevant dimensions. J Tissue Eng Regen Med. 2017;11:1574–87.

Schuurman W, Khristov V, Pot MW, van Weeren PR, Dhert WJ, Malda J. Bioprinting of hybrid tissue constructs with tailorable mechanical properties. Biofabrication. 2011;3:021001. (7 pages)

US Food and Drug Administration. Technical considerations for additive manufactured devices. 2016. www.fda.gov/BiologicsBloodVaccines/GuidanceComplianceRegulatoryInformation/Guidances/default.htm.

Wong KC, Kumta SM, Geel NV, Demol J. Onestep reconstruction with a 3D-printed, biomechanically evaluated custom implant after complex pelvic tumor resection. Comput Aided Surg. 2015;20:14–23.

Zein NN, Hanouneh IA, Bishop PD, Samaan M, Eghtesad B, Quintini C, Miller C, Yerian L, Klatte R. Three-dimensional print of a liver for preoperative planning in living donor liver transplantation. Liver Transpl. 2013;19:1304–10.

Zeng C, Xing W, Wu Z, Huang H, Huang W. A combination of three-dimensional printing and computer-assisted virtual surgical procedure for preoperative planning of acetabular fracture reduction. Injury. 2016;47:2223–7.

Chapter 9
Augmenting Behavioral Healthcare: Mobilizing Services with Virtual Reality and Augmented Reality

Brenda K. Wiederhold, Ian Miller, and Mark D. Wiederhold

Abstract From tools for hunting and harvesting and monumental inventions of the industrial revolution that have propelled us into today's ubiquitous information-age, innovative technologies and technological applications have transformed human-based experience. Abounding seemingly overnight, advanced technological applications have revolutionized the healthcare industry by mobilizing treatment and intervention services. While the advent of technologically driven mobile healthcare may appear to some as an emerging field, researchers, clinicians, and practitioners have been implementing contemporary technologies, such as virtual reality (VR), into their mental healthcare practices for over two decades. Clinically validated treatments for anxiety, phobias, pain distraction, posttraumatic stress disorder (PTSD), stress management and prevention, and rehabilitation are only a handful of ways that this immersive technology transforms behavioral healthcare. Via immersive environments, clinicians are better able to expose patients to feared stimuli than traditional imaginal techniques, providing greater effectiveness in treatments and significant improvements in patients' overall wellbeing. Additionally, the mobilization of healthcare to smartphones and other devices facilitates the migration of services beyond the walls of the traditional doctor's office and into the homes and everyday lives of those who need it most. Ultimately, innovative applications by researchers, clinicians, and practitioners prove VR and augmented reality (AR) technologies as effective, efficient, and widely accessible tools in mental healthcare interventions.

Keywords Virtual reality • Augmented reality • Behavioral healthcare • Advanced technologies • Pain • Anxiety • Phobia • Posttraumatic stress disorder • Stress management • Rehabilitation

B.K. Wiederhold (✉) • I. Miller • M.D. Wiederhold
Interactive Media Institute, Virtual Reality Medical Center,
6540 Lusk Blvd., Suite C115, San Diego, CA 92121, USA
e-mail: b@vrphobia.eu

© Springer International Publishing AG 2018
H. Rivas, K. Wac (eds.), *Digital Health*, Health Informatics,
https://doi.org/10.1007/978-3-319-61446-5_9

9.1 Augmenting Mental Healthcare: Mobilizing Services with Virtual Reality

For centuries, technological advancements have improved the quality of life across our world and progressed humankind. From tools for hunting and harvesting and monumental inventions of the industrial revolution that have propelled us into today's ubiquitous information-age, innovative technologies and technological applications have transformed human-based experience. Continuously evolving and advancing high-tech developments have dramatically increased quality of life by way of healthcare enhancements and the creation of interconnected networks around the world. Consequently, accessibility and availability of healthcare continues to grow, leading the way to greater networks and services worldwide. Today, ground-breaking technologies embolden healthcare professionals to approach their practices in continuously evolving ways, driving their services to previously unknown frontiers. Now, providers can serve more effectively, collaborate globally, and impact distant communities via mobile, internet-based, and virtual platforms.

This mass proliferation of digital services is utilized in a variety of ways, peaking interest about the impact of such tools on people's well-being. Consequently, the emergence of these omnipresent information and communication technologies (ICTs), compounded with innovative technological approaches in healthcare intervention, is generating unique clinical research and health service applications. Riva et al. (2012) address this feature in referencing the emerging discipline of Positive Psychology. Focusing on and studying factors that promote quality of life and human flourishing, this discipline emphasizes optimizing functions that enable individuals to "build the best in life" (Riva et al. 2012). Therein lies a junction between technology and the ongoing promotion of human prosperity, termed "positive technology"—a discipline focused on applying technology to manipulate the features and improve the quality of our personal experiences (Riva et al. 2012; Botella et al. 2012).

To date, researchers and clinicians have proven the utility of positive technology in psychological treatment by way of unique patient-provider interaction in computer-aided therapy, immersive, fully controllable environments via virtual reality (VR) and augmented reality (AR), and an intelligent, semantic, immersive, and interconnected Internet (Botella et al. 2012). Of these developments, VR poses some of the most promising potential to elicit transformative approaches to elevate quality of life. Established and effective, VR has been implemented in treatment for psychological and physiological pain, anxiety, phobias, stress disorders, and stress management. Although VR technology has only recently garnered widespread commercial attention, the advent of its healthcare applications, specifically virtual reality therapy (VRT), is nothing new to researchers, clinicians, and other professionals.

Explored in areas such as anxiety disorders, phobias (Wiederhold 2003), stress disorders and education (Psotka 1995), VR has a proven track record as an effective and efficient positive technology (Wiederhold and Wiederhold 2005; Wiederhold and Bouchard 2014). With the capability to immerse an individual into a three-dimensional environment that the brain perceives as real, VR poses distinctive opportunities for control of environments, enhanced magnitude of stimuli, and custom tailoring to individuals' needs (Psotka 1995; Wiederhold and Wiederhold 2005; Wiederhold and Bouchard 2014; Bailenson et al. 2003). Previous literature upholds the efficacy of VR as an exposure technique in comparison to in vivo exposure and/or cognitive behavior therapy (CBT) in treating anxiety (Powers and Emmelkamp 2008), stress and trauma (Mosso-Vázquez et al. 2014). VR treatments provide patients unprecedented access to feared stimuli that they might otherwise be unable to access via visualization or imaginal exposure, making it a suitable option for stress and anxiety disorders.

Success in these treatments depends on numerous factors, one of which is immersion. Referring to the objective level of sensory fidelity, immersive VR is an integral piece of VR therapy because it affords a user the ability to experience virtual worlds as if they were real. For phobias, immersive VR allows a patient to be sufficiently exposed to feared stimuli by triggering the same brain structures as if they were physically present. For uses like military training, immersive virtual environments allow infantrymen to experience combat situations with a level of realism not possible to achieve in other training environments (Bowman and McMahan 2007). Alongside evolving technologies, however, VR immersion continues to improve. In a 2009 study (Hirose et al. 2009), researchers investigated how different levels of immersion effected performance. Results indicate elevated immersion constantly increased performance. Thus, as we explore the crossroads between evolutions of VR technology and healthcare interventions, it is vital to acknowledge the growing capabilities of developing more immersive VR.

Rapid advancements in small, powerful computer technologies, decreasing prices, and the ubiquity of portable devices continually evolve VR applications, effectively modernizing mental healthcare services. The Virtual Reality Medical Center (VRMC) has dedicated over 20 years of expertise and clinical practice to transforming behavioral healthcare services toward positive, wellness-based programs enhanced by VR and biosensors. Of particular importance is the paradigm shift from a disease-based model—intervening and treating individuals with pre-existing conditions—to a more holistic wellness model, honing in on the prevention of conditions like PTSD, phobias, stress, anxiety and pain. Treatment methods have progressed through a variety of research and clinical validation trials, drawing on the development and evolution of new, innovative, and increasingly portable technologies.

The impact of this healthcare technology evolution is significant. Beginning with large, cumbersome devices, necessarily stationed within professionals' offices, VR equipment was not considered a portable device available to the general public. Not only did these expensive immobile Goliaths limit who could use them, but limitations in graphics and usability features stymied their effective dissemination early on. Nonetheless, technological improvements are ameliorating these issues and enabling the production of more user-friendly, realistic virtual environments with reduced sensory conflict between visual and vestibular systems (Mousavi et al. 2013). As advanced simulation technologies like VR and AR become more user friendly, in cost, complexity, and size, they have initiated a healthcare movement beyond the traditional doctor's office by providing greater mobile access for patients (Wiederhold et al. 2013). Accordingly the newfound accessibility and usability grants novel capabilities for enhancing the lives of millions of people.

Technological progression has propelled our innovative approaches to distribute health and wellness services to an expansive audience. Coinciding with this migration, we have moved treatments from expensive, in-clinic interventions, to fully immersive and cost-effective technology in patients' homes. This mobilization of services via smartphones, apps, and portable, inexpensive VR equipment has facilitated our research and practice in areas such as procedural pain distraction and prevention, alleviation of anxiety, chronic pain, phobias, and stress, treatment of PTSD, and even cognitive and physical rehabilitation.

9.2 Pain

Modern technological innovations and new applications of VR are changing the way clinicians, practitioners, and researchers approach healthcare treatment for pain management. Perceived through emotions, cognition, and attitudes, pain syndromes can be effectively alleviated by shifting negative thoughts to positive ones using cognitive behavioral therapy (CBT) (Wiederhold and Wiederhold 2014a). These negative thoughts can give way to psychological stress and anxiety which can cause unintended complications, such as more physical pain. VR distraction can aid in decreasing anxiety to enhance one's ability to cope with pain, or even be created to provide leisure activities for those without physical capability for them (e.g. those confined to a wheelchair, those with breathing difficulties, etc.). In addition, real-time biofeedback provides the practitioner with all of a patient's vital signs, e.g. heart rate, heart rate variability, respiration, skin conductance, and peripheral skin temperature (McLay et al. 2011). The application of VR distraction has been documented in medical procedures (Mosso-Vázquez et al. 2014; Wiederhold et al. 2014a). While pain seems to manifest itself physically, its perception is largely psychological and distraction has been found to take a patient's attention away from pain (Wiederhold et al. 2014a). Studies have also shown VR to be effective in reducing patient pain in procedures such as chemotherapy, burn wound dressing changes, physical therapy, and surgery (Wiederhold et al. 2014a; Vázquez et al. 2013, 2006; Wiederhold and Wiederhold 2012; Mühlberger et al. 2007; Mott et al. 2008). Funded by the National Institute for Drug Abuse, National Institutes of Health, VRMC designed and developed VR/AR worlds to be used as a form of distraction during dental procedures. Tested at the Scripps Center for Dental Care in La Jolla, California adult patients navigated through relaxing nature worlds such as beaches, forests, and mountains while receiving their dental treatment. Findings support VR therapy as a successful approach to controlling fear and anxiety during dental procedures (Wiederhold et al. 2014a). Another study found a positive correlation between breathing rate and subjective pain reports, verifying that VR is an effective tool for lowering pain and stress both subjectively (self-report) and objectively (physiologically) in patients (Wiederhold et al. 2014a; Vázquez et al. 2013).

While more research has been conducted on VR during medical and dental procedures, an article in the special issue of *Cyberpsychology, Behavior, and Social Networking* Journal *17(6)* on VR and pain (Wiederhold et al. 2014b) explored the use of VR as a distraction technique in chronic pain patients. A newer area of investigation, this study supports the efficacy of VR as a tool to relieve patients' subjective ratings of pain as well as objective physiological measures (Wiederhold et al. 2014c). In another article from this journal, researchers advocate for the potential use of mobile phones as a way of delivering an easily accessible, immersive virtual experience. In this 31 participant controlled study, Wiederhold, Gao, and Wiederhold (2014d) found mobile devices to be effective instruments to display immersive environments and sufficiently deliver pain distraction.

Historically, VR technology has been expensive and inaccessible to anyone other than researchers, academicians and gaming aficionados (Li et al. 2011). Despite this, for the past 22 years, Interactive Media Institute, a 501c3 non-profit based in San Diego, California has focused on universalizing access to platforms and other resources that aid in promoting the highest possible quality of life. Because pain manifests in multiple forms, patients can develop intolerance to treatments. An opportunity to merge both VR and appropriate pain relieving medications for patient treatment would provide another important mechanism for pain relief. VR environments can be programmed to change in response to patient pain. For example, a clinician can increase the "dosage" of stimuli as more relief is needed and vice versa. This ability to control the "CyberDose©" may be useful as patients administer more self-care in their homes (Wiederhold et al. 2014e).

9.3 Anxiety and Phobias

According to the *Anxiety and Depression Association of America*, nearly 75 million people in the United States alone suffer from anxiety and depression related disorders (Facts & Statistics|Anxiety and Depression Association of America, ADAA 2016). Traditionally, treating these psychological disorders has included exposure therapy (attempting to overcome a fear by gradually exposing oneself to it either in vivo or via mental imagery), traditional cognitive behavior therapy (CBT), or psychotherapy in conjunction with medications. Treatment at VRMC uniquely facilitates both enhanced versions of traditional therapies as well as innovative applications made possible by the clinicians and researchers at the clinic. A major drawback to traditional interventions is the inability to successfully elicit visual stimuli in imaginal therapies. Technological advances in VR and related technologies, like biofeedback, have made treatment for anxiety and phobias possible for those who have previously tried imaginal therapy without avail. For some, traditional therapies offer little comfort. Individuals who are too overwhelmed solely at the thought of driving on a real freeway or taking a 30-min flight may be too afraid to even attempt any type of treatment. VR-enhanced cognitive behavioral therapy (VR-CBT), however, allows patients to slowly and systematically be exposed to stimuli that they might have trouble mentally imagining and/or are too phobic to attempt or confront in real life.

Another drawback to traditional treatments for anxiety and phobias is the reliance on face-to-face patient-client interaction, forcing patients to take time out of a busy schedule to travel to a clinician's office for an appointment. Having completed the first randomized clinical trial to use VR Exposure Therapy to treat fear of flying, we have continued for over 20 years to try and decrease these requirements and move towards independent, mobilized treatment for a variety of scenarios. Although our in-clinic success rate for treating phobias with VR-CBT is 92% (Wiederhold and Wiederhold 2003), more individuals may be able to experience this treatment through mobile platforms. The constant evolution of VR continues to make this possible. Current platforms such as Samsung's *GearVR*, the *Oculus Rift*, the *HTC Vive* and *Google Cardboard* provide tremendous opportunity for clinicians to inexpensively and remotely treat patients with phobias and anxiety disorders. This migration away from the office and into the homes of patients accompanied by increasing access to mental health care is a movement called "telepsychology". Thus, the omnipresence of information and communication technologies provides growing opportunities for clinicians and practitioners to aid those in need, both at home and in the clinic.

Although virtual reality interventions might seem new, our experience in their applications dates back over two decades. From fears of enclosed spaces, to a fear of driving, flying, public speaking, and social phobia, we have found VR-enhanced CBT to be more effective and efficient in the treatment of many anxiety and stress-related disorders (Wiederhold, 2003). The migration of technology throughout the past 20 years has been an essential aspect to the development of adequate VR treatment for phobias and anxiety disorders. Increasingly realistic graphics, reduction of cybersickness, and a shift toward more user-friendly interfaces have all facilitated the development of exceptionally immersive environments and consequently more effective clinical interventions. Accordingly, clinicians have begun to adopt telepsychology as a proven, cost-effective, approach to the treatment of many anxiety disorders and phobias.

In-home care significantly reduces treatment costs for patients because they do not need a therapist to be physically present or transportation to the clinic or doctor's office. Additionally, the use of VR and web-based platforms for treatment facilitates increased accessibility to feared stimuli and greater confidentiality for a patient, another improvement over traditional techniques. Botella and colleagues (2000) reference a treatment program for public speaking phobias and its advantages. First, costs for the user decrease, as he/she does not need the physical presence of a therapist. Second, the feared event, public speaking, is more readily available in a virtual environment than it is in real life. Thus, with VR and Internet access, a phobic individual can access the feared stimuli at their convenience, emphasizing how telehealth can allow for self-management of a disorder (Botella et al. 2000). In total, decreasing costs and greater accessibility make VR telepsychology a desirable option, while their convenience and ease of use allow a greater number of individuals to seek help. This proves that in-clinic interventions are not the sole source of help however. Another platform accessible to anyone with a computer and Internet access, the virtual world *Second Life*, serves as a free program for individuals to socialize, connect, and create in a three dimensional virtual world. In assessing the feasibility and effectiveness of *Second Life* to aid in treating social phobias, researchers discovered significantly greater improvements in social anxiety symptoms, depression, and quality of life in comparison to a control group (Yuen et al. 2013). This underlines the ability of open-access virtual worlds to contribute to self-care healthcare across our world.

The transformation of treatments and interventions for anxiety disorders and phobias is well underway. The ability of VR to positively elicit distress and emotional responses make it a unique alternative to traditional CBT (Owens and Beidel 2015; Anderson et al. 2013). Moreover, VR's effectiveness can be enhanced when used adjunctively with pharmacological treatments such as cortisol (Dominique et al. 2011). While future advancements in technology will continue to push this field forward and heighten its ability to affect change, the current ability of VR to lower anxiety both subjectively and physiologically have proven to be an effective tool for the treatment of other disorders.

9.4   Posttraumatic Stress Disorder

Whether an individual is returning home from psychologically harmful combat situations, has experienced a gruesome car accident, been sexually or physically assaulted, experienced a natural disaster, or received a diagnosis of a life-threatening illness, they can be at risk of developing PTSD. Defined as a mental health condition that develops in some individuals who have experienced a shocking or dangerous event, PTSD affects hundreds of millions of people worldwide and nearly 8% of the U.S. population annually, with certain groups, such as military members, at a much higher rate (Bagalman 2011). Over half of the individuals who suffer from PTSD smoke, while others may become dependent on alcohol or prescription drugs (Bagalman 2011). Not only does PTSD detrimentally affect psychological wellness, but it can have deleterious physical health effects as well, including increased risk of cardiovascular disease. Due to its varied symptoms, PTSD can be difficult to treat and often requires a combination of methods. Medications for anxiety and depression, support from loved ones, and exposure therapy are just a few factors that can aid in recovery. However, these approaches have subpar success rates. Conversely, supported in earlier discussions on anxiety and phobias, as advances in medical technology proliferate, the application of VR for exposure therapy is rightfully gaining traction. Consequently, researchers and clinicians agree that exposure therapy is the most effective treatment for PTSD to date. Prior to the application of VR technology, imaginal exposure therapy, in which a patient would gradually and repeatedly "relive" the traumatic event, was the standard of care. Problematically, patients have a pervasive tendency to willingly or unwillingly avoid reliving the traumatic event. A failure to engage visually or emotionally, then, makes it difficult to alter any fear structures that exist in a patient, potentially resulting in an ineffective treatment outcome.

For the last two decades, VR therapy has continually improved treatment efficacy for individuals with PTSD. A virtual reality environment can be used to present both general and specific stimuli to patients in order to assist them in reducing reactivity to these stimuli. For individuals in the military, a general VR environment (e.g. Iraqi village) is often sufficient to elicit a reminder of the typical arousal one experienced during deployment. As a result of being placed in a virtual environment in which a trauma has occurred (in war veterans, it could be a virtual combat setting; in armed conflict survivors, a virtual countryside under attack) and then slowly experiencing that situation in a controlled way, patients ultimately experience less arousal and begin to reassess the initial situation that produced the PTSD. In turn, this facilitates emotional processing and may alleviate the intrusive memories and disconcerting symptoms PTSD sufferers experience. Traditional treatments, like in vivo therapy, are often hindered by access to the stress-inducing stimuli. In the case of war veterans, this type of therapy is nearly impossible and wholly impractical. In contrast, VR enables patient interaction with anxiety-inducing scenarios in the safety and confidentiality of the therapy room. Since its inception, positive response rates to VR exposure therapy have been as high as 88% for PTSD due to motor vehicle accidents and 80% for PTSD due to military situations (Wiederhold and Wiederhold 2010). Resultantly, there has been a growth in interest and support for further applications of VR to treat PTSD and other stress disorders. In October 2009, the North Atlantic Treaty Organization (NATO) funded an Advanced Research Workshop titled *Wounds of War II: Addressing Posttraumatic Stress Disorder (PTSD) in Peacekeeping and Combat Troops*, organized by Interactive Media Institute (IMI). With additional support provided by the Austrian Ministry of Defence, U.S. Army Medical Research and Materiel Command, Virtual Reality Medical Center and Croatian Ministry of Health and Social Welfare, the think tank assembled a small group of the world's experts to discuss the evolution of past, present, and future treatment plans for PTSD with an emphasis on innovation (Wiederhold 2013).

Although imaginal therapy can be helpful, nearly 85% of patients demonstrate an inability to appropriately and effectively visualize situations and become physiologically aroused. By providing immersive VR therapy, a patient is better able to relive a traumatic experience in the safety and comfort of a therapy room at his or her individual pace as the ability to tolerate the stimuli increases. Although technology has steadily improved video graphics and VR in particular, it is not necessary that the virtual environment be entirely "realistic." In fact, it may be undesirable to fully match the level of realism from a physical environment that a patient was exposed to during the actual trauma. It is important and useful for therapy to have some distance from the actual trauma. Even if the virtual environment is only 50% realistic it may be sufficient to trigger internal memories of the trauma and their corresponding emotional responses, if the right cues are included in the VR world (Gaggioli et al. 2014). With funding from the Office of Naval Research, VRMC conducted the first randomized controlled clinical trial using VR exposure therapy and biofeedback to treat active duty service members with combat related PTSD. First focus groups were held and then VR worlds were designed, developed and clinically validated in a pilot study followed by a randomized trial (McLay et al. 2011). The VR systems and accompanying protocols were then disseminated to other Active Duty hospitals and Veterans Administration hospitals as well as to NATO coalition partners. Therapists were given an APA-accredited training course on the use of the equipment within a standard cognitive behavior therapy protocol. Additionally, in an attempt to facilitate earlier intervention, researchers mobilized a treatment center to the combat theater of Fallujah, with those treated showing higher success rates in resolution of symptoms (McLay et al. 2010). This underlines the capability of VR to treat PTSD safely and effectively in controlled settings, to incite innovation, and to underscore the ways of progressing alongside technological evolution. An obvious extension of this work is into PTSD from other causes, demonstrating continuing evolution alongside rapid high-tech developments and taking an even greater step toward the transformation and mobilization of healthcare.

Thus, we revisit a model previously described: transitioning healthcare beyond the doors of the doctor's office, ubiquitizing access, and making treatment available at the touch of a finger. Researchers at VRMC have developed a mobile phone application, *iMAT* (Mental Armor Training), comprised of a series of short exercises designed to enhance soldiers' judgment during stressful situations. Ultimately, this application aids in troop evaluation, identifying PTSD and TBI risk, and diagnosing cases anytime, anywhere. As the progression of healthcare moves toward this type of mobile treatment, we have simultaneously extended our reach by adopting an entirely new model of care focused on the wellness of individuals and even inhibiting the development of stress and anxiety disorders.

9.5 Stress Management

In the past, the model of care focused on the treatment of disorders such as pain, anxiety, phobias, and stress-related disorders. As technology has progressed, however, we have shifted away from a disease model to a wellness model. That is, we have shifted from treating a phobia, stress, or anxiety disorder *after* it manifests to preventing such disorders *before* they take hold of a person's life. For example, a program created to better equip first responders by simulating battle injuries as realistically as possible was developed as VR stress inoculation training (SIT) for stressful situations. As it sounds, SIT is an approach taken to "inoculate" an individual against potentially traumatizing stressors. We realized from past studies on phobias and peak performance training for athletes, that by providing SIT, or "stress hardening", prior to sending individuals into potentially stressful situations, we may be able to provide some protection from the development of PTSD. Our study on SIT and combat medic training illustrates how VR can be a useful technology in helping to prevent stress-related reactions (Wiederhold and Wiederhold 2014b).

While researchers and clinicians at VRMC approach preventative treatments, our focus on management of preexisting conditions also remains.

The proven efficacy of VR to elicit emotional responses is a powerfully influential discovery. The gradual adoption of VR as part of an anxiety or stress inducing protocol lends credence to its use to facilitate relaxation processes in anxious individuals (Gorini and Riva 2008; Pallavicini et al. 2013; Gorini et al. 2010). The presentation of relaxing images can eventually lead to an individual's mastery of relaxation by enhancing their own immersion and feelings of empowerment in an environment, making it superior to similar processes in mental imagery (Pallavicini et al. 2013). In reference the corresponding advances in healthcare technologies alongside the migration of treatments toward mobile platforms, Gorini et al. (2010) conducted a study using VR, biofeedback, and mobile phones to improve treatments of generalized anxiety disorder. Researchers conducted VR relaxation training in a clinical setting and instructed patients to supplement with daily relaxation practice on mobile phones. Findings indicate adjunctive use of mobile phones with relaxation significantly reduced anxiety scores through an eight-session treatment period (Gorini et al. 2010). In its relatively short-lived existence, VR has already transformed healthcare. From its inception as an adjunctive in-clinic reality-enhancement technique for pain management and phobias, to its uses as an auxiliary in-home tool for stress management, VR continues to revolutionize healthcare services.

In a further step in technological and treatment evolution, researchers exploring "Interreality" again demonstrated progression along this continuum of wellness-based electronic health (Riva et al. 2010). In an attempt to lessen the effects of psychological stress and burnout in schoolteachers and nurses, we took part in the 3-year INTERSTRESS project, funded by the European Commission (DG Connect), and addressed limitations of traditional CBT protocols in this treatment area. Instead of using imagination and/or exposure to evoke emotional responses that can be changed through reflection and relaxation, as in traditional CBT, the INTERSTRESS protocol bridges virtual experiences, used to learn coping skills, with real experiences using advanced technologies like VR, biofeedback, and smartphones to provide more personalized, accessible, and effective stress management interventions. This strategy allows behaviors in the physical world to influence an experience in the virtual one while providing an opportunity for mobile treatment. For example, if emotional regulation during the day was poor, some new experiences in the virtual world would be unlocked to address this issue. Or, if coping skills in the virtual world (in the therapist's office) were subpar, patients might receive additional homework assignments to complete for the next session (McLay et al. 2011; Riva et al. 2010). The consensus on this type of stress management protocol is encouraging because it enhances the quality of treatment by fusing together the best aspects of both physical and virtual world experiences. Not only does it offer enhanced efficacy over CBT, but its application of mobile devices and Internet communication place it in a promising position in today's age of omnipresent ICTs.

9.6   Rehabilitation

In conjunction with preventative measures, we have also dedicated research to physiologically driven rehabilitation in a variety of areas while adapting to advances in technology. In 2003, VRMC participated in a research study exploring the use of VR to help stroke and traumatic brain injury (TBI) patients regain the ability to carry out activities of daily living (ADL), such as shopping at a supermarket (Lee et al. 2003). Overall, the study demonstrates that VR can be applied as a rehab technique for ADLs. In an effort to improve cognitive functioning and decrease abnormal behaviors caused by cerebrovascular accidents, like stroke or traumatic brain injuries (TBIs), we have also created a mixed reality rehabilitation system (MRRS) designed to improve cognitive deficits in warfighters (Salva et al. 2009a). Mixed reality, often synonymous with AR, provides an interactive, engaging rehabilitation tool for these patients (Salva et al. 2009a, b). The MRRS generated two types of mixed reality scenarios focusing on (1) trying to regain and improve a patient's memory and (2) seeking to improve a patient's independence by retraining them in ADLs. This system helps counteract some of the limitations associated with traditional rehabilitation processes like plateauing after an initial period of recovery, limited resources, and low levels of interest and subsequent participation. It is also an improvement on the 2003 study, which solely used VR. Additional studies from other institutions highlight the effectiveness of VR/AR systems to help TBI and CVA patients regain functioning in their daily and vocational lives (Lee et al. 2003; Salva et al. 2009a, b).

Even further along the continuum of innovation, we are applying advanced medical technologies to enable greater efficacy of VR interventions. Objective measures, like biofeedback, have greatly improved our understanding and application of VR technology in healthcare. However, understanding what is occurring in the brain during VR exposure may allow us to more fully exploit VR's full potential. As a result, Wiederhold and Wiederhold (2008) explored applications of functional magnetic resonance imaging (fMRI) to study how the brain itself reacts to VR. In reviewing literature on these studies, the team identified that VR not only causes patients to feel like they are in a virtual world, but that it actually causes areas in their brains reserved for movement in response to physical stimuli to actually activate (Wiederhold and Wiederhold 2008). In relation to rehabilitation, this type of technology has shown researchers that VR is able to "trick" the brain into perceiving a physical movement, thereby creating positive neuroplastic changes in deficient areas of the brain, and enhancing cognitive and/or motor functioning (Wiederhold and Wiederhold 2008).

In 2007, researchers developed a mobile application for neuropsychological assessment for combat PTSD (Reeves et al. 2007). *BrainCheckers*, is a system that utilizes the clinically validated Automated Neuropsychological Assessment Metrics (ANAM) and a Combat Stress Assessment (CSA) to precisely measure cognitive processing efficiency in a variety of contexts. This approach to mobile assessment, then, allows for more ubiquitous access and use as a screening and serial testing instrument (Reeves et al. 2007).

9.7 Conclusion

Despite the newfound interest in these revolutionary technologies for entertainment, applications of virtual and augmented reality in healthcare have existed for over two decades. VR has evolved from using simple virtual worlds and clunky, cumbersome devices to virtual environments accessible through no more than a pair of glasses or a phone screen. With the resulting emergence of positive technology and psychology, the number of technological approaches for increasing quality of life and well-being has grown and stimulated significant interest. Enhancements in information and communication technologies, graphic qualities, immersion levels, and decreases in vestibular system conflicts and overall costs of technology have driven researchers and clinicians to evolve approaches and application techniques that continue to provide new insights for clinical innovation. From the use of VR as a distraction tool for pain management during medical procedures to its implementation as wellness based technology for stress management and rehabilitation, researchers have been able to benefit from rapid advances in computer hardware, software, and image processing. In its uses for treatment of PTSD and as a stress hardening tool in stress inoculation training, transitioning to battlefield interventions can improve outcome. It is also worth noting the efficacy of VR used in conjunction with pharmacological agents. Combined therapies is a very rapidly advancing concept which needs continued research and clinical studies. While we have developed tools and protocols that effectively use non-invasive sensors for guiding therapy, understanding brain function in real time is a more important goal. Advances in technology have not only transformed clinical practice and research, but they have begun a migration of treatment and intervention away from the hospitals, out of the doctor's office, and into the homes and lives of individual patients.

Mobilized treatments are becoming increasingly popular in today's information and communication technology driven environment. Via relaxation worlds, games, and specifically tailored environments on mobile devices, treatments of anxieties, phobias, stress disorders and other important conditions are gaining popularity because they are convenient and easy to use. In conjunction, by exporting healthcare beyond the traditional boundaries of hospitals or clinics, researchers, developers, and healthcare providers are raising awareness about wellness-based services and access to self-help. A transformation is occurring in real time with the development of mobile device applications centered on improving human existence. The evolution of information and communication technologies have modernized treatments, interventions, and rehabilitation approaches across medical and scientific disciplines. Each new year, the omnipresent sharing and transferring of information increases technological advancements exponentially. It is especially important that technology developers continue to work closely with healthcare providers and with end users so that effective and clinically validated solutions can be made available to disparate groups of patients. As we move forward, we may need to consider some form of evaluation by subject matter experts to guide patients through the multitude of available apps and software solutions. As well, clinicians may need continued training and certification to incorporate these new tools and technologies into their established treatment regime. And finally, to provide wider dissemination in a cost-effective manner, we may need to consider cloud-based solutions. Transforming healthcare through technology is within our grasp.

References

Anderson PL, Price M, Edwards SM, Obasaju MA, Schmertz SK, Zimand E, Calamaras MR. Virtual reality exposure therapy for social anxiety disorder: a randomized controlled trial. J Consult Clin Psychol. 2013;81(5):751.

Bagalman E. Suicide, PTSD, and substance use among OEF/OIF veterans using VA health care: facts and figures. Washington, DC: Congressional Research Service, Library of Congress; 2011.

Bailenson JN, Blascovich J, Beall AC, Loomis JM. Interpersonal distance in immersive virtual environments. Pers Soc Psychol Bull. 2003;29(7):819–33.

Botella C, Banos R, Guillén V, Perpiñá C, Alcañiz M, Pons A. Telepsychology: public speaking fear treatment on the internet. Cyberpsychol Behav. 2000;3(6):959–68.

Botella C, Riva G, Gaggioli A, Wiederhold BK, Alcaniz M, Banos RM. The present and future of positive technologies. Cyberpsychol Behav Soc Netw. 2012;15(2):78–84.

Bowman DA, McMahan RP. Virtual reality: how much immersion is enough? Computer. 2007;40(7):36–43.

de Quervain D, Bentz D, Michael T, Bolt OC, Wiederhold BK, Margraf J, Wilhelm FH. Glucocorticoids enhance extinction-based psychotherapy. Proc Natl Acad Sci. 2011;108(16):6621–5.

Facts & Statistics|Anxiety and Depression Association of America, ADAA [Internet]. Adaa.org. 2016. http://www.adaa.org/aboutadaa/press-room/facts-statistics.

Gaggioli A, Pallavicini F, Morganti L, Serino S, Scaratti C, Briguglio M, Crifaci G, Vetrano N, Giulintano A, Bernava G, Tartarisco G, Wiederhold B, Riva G. Experiential virtual scenarios with real-time monitoring (interreality) for the management of psychological stress: a block randomized controlled trial. J Med Internet Res. 2014;16(7):167.

Gorini A, Riva G. The potential of virtual reality as anxiety management tool: a randomized controlled study in a sample of patients affected by generalized anxiety disorder. Trials. 2008;9(1):1.

Gorini A, Pallavicini F, Algeri D, Repetto C, Gaggioli A, Riva G. Virtual reality in the treatment of generalized anxiety disorders. Stud Health Technol Inform. 2010;154:39–43.

Hirose M, Schmalstieg D, Wingrave CA, Nishimura K. Higher levels of immersion improve procedure memorization performance. Proceedings of the 15th Joint Virtual Reality Eurographics Conference on Virtual Environments, 2009, pp. 121–128.

Lee JH, Ku J, Cho W, Hahn WY, Kim IY, Lee SM, Kang Y, Kim DY, Yu T, Wiederhold BK, Wiederhold MD. A virtual reality system for the assessment and rehabilitation of the activities of daily living. Cyberpsychol Behav. 2003;6(4):383–8.

Li A, Montaño Z, Chen VJ, Gold JI. Virtual reality and pain management: current trends and future directions. Pain. 2011;1(2):147–57.

McLay RN, McBrien C, Wiederhold MD, Wiederhold BK. Exposure therapy with and without virtual reality to treat PTSD while in the combat theater: a parallel case series. Cyberpsychol Behav Soc Netw. 2010;13(1):37–42.

McLay RN, Wood DP, Webb-Murphy JA, Spira JL, Wiederhold MD, Pyne JM, Wiederhold BK. A randomized, controlled trial of virtual reality-graded exposure therapy for post-traumatic stress disorder in active duty service members with combat-related post-traumatic stress disorder. Cyberpsychol Behav Soc Netw. 2011;14(4):223–9.

Mosso-Vázquez JL, Gao K, Wiederhold BK, Wiederhold MD. Virtual reality for pain management in cardiac surgery. Cyberpsychol Behav Soc Netw. 2014;17(6):371–8.

Mott J, Bucolo S, Cuttle L, Mill J, Hilder M, Miller K, Kimble RM. The efficacy of an augmented virtual reality system to alleviate pain in children undergoing burns dressing changes: a randomised controlled trial. Burns. 2008;34(6):803–8.

Mousavi M, Jen YH, Musa SN. A review on cybersickness and usability in virtual environments. Adv Eng Forum. 2013;10:34.

Mühlberger A, Wieser MJ, Kenntner-Mabiala R, Pauli P, Wiederhold BK. Pain modulation during drives through cold and hot virtual environments. Cyberpsychol Behav. 2007;10(4):516–22.

Owens ME, Beidel DC. Can virtual reality effectively elicit distress associated with social anxiety disorder? J Psychopathol Behav Assess. 2015;37(2):296–305.

Pallavicini F, Gaggioli A, Raspelli S, Cipresso P, Serino S, Vigna C, Grassi A, Morganti L, Baruffi M, Wiederhold B, Riva G. Interreality for the management and training of psychological stress: study protocol for a randomized controlled trial. Trials. 2013;14(1):1.

Powers MB, Emmelkamp PM. Virtual reality exposure therapy for anxiety disorders: a meta-analysis. J Anxiety Disord. 2008;22(3):561–9.

Psotka J. Immersive training systems: virtual reality and education and training. Instruct Sci. 1995;23(5-6):405–31.

Reeves D, Elsmore T, Wiederhold MD, Wood D, Murphy J, Center C, Spira J, Wiederhold BK. Handheld computerized neuropsychological assessment in a virtual reality treatment protocol for combat PTSD. Annual review of cybertherapy and telemedicine, vol. 5. Washington, DC: IOS Press; 2007. p. 151–6.

Riva G, Raspelli S, Algeri D, Pallavicini F, Gorini A, Wiederhold BK, Gaggioli A. Interreality in practice: bridging virtual and real worlds in the treatment of posttraumatic stress disorders. Cyberpsychol Behav Soc Netw. 2010;13(1):55–65.

Riva G, Banos RM, Botella C, Wiederhold BK, Gaggioli A. Positive technology: using interactive technologies to promote positive functioning. Cyberpsychol Behav Soc Netw. 2012;15(2):69–77.

Salva AM, Alban AJ, Wiederhold MD, Wiederhold BK, Kong L. Physiologically driven rehabilitation using virtual reality. International Conference on Foundations of Augmented Cognition. Berlin: Springer; 2009a. p. 836–45.

Salva AM, Wiederhold BK, Alban AJ, Hughes C, Smith E, Fidopiastis C, Wiederhold MD. Cognitive therapy using mixed reality for those impaired by a cerebrovascular accident (CVA). Annual review of cybertherapy and telemedicine, 2009. Advanced technologies in the behavioral, social, and neurosciences, vol. 144. Washington, DC: IOS Press; 2009b. p. 253.

Vázquez JL, Rizzo S, Wiederhold B, Lara V, Flores J, Espiritusanto E, Minor A, Santander A, Avila O, Balice O, Benavides B. Cybertherapy--new applications for discomfort reductions. Surgical care unit of heart, neonatology care unit, transplant kidney care unit, delivery room-cesarean surgery and ambulatory surgery, 27 case reports. Stud Health Technol Inform. 2006;125:334–6.

Vázquez JL, Santander A, Mosso JL, Gao K, Wiederhold BK, Wiederhold MD. Using cybertherapy to reduce postoperative anxiety in cardiac recovery intensive care units. J Anesth Clin Res. 2013;4:363.

Wiederhold BK. Conquering panic, anxiety and phobias: achieving success through virtual reality and cognitive-behavioral therapy. San Diego, CA: Virtual Reality Medical Center; 2003.

Wiederhold BK. New tools to enhance posttraumatic stress disorder diagnosis and treatment: invisible wounds of war. Washington, DC: NATO Science for Peace and Security Series-E: Human and Societal Dynamics, IOS Press; 2013.

Wiederhold BK, Bouchard S. Virtual reality for posttraumatic stress disorder. Advances in virtual reality and anxiety disorders. New York, NY: Springer; 2014.

Wiederhold BK, Wiederhold MD. A new approach: using virtual reality psychotherapy in panic disorder with agoraphobia. Psychiatric Times. 2003;20(7).

Wiederhold BK, Wiederhold MD. Virtual reality therapy for anxiety disorders: advances in evaluation and treatment. Washington, DC: American Psychological Association; 2005.

Wiederhold BK, Wiederhold MD. Virtual reality with fMRI: a breakthrough cognitive treatment tool. Virtual Real. 2008;12(4):259–67.

Wiederhold BK, Wiederhold MD. Virtual reality treatment of posttraumatic stress disorder due to motor vehicle accident. Cyberpsychol Behav Soc Netw. 2010;13(1):21–7.

Wiederhold BK, Wiederhold MD. Managing pain in military populations with virtual reality. In: Pain syndromes—from recruitment to returning troops, B. Wiederhold (editor), vol. 91. Washington, DC: NATO Science for Peace and Security Series-E: Human and Societal Dynamics, IOS Press; 2012. p. 75–93.

Wiederhold BK, Wiederhold MD. A continuum of care: virtual reality as treatment of posttraumatic stress disorder (PTSD) and other pain syndromes. Int Rev Armed Forces Med Serv. 2014a;87(3):47–52.

Wiederhold MD, Wiederhold BK. A continuum of care: pre-deployment medical and tactical stress inoculation training using virtual reality. Int Rev Armed Forces Med Serv. 2014b;87(3):39–45.

Wiederhold BK, Riva G, Graffigna G. Ensuring the best care for our increasing aging population: health engagement and positive technology can help patients achieve a more active role in future healthcare. Cyberpsychol Behav Soc Netw. 2013;16(6):411–2.

Wiederhold MD, Gao K, Wiederhold BK. Clinical use of virtual reality distraction system to reduce anxiety and pain in dental procedures. Cyberpsychol Behav Soc Netw. 2014a;17(6):359–65.

Wiederhold BK, Riva G, Wiederhold MD. How can virtual reality interventions help reduce prescription opioid drug misuse? Cyberpsychol Behav Soc Netw. 2014b;17(6):331–2.

Wiederhold BK, Gao K, Sulea C, Wiederhold MD. Virtual reality as a distraction technique in chronic pain patients. Cyberpsychol Behav Soc Netw. 2014c;17(6):346–52.

Wiederhold BK, Gao K, Kong L, Wiederhold MD. Mobile devices as adjunctive pain management tools. Cyberpsychol Behav Soc Netw. 2014d;17(6):385–9.

Wiederhold BK, Soomro A, Riva G, Wiederhold MD. Future directions: advances and implications of virtual environments designed for pain management. Cyberpsychol Behav Soc Netw. 2014e;17(6):414–22.

Yuen EK, Herbert JD, Forman EM, Goetter EM, Comer R, Bradley JC. Treatment of social anxiety disorder using online virtual environments in second life. Behav Ther. 2013;44(1):51–61.

Chapter 10
How *Serious Games* Will Improve Healthcare

Maurits Graafland and Marlies Schijven

Abstract Games have the potential to attract large numbers of players and bring to them a specific understanding, skill, or attitude. The classic image of videogaming—socially deprived youngsters killing mystical monsters in their parents' basement—has evolved into a highly social, everyday activity that attracts all age groups to play games in the family living room. *Serious games*, therefore, are increasingly recognized as methods to promote health, treat patients, and train healthcare professionals. Whereas the technological developments in software, platforms, and wearable sensors are moving at high speed, the number of potential applications is rising and so is their use. This chapter aims to give an overview of underlying game mechanisms, main healthcare-related purposes, and the evidence supporting their effectiveness. We conclude that although the field is maturing in terms of diversification and evidence, more high-quality trials are needed to gain insight into the effectiveness of individual games as well as methods to improve transparency for individual users and clinicians.

Keywords Videogame • Education • Medical • Smartphone • Telemedicine • Mobile health • Rehabilitation • Wearable technology

10.1 Introduction

In 2002, the United States Army launched *America's Army*, a massive multiplayer online videogame simulating combat situations. The army originally designed it to be a "strategic communication platform" that would reach out to American

M. Graafland, M.D. Ph.D. (✉) • M. Schijven, M.D., Ph.D., M.H.Sc.
Department of Surgery, Academic Medical Centre,
PO Box 22660, Amsterdam 1100, The Netherlands
e-mail: maurits.graafland@gmail.com

youngsters. The game was played for over 40 million hours by 2.4 million registered users between July 2002 and November 2003 (Davis 2004). Because it encompassed highly realistic combat simulations, field commanders soon started to use it as a training and selection tool for new recruits (Zyda 2005).

This example perfectly illustrates the impact that well-designed *serious games may* have. Serious games can be defined as the application of (digital) games to improve users' skills, knowledge, or attitudes in real life (Michael and Chen 2006). In games, players are motivated by challenges, narrative, rules, and competitions to actively display a particular behavior or solve a problem. That games are able to trigger a player's intrinsic motivation can be of particular use and significance in the field of healthcare. This has been proven by the serious game *Re-mission* (HopeLab, Palo Alto, CA, 2006), a freely available online videogame designed to help teenage leukemia patients fight their disease. In this game, players virtually travel the blood vessels and combat malignant cells. A randomized controlled trial shows an increase in self-determination and drug adherence in patients playing the videogame, whereas these individuals are typically exceptionally difficult to motivate to adhere to medical treatment regimens (Kato et al. 2008).

Developments in the serious game industry have progressed rapidly in the past decade. Adaptation in healthcare, however, has proved to be slow. As with any healthcare innovation, the major concerns are safety and efficacy against costs for development and maintenance. However, the field may well have bypassed the initial peaks and disillusionments that many tech hypes experience. This chapter aims to give an overview of serious games applied to the field of medicine, evidence, and future issues to be resolved.

10.1.1   Homo Ludens

Using games to enhance skills acquisition is not a new phenomenon. The Russian Czar Peter the Great was known to build simulation armies to try out different military scenarios and strategies (Konstam 1993). In the 1990s, the first educational videogames were introduced in high schools, sometimes referred to as "edutainment" programs—mostly with little success (Susi et al. 2007). As the videogame industry developed into a multibillion-dollar industry and computers became powerful enough to create complex simulations, the possibilities for creating more immersive and purposeful serious games have increased greatly. New generations of serious games differ from edutainment in that they first and foremost attempt to attract and immerse the player into the gameplay while simultaneously incorporating purposeful content in a subtle, stealthy way (Susi et al. 2007; Sharp 2012).

User groups and their behavior have changed dramatically too. The common perception of average *gamers* being overweight anti-social teenage boys spending their days in their parents' basement killing off monsters is long gone. The average gamer to date is 35-years-old: 73% of all gamers are over 18-years-old and about 41% of them are female. About 77% of gamers play at least 1 h per week, 48% play games socially, and 36% play games on their smartphones (Entertainment Software Association 2016).

10.2   Learning Through Challenge and Fun

10.2.1   Flow Experiences

In well-designed games, interaction with the gameplay captivates the player. Series of causally linked challenges keep a player motivated and engaged throughout the game and, ideally, longing for more after he or she has quit playing. Gameplay depends on the interaction between the player and a series of challenges presented by the game, following specific (predictable or sometimes unpredictable) rules. Good games evoke emotions and surprise, creating a positive experience in players. Games are most effective when the player enters a state of *flow* (Kiili 2005). In this state of mind, players become completely absorbed in the challenges presented to them, ignoring all surroundings and focusing solely on playing. Flow experience (Fig. 10.1) results from an optimal balance between the game's challenges and the player's abilities as illustrated by Csiksentmihalyi's flow channel (Csikszentmihalyi 1975). Various factors are recognized to generate flow experience, such as clearly defined goals, immediate and appropriate feedback, playfulness, surprise, usability, and speed. Above all, players must sense that the challenges in the game match their abilities as well as a level of control to avoid them from opting-out (Kiili 2005). A player absorbed in a state of *flow* will learn more from the game, explore further, display a more positive attitude toward the subject and feel more in control (Kiili 2005; Schüler 2007; Skadberg and Kimmel 2004).

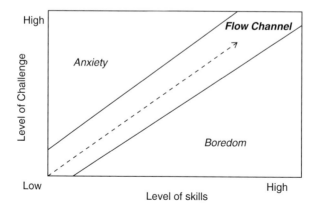

Fig. 10.1 Csikszentmihalyi's *flow* channel shows the relation between challenges and player skills in order to create an optimum experience in goal-driven activities (Schüler 2007)

10.3   Physical and Functional Fidelity

Games are ideal for problem-based learning as long as gameplay and educational goals are sufficiently balanced (Kiili 2005; Rollings and Adams 2003). Individuals learn from gaming experiences through abstract conceptualization and forming hypotheses, subsequently refining them in later experiences (Kolb 1984). If challenges, rules, and actions in the gameplay sufficiently cohere with real-life situations, the transfer of knowledge and skills to reality will occur (Kiili 2005). This is referred to as a game's *fidelity*. In the past, a lot of effort has been put into creating simulations that bare high *physical* fidelity to reality (i.e., the degree to which the physical appearance replicates the real task), whereas it was thought that only perfect physical recreation of the task leads to learning. Therefore, much effort was put into creating *simulators* in medical education, such as the virtual reality simulators in laparoscopic surgery. However, it has become clear that for a game (or simulator) to lead to skills transfer, its *functional* fidelity is most important. This refers to the degree to which the instrument replicates specific cues on which decisions in reality are based (Maran and Glavin 2003; Alexander et al. 2005). As long as problem-solving in a serious game follows the same rules as the real-life situation it is meant to support, the game's contexts and graphical appearance are secondary to the learning result and can be adjusted to optimize the player's immersion and flow.

10.4   Games for Health

The earliest and most obvious goal for use of serious games in healthcare is to change individuals' behavior in order to promote health. These "health games" can be specifically designed to promote healthy behavior, but may also be commercial games that serve general goals. These games fall in a wide range, including action or sports games, played on platforms that can detect motion (e.g., Nintendo Wii™ or Kinect™), but can also include actions, role-playing, or puzzle games with an element of strategy on mobile phones such as *Pokémon Go*™ (Niantic I 2016). Health games were originally developed mostly for the younger generations as it was believed to be most in line with their digital style of learning. Nowadays, they come in many forms for all generations and cater to specific interests.

Systematic literature reviews summarize a large number of potential applications for games in health education, promotion, and management (Table 10.1). They are applied to promote physical fitness (*Exergames*), for cognitive training (*Brain* games), to promote knowledge and self-management in chronic diseases and conditions (including asthma, diabetes, and obesity), and to reduce psychological conditions and stress related to treatment (e.g., low self-esteem, anxiety, and pain). Recently, Charlier et al. performed a systematic review of serious games directed specifically at improving adolescents' health behavior and self-management in the context of chronic illness. They included nine randomized

Table 10.1 Summary of systematic reviews on the effectiveness of games for health

Article	Game purpose	No. of articles	No. of games	Study types included	Meta-analysis	Conclusions
Charlier et al. (2016)	Health education and self-management in adolescents	9	7	RCTs only	Yes	Significant positive effect of serious games on health education and self-management in adolescents.
Kueider et al. (2012)	Cognitive training in older adults	8	22	RCTs, cohort studies	No	Videogames appear to be an effective means of enhancing reaction time, processing speed, executive function, and global cognition in older adults. Low-quality evidence.
Primack et al. (2012)	Promoting health and/or improving health outcomes	38	NR	RCTs only	No	Potential health-related benefits of serious games. Low-quality evidence.
Guy et al. (2011)	Combat childhood obesity	34	21	All	No	Action videogames use can elicit light to moderate physical activity among youth and increase nutrition-related knowledge. Evidence remains limited.
DeShazo et al. (2010)	Diabetes education	9	8	RCT, cohort	No	Games hold great potential as an alternative modality for diabetes education. Games described are exclusively for children. Evidence remains limited.

(continued)

Table 10.1 (continued)

Article	Game purpose	No. of articles	No. of games	Study types included	Meta-analysis	Conclusions
Adams (2010)	Healthcare in general	51	12	All	No	May be used for health education and training. Evidence remains limited.
Papastergiou (2009)	Health education and physical education	34	NR	All	No	Games may positively influence young people's knowledge, skills, attitudes and behavior in relation to health and physical exercise. Evidence remains limited.

NR = not reported, RCT = randomized controlled trial

controlled trials in a meta-analysis in which seven serious games were applied for the management of asthma: Asthma Command (Rubin et al. 1986; Homer et al. 2000); Watch, Discover, Think, and Act (Bartholomew et al. 2000; Shegog et al. 2001); Wee Willie Wheezie (Huss et al. 2003); The Asthma Files (McPherson 2006); juvenile diabetes (DiaBetNet) (Kumar et al. 2004); Packy and Marlon (Brown et al. 1997): and leukemia (Re-mission) (Kato et al. 2008). Results show a combined significant effect size of 0.361 (Hedges' gu, 95% confidence interval 0.098–0.624) on improving knowledge of the game groups versus the control groups that received mostly written knowledge. On improving self-management behavior, the effect size was 0.361 in favor of the game group (Hedges' gu, 95% CI 0.122–0.497) versus control groups that did not receive any education (Charlier et al. 2016). This study is the first to prove that serious games can improve the treatment of chronic disease in adolescents at the highest level of evidence (Grade A recommendation, level 1a).

10.5   Rehabilitation

Because of the strong motivation and immersion that videogames exert on their players, clinicians see them as interesting adjuncts to conventional physical rehabilitation in patients suffering from injury or disability. The spectrum varies from complex immersive virtual reality systems (van Kerckhoven et al. 2014) to commercially available games played on off-the-shelf game consoles (Saposnik et al. 2016). Rapid developments in motion detection systems in these consoles will make these games easily accessible for large groups of patients in need for rehabilitation on a global scale.

Saposnik et al. published a systematic review of the medical literature on the effectiveness of virtual reality (VR) rehabilitation systems (including both immersive VR systems and commercial videogames) for recovery of upper extremity motor function after stroke (Saposnik et al. 2011). The authors describe 12 clinical trials and observational studies in which technology was applied to detect movement through cameras and motion detection software or wearable devices with motion sensors. Limb function is then improved by through VR exercises ($n = 9$) or (commercial) videogames ($n = 3$). Data from five RCTs were pooled in a meta-analysis that showed a significant effect in favor of VR rehabilitation (OR 4.86, 95% CI 1.31–18.3, $p < 0.02$). The authors view the lack of trials *combining* VR with conventional therapy as a major shortcoming in current clinical practice (Saposnik et al. 2011).

Apart from rehabilitation in chronic conditions (e.g., cerebral palsy, multiple sclerosis, stroke, and Parkinson's disease), evidence is accumulating that also short- and medium-term rehabilitation after trauma or orthopedic surgery is achievable using serious games (Fig. 10.2). Rehabilitation after burn injury using videogames was shown to be equally effective as standard therapy, whereas videogame play even resulted in less pain experienced (Parry et al. 2015). This may be the result of a higher level of motivation and/or immersion, which perfectly exemplifies the major benefit of videogames in this context. Videogames have great potential as (adjuncts to) rehabilitation therapy in terms of cost reduction and effectiveness. The rapid advances in VR and wearable technology are likely to boost their application in the foreseeable future.

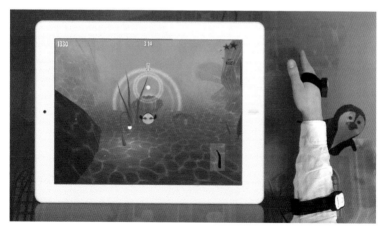

Fig. 10.2 In *Revalidate*™ (Motek (Amsterdam, The Netherlands)), in cooperation with Virtual play (Utrecht, The Netherlands), a player trains his or her wrist function after trauma or surgery. The controller attached to the player's hand measures its posture, allowing the player to control the turtle in the game to follow a specific course and score points. By introducing a fun and challenging aspect to rehabilitation, the producers hope to improve patients' functional outcome after trauma

10.6   Crowdsourcing Science

Online multiplayer gaming communities often spend a vast number of hours playing one single game—often in a social context (Entertainment Software Association 2016). The scientific community has been trying to capitalize on this phenomenon, attempting to use these massive amounts of human brainpower to solve complex or large-scale problems for healthcare-related purposes such as unraveling complex three-dimensional structures of specific proteins, DNA, and RNA. *Foldit* was developed by the University of Washington's Center for Game Science to allow non-scientists help unfold protein structures (Cooper et al. 2010). In the serious game, players can improve their scores by optimizing a given protein's structure or reducing the amount of intrinsic energy required, which is computed by a structure prediction model. One protein is presented at a time, allowing multiple players to attempt to solve the puzzle, automatically checking each other's efforts. *Foldit* has over 300,000 registered users who already delivered over 5400 protein recipes (Khatib et al. 2011). The players' efforts have resulted in real-world improvements in computational enzyme design (Eiben et al. 2012). In a survey dispersed by the developers, players give the game's competitive elements, social interaction through chat and web community, as well as the possibility to unravel scientific problems as main reasons to participate (Cooper et al. 2010).

Eyewire, developed by the Brain & Cognitive Sciences Department of the Massachusetts Institute of Technology, is a multiplayer online puzzle game that involves over 100,000 "citizen neuroscientists" in unraveling the structures of the mammalian retina. A dataset containing 3D electron micrographs of a mouse retina is chopped into little puzzle pieces and the players have to color subsets of individual neurons. The scoring system rewards agreements between players coloring the same neurons. Using this approach, "real" scientists were then able to reconstruct a connectivity model of the mouse retina (Kim et al. 2014). Other scientific problems addressed by crowdsourcing games are DNA multiple sequence alignment (*Phylo*) (Kawrykow et al. 2012), RNA structure design (*EteRNA*) (Lee et al. 2014), gene–disease associations (*Dizeez*) (Loguercio et al. 2013), and issues related to quantum physics (*Quantum Moves*) (Sørensen et al. 2016).

10.7   The Gaming Doctor

In the last decade, the availability of serious games developed to train or educate health professionals has increased rapidly. As Wang et al. (2016) showed in a systematic review, the number has increased from 4 in 2007 (including two different genres) to 42 in 2014 (including eight different genres) (Wang et al. 2016). The scope has widened from merely surgically oriented simulation games to almost all disciplines: internal medicine, neurology, geriatrics, intensive care, emergency medicine, general surgery, urology, obstetrics, pediatrics, pharmacy, nursing, pathology, and preclinical medical education. Game types include simulations, quizzes, puzzles, adventure games, and board games. The following three examples of educational serious games

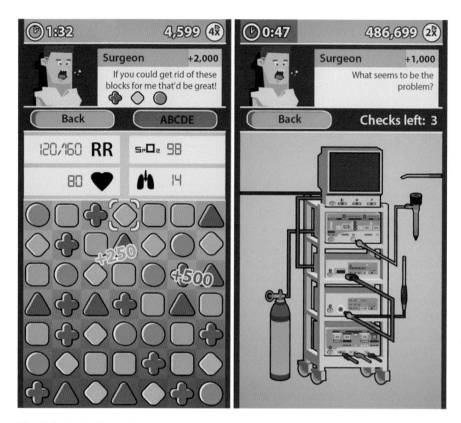

Fig. 10.3 In *Dr. Game: Surgeon Trouble*™ (Weirdbeard, Co., Amsterdam, The Netherlands), the trainee plays an amusing game on their smartphone (*left*) in which sudden changes may occur resembling equipment-related problems during laparoscopic surgery. The player has to solve the problem in a pop-up screen (*right*). The player learns surgical problem-solving skills while playing an amusing game (©Weirdbeard Co.)

give insight into the wide range of goals and design features. *GeriatriX*™ is a management simulation game aimed at teaching medical students how to deal with cases in geriatric medicine in which cost consciousness, end-of-life decisions, and psychosocial factors play a significant part (Lagro et al. 2014). *Dr. Game, Surgeon Trouble*™, is a simple arcade-type game (resembling *Bejewled*), in which equipment-related malfunctions typical to laparoscopic surgery are concealed (Fig. 10.3). The purpose of the game is to train the surgeon's situational awareness in a subtle, stealthy way while they play an amusing arcade game (Graafland et al. 2014a). In the serious game *Underground*™, the player has to build and manage an underground society of trolls using Nintendo Wii™ controllers adjusted to resemble laparoscopic surgical instruments (Fig. 10.4). While playing a game that has seemingly little to do with surgery itself, one acquires dexterity skills that can be translated to real-life laparoscopic surgery (Jalink et al. 2014a). All three serious games were the product of a collaboration of medical educators and game designers.

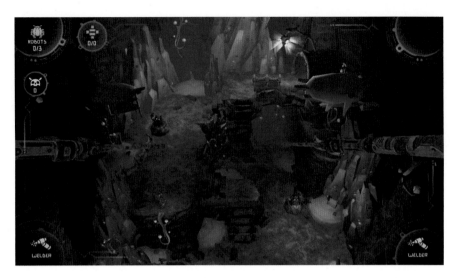

Fig. 10.4 In *Underground*™ (Grendel Games, Leeuwarden, The Netherlands), the trainee controls an underground society of trolls with two handles (depicted *left* and *right*) that resemble laparoscopic surgical instruments attached to a Nintendo Wii™ game console. While playing a game that has seemingly nothing to do with surgery, the player develops complex laparoscopic dexterity skills (©Grendel Games) https://www.undergroundthegame.com/

   Healthcare professionals will only accept games as tool for training or treatment if their effectiveness has been scientifically scrutinized. In their systematic review, Wang et al. found that 33/42 serious games were subjected to (at least) one study evaluating their efficacy as teaching intervention (Wang et al. 2016). They found a high heterogeneity in study design, with mainly positive results (only 11% of the studies found a negative result). Moreover, overall study quality was low (10.5 out of 18 points on the MERSQI score (Reed et al. 2008)). This more or less coincides with earlier systematic reviews, showing similar study quality and a limited amount of randomized controlled trials (Graafland et al. 2012; Akl et al. 2013). To answer the question of whether serious games are effective in general, one can merely conclude that there is sufficient evidence that *some* serious games have a significant effect on learning outcomes for healthcare professionals (level 2, Grade B). However, these studies did not research skills transfer to real-life (clinical) performance. Moreover, evidence of long-term learning retention is limited (Wang et al. 2016; Graafland et al. 2012; Akl et al. 2013).

10.8   Games in Official Medical Programs: *Seriously*?

10.8.1   Validity

It needs to be emphasized that the overall effect of serious games in clinical education or health promotion for individuals must not be confused with the effectiveness of individual games (Schijven and Jakimowicz 2005). Because of the heterogeneity in

Table 10.2 Validity of research process

Validity type	Description	Criteria for achievement
Content validity	The degree to which a game content adequately covers the dimensions of the medical construct it aims to educate (or is associated with).	Uniform and positive evaluation of game content and associated testing parameters by expert medical specialist panel.
Face validity	Degree of resemblance between medical constructs featured in gameplay and in reality, as assessed by novices (trainees) and experts (referents).	Uniform and positive evaluation of the game as a valuable learning environment among novice and expert medical specialists.
Construct validity	Inherent difference in outcomes of experts and novices on gameplay outcome parameters.	Outcome differences considered to be of significance between players being of different medical specialist levels of skill.
Concurrent validity	Concordance of study results using a concept instrument (e.g., game) and study results on an established instrument or method, believed to measure the same medical theoretical construct.	Outcome parameters show correlation considered to be significant between game and an alternative, established training method.
Predictive validity	The degree of concordance of a concept instrument (e.g., game) outcome and task performance in reality based on a validated scoring system.	Metrics show correlation considered to be significant between outcome parameters of a game and performance results on the medical construct featured in the game in real life after performers are trained using the game.

Adapted from Graafland et al. (2012)

design aspects, target groups, and purposes, every newly developed game will require a *separate* evaluation process—the gravity of which should be in accordance with the game's application. For instance, when applied to treating a sick patient or assessing a surgeon before he or she will perform a real-life operation, a game's assessment system should be more rigorously tested than when used as an adjunct to promote fruit and vegetable consumption in 5-year-old, otherwise healthy individuals. Consensus on the level of evidence required for specific games is an ongoing topic of discussion (Graafland et al. 2014b). However, there is a general need for *systematic* assessment strategies to prevent false and incomplete claims of effectiveness.

A useful concept in this systematic approach is *validity*. Validity research is a stepwise approach to evaluate various aspects of an instrument's resemblance to a real-life skill or performance parameter. The highest form of validity is *predictive validity*—an instrument's ability to improve skills in reality (Schijven and Jakimowicz 2005; Gallagher et al. 2003; Youngblood and Dev 2005). Table 10.2 shows the steps in the classical validity research processes applied most widely, although the concept itself is the subject of ongoing debate (Cook et al. 2014).

For example, one cohort study compared the speed and movement efficiency of experienced surgeons playing *Underground*™ to novices ($n = 30$) and found their result to be significantly faster (111%), thus proving its effectiveness in measuring competence on this specific skill (Jalink et al. 2014a). A second cohort study found that 97% of 34 pediatrics residents found the *Bronx Jeopardy*™ quiz game an easy-to-use and effective learning tool through a questionnaire (Jirasevijinda and Brown 2010), proving the likelihood that residents are likely to accept it as a training modality. However, the study setup and research purpose leads to the conclusion that *Underground*™ can be regarded as a more reliable or valid training instrument than *Bronx Jeopardy*™. In the first case, the game shows to have clear *construct* validity, whereas the second shows to have reasonable *face* validity.

10.9   Games in Skills Training Outside the Operating Room

Achieving an expert level in complex medical tasks requires prolonged *deliberate practice*. This is more than mere repetition, which in itself leads to arrested development over time. In deliberate practice, trainees require a well-defined goal, motivation to improve, feedback, and ample opportunity to repeat and refine their performance (Ericsson 2006). Surgical postgraduate curricula aim to create professionals who are *competent*, and preferably *proficient*, in essential surgical procedures within approximately 1200 h of operating time. Even though including the time performing non-essential procedures approximately doubles this number, it can be considered rather limited (Bell 2009; Chung 2005). Simulation and serious gaming could play a significant role in training and assessing performance in individual procedures or activities, limiting the number of "flying hours" required inside the surgical theatre (Bell 2009; Smith et al. 2009). Ideally, the objective measurement of skills and progress within simulators and serious games could lead to a system of accreditation and awarded responsibility. From this perspective, serious games and simulators should not be regarded as two different entities, but rather as two extremities from the same continuum of VR-enhanced training.

Virtual reality simulations have been developed and evaluated extensively for use in medical training (Dawe et al. 2014; Cook et al. 2011). Well-known examples include the minimally invasive surgical (MIS) simulators, developed for improving visuospatial skills and dexterity. Simulators are able to produce standardized, reproducible virtual surgical procedures. Their range encompasses basic task exercises (e.g., knot-tying or artery clipping) to complete MIS procedures with distinct patient scenarios (Schreuder et al. 2011). Surgical residents training on VR simulators work more efficiently and make fewer errors than residents not trained using VR simulators (Gurusamy et al. 2008; Ahlberg et al. 2007; Larsen et al. 2009). Simulators are able to give high-fidelity procedural training, measure skills progression, and deliver direct feedback to the trainee (Lamata de la Orden 2004). Thus, they are effective stand-alone training instruments and incorporated in residency training curricula in many developed countries (Dutch Society for Endoscopic Surgery 2009; Hamming et al. 2009).

However, apart from basic dexterity training for various surgical procedures and crew resource management in emergency situations, the integration of virtual reality (VR)-enhanced simulation in medical and surgical training curricula has been rather limited (Zevin et al. 2014). Lack of financial investments and manpower form practical hurdles in many hospitals. Next, the lack of structured, proficiency-based training curricula hinders the integration of simulation in the competency-based training curricula (Zevin et al. 2014; Schijven and Bemelman 2011). Finally, most commercially available VR simulators are frequently not seen as very motivating by their users (van Dongen et al. 2008; Chang et al. 2007). One can imagine that repeating *peg transfer* in a box trainer will not trigger a busy adult healthcare professional's interest for long.

This is where gamification, serious games, and VR headset solutions—the second wave of VR-enhanced learning—can play a major role. First, gamifying existing VR simulators, such as adding competitions and leaderboards, significantly increases its use by trainees (Verdaasdonk et al. 2009). Second, the design features and game mechanisms discussed above will assist the development of immersive, challenging educational instruments, tailored to a trainee's specific level and requirements (Dankbaar et al. 2014). Third, a new generation of VR head-mounted displays and systems capable of overlaying the real world with digital features are coming into play, varying from expensive headsets (e.g., Oculus Rift™, Samsung Gear VR™) and simple cardboard headset boxes holding a smartphone (Google Cardboard™) (Allaway 2015). These have great potential for creating complex and blended simulations in medical postgraduate education.

10.10 Financial and Ethical Aspects

Various financial reimbursement strategies have been applied in medical serious games in recent years. The most common model is where one or more health institutions present as the sponsor of a game, making the investment necessary for its production. The sponsor then distributes the game among patients or trainees (e.g. Dr. Game, Surgeon Trouble™). The main disadvantage of this strategy is that the sponsor may ultimately lose its interest or budget in the long run, threatening the game's development or maintenance.

A second model is when the game designer himself makes the investment for production and distributes the game to clients (e.g. Underground™). This model will naturally lead to better, high-quality products on the long term, but requires a significant investment from -often-small design companies. The designer runs the risk of the game failing to produce the desired effectiveness or popularity. Furthermore, designers often do not have the time or the budget to conduct scientific research.

A third model is when a non-profit organization (university, hospital or governmental organization) produces the game for free use to the public (e.g. Foldit™, Re-Mission™). This model is mostly applied when the use of the game has a common public interest and/or charitable objective.

In order for the medical serious game market to become more mature and independent on the long term, more rigid reimbursement models should be implemented. Opportunities lie in involving the main stakeholders in the development process, such as health insurance companies, patient organizations and (inter-)national federations charged with training and education of medical professionals.

From an ethical perspective, it is important that serious games do not lead to injuries or exacerbate diseases to their clients. Jalink et al. (2014b) published a systematic review on injuries caused by using the Nintendo game system. Apart from bizarre injuries such as haemothorax by falling from a couch during gameplay, most injuries described are relatively mild and non-specific. The authors conclude that videogames do not appear to be a serious health threat. However, when specific serious games are designed to treat specific patients, rigorous testing and/or FDA approval may be necessary before introduction to the market.

10.11 Discussion

Many tech hypes experience a period of disillusionment after an initial period of rapid growth, whereas the field of serious games in healthcare may be well have bypassed this stage. The field has diversified substantially and evidence on the effectiveness of serious games is mounting among a variety of applications and target groups. The technological advances continue to stride forward. For example, the use of optical head-mounted displays can significantly enhance the level of immersion and fidelity of serious games in the near future. Wearable sensors combined with motion detection software are already altering the field of rehabilitation. Applications that may render a virtual reality "layer" over the real world (*augmented reality*) are available in smart visors (Hololens™, Google Glass™, Vuzix™, etc.) but also on smartphones (Layar™). Combined with videogames, augmented reality will lead to holistic, immersive, diversified experiences that can be used to educate patients and professionals (Schreinemacher et al. 2014).

Although the future perspective for serious games is hopeful, there is still a multitude of challenges to be overcome before they will become common clinical applications. First, healthcare professionals are—for good reasons—hard to convince of the (cost-)effectiveness of new technologies. In contrast, the gaming industry is pushing for rapid adaptation from a business point of view. Although game designers and early medical adapters are starting to understand the importance of testing and validating new serious games, the evidence still remains rather thin. The systematic reviews discussed in this chapter all conclude that the quality of present clinical studies is moderate at best. There is a lack of randomized clinical trials and there are few negative studies, indicating some form of publication bias. Second, no evidence has been produced on the cost-effectiveness of game-enhanced therapies and training. In the age of cost reductions in healthcare across many developed countries, this potential benefit of videogames requires more emphasis. Third, our understanding on *what* motivates individuals to interact with a game remains very limited. It is important to know what aspects trigger specific user groups in order to predict the long-term effectiveness of games. In this context, so-called *super-users*, players that spend an unusual amount of time and effort playing digital applications, are thought to blur outcome statistics (van Mierlo et al. 2012).

Next to these scientific hurdles, practical issues need to be overcome as well. For example, most "mainstream" clinicians and patients remain simply unaware of the existence of relevant games let alone of the evidence supporting their use. Relevant information on games and mHealth applications is often hard to find in disorganized app stores and claims of effectiveness are hard to judge. This will cause caution and possibly even distrust among clinicians. Moreover, most clinicians are currently unequipped to judge the validity of serious games.

The establishment of scientific conferences and journals directed at serious games for healthcare purposes, such as Games for Health Journal (Baranowski n.d.), BMJ innovations (Jha n.d.), and JMIR Serious Games (Eysenbach n.d.), have greatly enhanced their visibility and awareness on importance to both the public and healthcare professionals. Efforts have been made to construct validation frameworks, to guide users in seeking the information necessary to judge a game's purpose, and effectiveness (Graafland et al. 2014b). To gain clinical exposure and reduce our dependency on disorganized app stores, we recommend some form of a publicly available library for medical serious games and comparable digital applications. Full transparency of serious games' benefits and limitations to both the public and healthcare professionals will ultimately facilitate their adaptation in treatment protocols and training curricula.

Acknowledgements *Disclosure*: The authors declare no conflicts of interest.

References

Adams SA. Use of "serious health games" in health care: a review. Stud Health Technol Inform. 2010;157:160–6.

Ahlberg G, Enochsson L, Gallagher AG, Hedman L, Hogman C, McClusky DA, et al. Proficiency-based virtual reality training significantly reduces the error rate for residents during their first 10 laparoscopic cholecystectomies. Am J Surg. 2007;193(6):797–804.

Akl EA, Kairouz VF, Sackett KM, Erdley WS, Mustafa RA, Fiander M, et al. Educational games for health professionals. Cochrane Database Syst Rev. 2013;3(3):CD006411.

Alexander AL, Brunyé T, Sidman J, Weil SA. From gaming to training: a review of studies on fidelity, immersion, presence, and buy-in and their effects on transfer in PC-based simulations and games. Proceedings from the 2005 Interservice/Industry Training, Simulation, and Education Conference (I/ITSEC). Arlington, VA; 2005. pp. 1–14.

Allaway T. Digital pulse [Internet]. PricewaterhouseCoopers Consulting (Australia) Pty Limited. 2015. https://www.digitalpulse.pwc.com.au/infographic-history-virtual-reality/.

Baranowski T. Games for Health Journal [Internet]. ISSN 2161-783X. http://www.liebertpub.com/g4h/.

Bartholomew LK, Gold RS, Parcel GS, Czyzewski DI, Sockrider MM, Fernandez M, et al. Watch, discover, think, and act: evaluation of computer-assisted instruction to improve asthma self-management in inner-city children. Patient Educ Couns. 2000;39(2–3):269–80.

Bell RH. Why Johnny cannot operate. Surgery. 2009;146(4):533–42.

Brown SJ, Lieberman DA, Germeny BA, Fan YC, Wilson DM, Pasta DJ. Educational video game for juvenile diabetes: results of a controlled trial. Med Inform. 1997;22(1):77–89.

Chang L, Petros J, Hess DT, Rotondi C, Babineau TJ. Integrating simulation into a surgical residency program: is voluntary participation effective? Surg Endosc. 2007;21(3):418–21.

Charlier N, Zupancic N, Fieuws S, Denhaerynck K, Zaman B, Moons P. Serious games for improving knowledge and self-management in young people with chronic conditions: a systematic review and meta-analysis. J Am Med Inform Assoc. 2016;23(1):230–9.

Chung RS. How much time do surgical residents need to learn operative surgery? Am J Surg. 2005;190(3):351–3.

Cook DA, Hatala R, Brydges R, Zendejas B, Szostek JH, Wang AT, et al. Technology-enhanced simulation for health professions education: a systematic review and meta-analysis. JAMA. 2011;306(9):978–88.

Cook DA, Zendejas B, Hamstra SJ, Hatala R, Brydges R. What counts as validity evidence? Examples and prevalence in a systematic review of simulation-based assessment. Adv Heal Sci Educ. 2014;19(2):233–50.

Cooper S, Khatib F, Treuille A, Barbero J, Lee J, Beenen M, et al. Predicting protein structures with a multiplayer online game. Nature. 2010;466(7307):756–60.

Csikszentmihalyi M. Beyond boredom and anxiety. 1st ed. San Francisco, CA: Jossey Bass; 1975.

Dankbaar MEW, Storm DJ, Teeuwen IC, Schuit SCE. A blended design in acute care training: similar learning results, less training costs compared with a traditional format. Perspect Med Educ. 2014;3(4):289–99.

Davis M, editor. America's Army: PC game vision and realization. San Francisco, CA: United States Army MOVES Institute; 2004.

Dawe SR, Pena GN, Windsor JA, Broeders JA, Cregan PC, Hewett PJ, et al. Systematic review of skills transfer after surgical simulation-based training. Br J Surg. 2014;101(9):1063–76.

DeShazo J, Harris L, Pratt W. Effective intervention or child's play? A review of video games for diabetes education. Diabetes Technol Ther. 2010;12(10):815–22.

van Dongen KW, van der Wal WA, Rinkes IHMB, Schijven MP, Broeders IAMJ. Virtual reality training for endoscopic surgery: voluntary or obligatory? Surg Endosc. 2008;22(3):664–7.

Dutch Society for Endoscopic Surgery (Nederlandse Vereniging voor Endoscopische Chirurgie). Minimally invasive surgery: plan for policy and approach. [Dutch] [Internet]. 2009. p. 1–74. www.nvec.nl.

Eiben CB, Siegel JB, Bale JB, Cooper S, Khatib F, Shen BW, et al. Increased Diels-Alderase activity through backbone remodeling guided by Foldit players. Nat Biotechnol. 2012;30(2):190–2.

Entertainment Software Association. Essential facts about the computer and videogame industry [Internet]. 2016. http://www.theesa.com/wp-content/uploads/2016/04/Essential-Facts-2016.pdf.

Ericsson KA. The influence of experience and deliberate practice on the development of superior expert performance. In: Ericsson KA, Charness N, Feltovich PJ, Hoffman RR, editors. The Cambridge handbook of expertise and expert performance. 1st ed. Cambridge: Cambridge University Press; 2006. p. 683–704.

Eysenbach G. JMIR Serious Games [Internet]. ISSN 2291-9279. http://games.jmir.org.

Gallagher AG, Ritter EM, Satava RM. Fundamental principles of validation, and reliability: rigorous science for the assessment of surgical education and training. Surg Endosc. 2003;17(10):1525–9.

Graafland M, Schraagen JMC, Schijven MP. Systematic review of serious games for medical education and surgical skills training. Br J Surg. 2012;99(10):1322–30.

Graafland M, Bemelman WA, Schijven MP. Prospective cohort study on surgeons' response to equipment failure in the laparoscopic environment. Surg Endosc. 2014a;28(9):2695–701.

Graafland M, Dankbaar M, Mert A, Lagro J, De Wit-Zuurendonk L, Schuit S, et al. How to systematically assess serious games applied to health care. JMIR Serious Games. 2014b;2(2):e11.

Gurusamy K, Aggarwal R, Palanivelu L, Davidson BR. Systematic review of randomized controlled trials on the effectiveness of virtual reality training for laparoscopic surgery. Br J Surg. 2008;95(9):1088–97.

Guy S, Ratzki-Leewing A, Gwadry-Sridhar F. Moving beyond the stigma: systematic review of video games and their potential to combat obesity. Int J Hypertens. 2011;2011:1–13.

Hamming J, Borel Rinkes IHM, Heineman E. Scherp: structured curriculum for surgery for reflective professionals (Structuur Curriculum Heelkunde voor Reflectieve Professionals). [Dutch]. Opleidingsplan Heelkunde [Internet]. Dutch Surgical Society (Nederlandse Vereniging voor Heelkunde); 2009. http://knmg.artsennet.nl.

Homer C, Susskind O, Alpert HR, Owusu MS, Schneider L, Rappaport LA, et al. An evaluation of an innovative multimedia educational software program for asthma management: report of a randomized, controlled trial. Pediatrics. 2000;106(1 Pt 2):210–5.

Huss K, Winkelstein M, Nanda J, Naumann PL, Sloand ED, Huss RW. Computer game for inner-city children does not improve asthma outcomes. J Pediatr Health Care. 2003;17(2):72–8.

Jalink MB, Goris J, Heineman E, Pierie JPEN, ten Cate Hoedemaker HO. Construct and concurrent validity of a Nintendo Wii video game made for training basic laparoscopic skills. Surg Endosc. 2014a;28(2):537–42.

Jalink MB, Heineman E, Pierie J-PEN, ten Cate Hoedemaker HO. Nintendo related injuries and other problems: review. BMJ. 2014b;349:g7267.

Jha P. BMJ Innovations [Internet]. ISSN 2055-8074. n.d. http://innovations.bmj.com.

Jirasevijinda T, Brown LC. Jeopardy!©: an innovative approach to teach psychosocial aspects of pediatrics. Patient Educ Couns. 2010;80(3):333–6.

Kato PM, Cole SW, Bradlyn AS, Pollock BH. A video game improves behavioral outcomes in adolescents and young adults with cancer: a randomized trial. Pediatrics. 2008;122(2):e305–17.

Kawrykow A, Roumanis G, Kam A, Kwak D, Leung C, Wu C, et al. Phylo: a citizen science approach for improving multiple sequence alignment. PLoS One. 2012;7(3):e31362.

van Kerckhoven G, Mert A, De Ru JA. Treatment of vertigo and postural instability using visual illusions. J Laryngol Otol. 2014;128(11):1005–7.

Khatib F, Cooper S, Tyka MD, Xu K, Makedon I, Popovic Z, et al. Algorithm discovery by protein folding game players. Proc Natl Acad Sci. 2011;108(47):18949–53.

Kiili K. Digital game-based learning: Towards an experiential gaming model. Internet High Educ. 2005;8(1):13–24.

Kim JS, Greene MJ, Zlateski A, Lee K, Richardson M, Turaga SC, et al. Space–time wiring specificity supports direction selectivity in the retina. Nature. 2014;509(7500):331–6.

Kolb D. Experiential learning: experience as the source of learning and development. Englewood Cliffs, NJ: Prentice Hall; 1984.

Konstam A. Peter the Great's Army (1): infantry. 1st ed. London: Osprey Publishing; 1993. 48 p.

Kueider AM, Parisi JM, Gross AL, Rebok GW. Computerized cognitive training with older adults: a systematic review. PLoS One. 2012;7(7):e40588.

Kumar VS, Wentzell KJ, Mikkelsen T, Pentland A, Laffel LM. The DAILY (daily automated intensive log for youth) trial: a wireless, portable system to improve adherence and glycemic control in youth with diabetes. Diabetes Technol Ther. 2004;6(4):445–53.

Lagro J, van de Pol MHJJ, Laan A, Huijbregts-Verheyden FJ, Fluit LCRR, Olde Rikkert MGMM. A randomized controlled trial on teaching geriatric medical decision making and cost consciousness with the serious game GeriatriX. J Am Med Dir Assoc. 2014;15(12):957.e1–6.

Lamata de la Orden P. Methodologies for the analysis, design and evaluation of laparoscopic surgical simulators. Universit de Louvain; 2004.

Larsen CR, Soerensen JL, Grantcharov TP, Dalsgaard T, Schouenborg L, Ottosen C, et al. Effect of virtual reality training on laparoscopic surgery: randomised controlled trial. BMJ. 2009;338:b1802.

Lee J, Kladwang W, Lee M, Cantu D, Azizyan M, Kim H, et al. RNA design rules from a massive open laboratory. Proc Natl Acad Sci. 2014;111(6):2122–7.

Loguercio S, Good BM, Su AI. Dizeez: an online game for human gene-disease annotation. Bajic VB, editor. PLoS One. 2013;8(8):e71171.

Maran NJ, Glavin RJ. Low- to high-fidelity simulation - a continuum of medical education? Med Educ. 2003;37(Suppl 1):22–8.

McPherson AC. A randomized, controlled trial of an interactive educational computer package for children with asthma. Pediatrics. 2006;117(4):1046–54.

Michael DR, Chen S. Serious games: games that educate, train, and inform. 1st ed. Boston, MA: Thomson Course Technology; 2006.

van Mierlo T, Voci S, Lee S, Fournier R, Selby P. Superusers in social networks for smoking cessation: analysis of demographic characteristics and posting behavior from the Canadian Cancer Society's smokers' helpline online and StopSmokingCenter.net. J Med Internet Res. 2012;14(3):e66.

Niantic I. Niantic Labs [Internet]. 2016. https://www.nianticlabs.com/blog/.

Papastergiou M. Exploring the potential of computer and video games for health and physical education: a literature review. Comput Educ. 2009;53(3):603–22.

Parry I, Painting L, Bagley A, Kawada J, Molitor F, Sen S, et al. A pilot prospective randomized control trial comparing exercises using videogame therapy to standard physical therapy. J Burn Care Res. 2015;36(5):534–44.

Primack BA, Carroll MV, McNamara M, Klem ML, King B, Rich M, et al. Role of video games in improving health-related outcomes. Am J Prev Med. 2012;42(6):630–8.

Reed DA, Beckman TJ, Wright SM, Levine RB, Kern DE, Cook DA. Predictive validity evidence for medical education research study quality instrument scores: quality of submissions to JGIM's Medical Education Special Issue. J Gen Intern Med. 2008;23(7):903–7.

Rollings A, Adams E. Gameplay. In: Rollings A, Adams E, editors. Andrew Rollings and Ernest Adams on game design. Berkeley, CA: New Riders Press; 2003. p. 199–238.

Rubin DH, Leventhal JM, Sadock RT, Letovsky E, Schottland P, Clemente I, et al. Educational intervention by computer in childhood asthma: a randomized clinical trial testing the use of a new teaching intervention in childhood asthma. Pediatrics. 1986;77(1):1–10.

Saposnik G, Levin M, Outcome Research Canada (SORCan) Working Group. Virtual reality in stroke rehabilitation: a meta-analysis and implications for clinicians. Stroke. 2011;42(5):1380–6.

Saposnik G, Cohen LG, Mamdani M, Pooyania S, Ploughman M, Cheung D, et al. Efficacy and safety of non-immersive virtual reality exercising in stroke rehabilitation (EVREST): a randomised, multicentre, single-blind, controlled trial. Lancet Neurol. 2016;4422(16):1–9.

Schijven MP, Bemelman WA. Problems and pitfalls in modern competency-based laparoscopic training. Surg Endosc. 2011;25(7):2159–63.

Schijven MP, Jakimowicz JJ. Validation of virtual reality simulators: key to the successful integration of a novel teaching technology into minimal access surgery. Minim Invasive Ther Allied Technol. 2005;14(4):244–6.

Schreinemacher MH, Graafland M, Schijven MP. Google glass in surgery. Surg Innov. 2014;21(6):651–2.

Schreuder HWR, Oei G, Maas M, Borleffs JCC, Schijven MP. Implementation of simulation in surgical practice: minimally invasive surgery has taken the lead: the Dutch experience. Med Teach. 2011;33(2):105–15.

Schüler J. Arousal of flow experience in a learning setting and its effects on exam performance and affect. Z Pädagog Psychol. 2007;21(3):217–27.

Sharp L. Stealth learning: unexpected learning opportunities through games. J Instr Res. 2012;1:42–8.

Shegog R, Bartholomew LK, Parcel GS, Sockrider MM, Mâsse L, Abramson SL. Impact of a computer-assisted education program on factors related to asthma self-management behavior. J Am Med Inform Assoc. 2001;8(1):49–61.

Skadberg YX, Kimmel JR. Visitors' flow experience while browsing a Web site: its measurement, contributing factors and consequences. Comput Human Behav. 2004;20(3):403–22.

Smith AJ, Aggarwal R, Warren OJ, Paraskeva P. Surgical training and certification in the United kingdom. World J Surg. 2009;33(2):174–9.

Sørensen JJWH, Pedersen MK, Munch M, Haikka P, Jensen JH, Planke T, et al. Exploring the quantum speed limit with computer games. Nature. 2016;532(7598):210–3.

Susi T, Johannesson M, Backlund P. Serious games – an overview. Elearning. 2007;73(10):28.

Verdaasdonk EGG, Dankelman J, Schijven MP, Lange JF, Wentink M, Stassen LPS. Serious gaming and voluntary laparoscopic skills training: a multicenter study. Minim Invasive Ther Allied Technol. 2009;18(4):232–8.

Wang R, DeMaria S, Goldberg A, Katz D. A systematic review of serious games in training health care professionals. Simul Healthc. 2016;11(1):41–51.

Youngblood P, Dev P. A framework for evaluating new learning technologies in medicine. AMIA 2005 Symposium Proceedings. 2005. p. 1163.

Zevin B, Aggarwal R, Grantcharov TP. Surgical simulation in 2013: why is it still not the standard in surgical training? J Am Coll Surg. 2014;218(2):294–301.

Zyda M. From visual simulation to virtual reality to games. Computer. 2005;38(9):25–32.

Chapter 11
Drones in Healthcare

Sharon Wulfovich, Homero Rivas, and Pedro Matabuena

Abstract Unmanned aerial vehicles (Drones) were first used in the 1990s by military organizations. However, the decline in cost due to technological advancements has allowed drones to become viable options for a diverse range of services including health services. Currently, health services and medical resources in underserved communities are limited to motor transportation and in-person interactions; however, drones may be a feasible option in providing these services in a more effective manner. Current research has explored the use of drones for natural disaster relief, search and rescue missions, and transfer units. However, there is limited research on how drones could be used as telemedicine and transfer units. This chapter discusses the current research on the use of drones in the health field and presents a pilot research project on drones as telemedicine and transfer units.

Keywords Unmanned aerial vehicles • Drones • Rural medicine • Telemedicine

11.1 Introduction

Drones have generated great interest in recent years due to their industrial, commercial, and recreational potential. Drones have locomotion capacities, the ability to move from one side to another. However, drones are differentiated from

S. Wulfovich (✉)
Stanford University, Stanford, CA, USA
e-mail: sharonws@stanford.edu

H. Rivas, M.D., M.B.A.
Stanford University School of Medicine,
300 Pasteur Ct, Suite H3680H, Stanford, CA 94305, USA
e-mail: hrivas@stanford.edu

P. Matabuena
Unmanned Aerial Vehicle Systems, Instituto Tecnológico Autónomo de México and Aidronix,
CDMX, Mexico
e-mail: pmatabuena@gmail.com

© Springer International Publishing AG 2018
H. Rivas, K. Wac (eds.), *Digital Health*, Health Informatics,
https://doi.org/10.1007/978-3-319-61446-5_11

other air vehicles in that they do not need to be manned by a human. Their remote pilots can control them from varying distances, dependent on their automation and autonomy. Therefore any unmanned aerial vehicle that has the capacity to be autonomous even with various functions and uses is considered a drone.

The most common term used in the media today to describe an "unmanned aerial vehicle" is a drone. Unfortunately the term drone often carries a level of stigma inherited from its controversial military applications on the battlefield. A more preferable and descriptive term used by proponents of the industry is unmanned aerial vehicle (UAV). Drones and UAVs are considered synonymous, although some argue that a drone can be differentiated by a level of automation that makes it flight dependent on pre programmed behaviors as opposed to a UAV that is a remotely piloted aircraft flown by "stick and rudder," with a pilot in control. This point of differentiation, however, remains debatable. On the other hand, unmanned aerial systems (UAS) is a term of reference that by definition is clearly distinguishable from a drone or UAV. A UAS is a description that encompasses the aircraft or the UAV, the ground controller, and the communication system that connects the two. In this chapter the term UAV and drones will be used interchangeably.

Current technological advancements have made drones more efficient. Drones contain cameras, GPS, and diverse sensors that allow greater autonomy and efficient flights (Scott and Scott 2017). Additionally, new lithium batteries are allowing drones to cover greater distance (Scott and Scott 2017). Furthermore, mobile phone or tablet software increases accuracy in tracking and navigation (Scott and Scott 2017). These mobile applications also make it increasingly intuitive and easy for all audiences to pilot a drone.

Civilian drones with commercial-grade low-cost technology have already been used for various rescue tasks and natural disasters around the world. However, this technology's potential has yet to be fully explored and used. In fact this technology's use is limited for public services around the world due to regulatory issues in airspace (DeBusk 2010). Although this technology is already available and ready to be used, technology advances much faster than the laws themselves. One of the main reasons that airspace regulatory agencies block or restrict certain uses of these aircrafts is to preserve air safety of manned aircrafts and people on the ground by gradually analyzing the risks and knowing the modes of operation and then slowly deciding restrictions and operating laws (DeBusk 2010). Due to these limitations, there is very limited research on the use of drones in the health industry. This chapter will present the current uses and research of drones in the health industry and then present a pilot study on the use of drones as telemedicine and transport units.

11.2   Drones and Natural Disaster Relief

The systems used in civilian-grade UAVs can provide effective assistance in natural disaster relief and make emergency response increasingly effective and timely (DeBusk 2010). The optimum design of aerial systems for these applications is regularly improving with the use of rapid prototyping techniques including 3D printing, laser cutting, and new light-weight and resistant materials (DeBusk 2010).

Successful examples of the use of drones in natural disaster relief are with tornados (DeBusk 2010). There are many regions in the world including Europe, the United States, and South America, where tornadoes are very active (DeBusk 2010). Drones can be used to advance tornado and storm warnings (DeBusk 2010). Different institutions have created diverse techniques and process to maximize the accuracy of storm warnings. A research study by Georgia Institute of Technology examined the use of micro-radars called MiniSAR (miniature synthetic aperture radar), a form of radar that is used to create images, to observe the shape and composition of the clouds in greater detail, and to analyze the atmosphere with greater precision (DeBusk 2010). Current micro-radar systems such as MiniSAR are small enough to be inserted into unmanned aerial vehicles as they weigh only a few hundred grams (DeBusk 2010), but advances in the near future could put radar systems in smaller aircrafts.

Climate monitoring is a key aspect of storm classification and early detection of tornadoes. Obtaining information about speed and direction of the wind directly from the source increases the accuracy of climate monitoring. Drones have the ability to get readings of wind speed and direction as the aircrafts can fly near the storms (DeBusk 2010). Drones use sensors that can distinguish the type and composition of clouds that then use software to process them as images (DeBusk 2010). Therefore drones provide more accurate readings compared to indirect traditional methods (DeBusk 2010). The type of drone that this data can be obtained from is a fixed wing (Figs. 11.2, 11.3, and 11.4); that is to say, it is an airplane very similar to those used in the aeromodelling but larger with dimensions ranging from 4 to 26 m of wingspan (DeBusk 2010). Making some structural modifications to the fixed-wing drone allows it to withstand rain, low temperatures, severe winds, and turbulence while caring the measuring instruments (DeBusk 2010). The current aircrafts that meet these technical specifications include Textron's "Aerosonde" and General Atomics' "Altair/Ikhana" (DeBusk 2010).

Additionally, drones can be used to respond to a natural disaster. For example, in Nepal after the earthquake (2015) and in the Philippines after typhoon Haiyan (2013), drones were used by humanitarian organizations to collect real-time information (Htet 2016). Specifically, these drones were used to evaluate the damage and map which areas were affected (Htet 2016). This information was used to assess what areas needed help and determine which roads were still okay to use (Htet 2016). This information proved to be useful responding to natural disasters and can be used in any emergency situation.

11.3   Drones as Search and Rescue Units

What if instead of sending personnel to dangerous situations, authorities could send a drone? The Autonomous Unmanned Aerial Vehicle Technology Laboratory at Linköping University in Sweden is conducting research on how to integrate artificial intelligence in distributed software architectural frameworks (Burdakov et al. 2010). This allows for greater autonomy and functionality in complex operational environments.

Other research at Linköping University in Sweden has focused on the combination of drones and human operators to provide emergency service assistance (Doherty and Rudol 2007). First, drones explore the affected areas and try to identify wounded individuals by means of specialized area photos (Doherty and Rudol 2007). Then, medical instruments and other resources (food, water, etc.) are delivered to the previously identified individuals (Doherty and Rudol 2007).

These drones use different video sensors including thermal and conventional RGB spectrum, which transmit the images captured to software involved in image recognition for detection and geo location of human bodies (Doherty and Rudol 2007). This is a complicated process as technology on these UAVs involves the development and manufacture of new flight hardware and aircraft design. The sensors that are continuously developing and improving are the vision sensors (Doherty and Rudol 2007). These sensors are crucial for the use of drones in search and rescue missions and are continuously being developed to provide advanced synthetic vision and offer a clearer picture of what is on the ground (Doherty and Rudol 2007). The incorporation of night and infrared spectrum vision allows these operations to extend at night and continue search operations in conditions with less visibility (Doherty and Rudol 2007).

11.4   Drones as Transfer Units

Currently, there are organizations in different parts of the world that have implemented and are continuing to develop uses for drones in the health sector. Organizations such as WeRobotics have made strategic alliances with robotics manufacturers, technology companies, and research institutes to co create, with local universities, non profits, community, or government innovation labs, drones called "Flying Labs" (We Robotics, 2017). These "Flying Labs" are implemented in developing countries and allow local communities to use robotics for their own improvement (We Robotics, n.d.). These labs provide training, equipment, data-processing experience, and other services depending on the community's identified needs (We Robotics, n.d.).

A research study by the Department of Pathology at Johns Hopkins University School of Medicine found that drone transportation of laboratory tests including chemistry, hematology, and coagulation testing did not affect the accuracy of the test results (Amukele et al. 2015). This provides evidence that there are no systematic differences between the laboratory test results of samples due to transportation (Amukele et al. 2015). This provides support for using drones as a means to transport laboratory tests.

Inexpensive drones (approximate cost of $10,000) can fly 20–60 miles with a 5-lb cargo load (Lippi and Mattiuzzi 2016). Drones can transport biological samples including blood derivatives and pharmaceutical specimens (Thiels et al. 2015). The transportation of medical devices and medical supplies can be valuable in natural disasters, when roads are blocked or when other forms of transport are unavailable or not timely. Although there is concern about the risk of collision, regulations for healthcare usage, and areas for safe takeoff and landing (Lippi and Mattiuzzi 2016), with technological advancements, research, and trials, these concerns can be minimized and outweighed by the benefits.

11.5 Drones as Telemedicine and Transfer Units

Drones can be used to facilitate access to medical care in marginalized communities. Drones are particularly useful in marginalized communities as these communities lack infrastructure and transportation to allow for the delivery of necessary health services and supplies in a time-effective manner. Drones are able to travel quickly with a speed of 40–60 miles/hour (Lippi and Mattiuzzi 2016) and can overcome topographic challenges that would be very challenging to overcome by other forms of transportation.

Currently, some organizations are attempting to develop drones that can deliver a range of health services to underserved communities. For example, Aidronix, Mexico (Aidronix, 2017), is developing a high-value light-duty unmanned aerial transport system, which aims to reach out to marginalized communities with medical assistance. One of the projects is to develop aerial bridges from distribution centers installed at strategic locations to supply medical supplies to rural communities. These distribution centers would load the drones with the supplies needed, and the drones would deliver them and return to the distribution center for more. The distribution centers can be built with shipping containers, camping trailers, or low-cost thermal booths and be equipped with all the necessary medical supplies including medications, vaccines, antibiotics, and antidotes (Fig. 11.1). Fixed-wing drones may be used for this project (Figs. 11.2, 11.3, and 11.4) due to their higher performance, carrying capacity, and speed compared to the multi-rotor drone (Fig. 11.5). These low-cost aircrafts are currently in the prototype stage, and further field testing is required. This would allow Aidronix to effectively supply rural communities with any medical supplies needed.

Additionally, Stanford University with funding provided by the Stanford Center for Innovation in Global Health and in collaboration with Aidronix will begin a study in 2017 to create and evaluate the feasibility of drone telemedicine units. This pilot study will be conducted in Mezquital, a highly marginalized municipality of Durango, Mexico (Fig. 11.6).

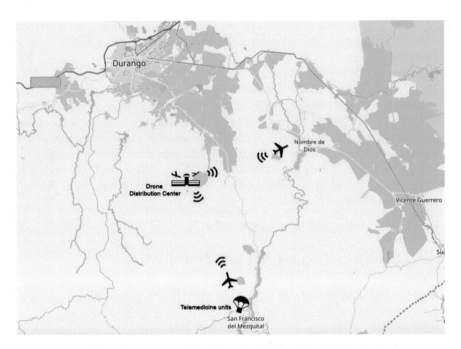

Fig. 11.1 *Map of distribution centers.* Map illustrating the idea of developing distribution centers. These distribution centers would load the drones with the supplies needed, and the drones would deliver them and return to the distribution centers for more. Map adapted from © OpenStreetMap contributors, and this data is available under the Open Database License

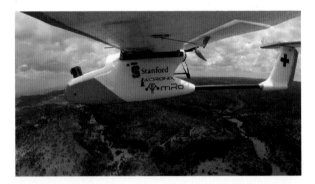

Fig. 11.2 *Fixed-wing drone.* Picture taken from the tip of the wing of a fixed-wing drone, during an aircraft test on stress, battery life, and carrying capacity. This unit is equipped with video cameras that transmit video to the remote pilot, so they can see where it is flying (first-person view, FPV) and at the same time sends the telemetry of the aircraft

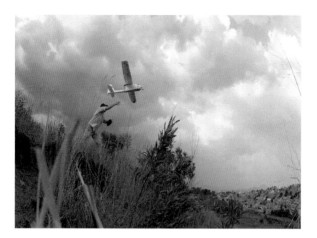

Fig. 11.3 *Manual launch of a fixed-wing drone.* Manual launch practice of a fixed-wing drone built by Aidronix. Manual launch of a drone can be very complicated as human error can compromise the aircraft. Additionally, the operator is at very close proximity to the propeller, which can be dangerous. In larger units this technique is impractical due to the total weight of the aircraft

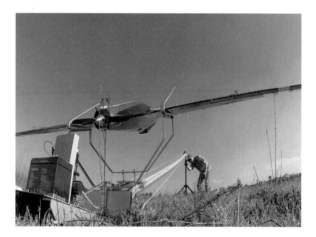

Fig. 11.4 *Delta fixed-wing drone.* This is a delta fixed-wing drone of 2-m wingspan. Due to its heavy weight, it is released by means of a catapult. This is one of the prototypes used to transport medical supplies to rural communities. Its approximate flight time is 45 min and cruising speed is 70 km/h

Geographically isolated areas have limited financial resources and low access to immediate medical care and specialized medical centers. Mexico is a clear example of a country where inequalities exist and provides a development platform for a disruptive solution. Durango is the fourth largest state in Mexico with the second lowest population density with a population of 1,754,754 in its 123,317 km^2 (National Institute of Statistics and Geography, n.d.). Durango is prone to inequalities in access

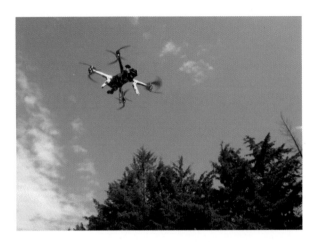

Fig. 11.5 *Multi-rotor drone.* This image was taken during the search for a missing person in a canyon in Mexico. This 8-motor multi-rotor drone incorporates a video camera that transmits to the operator. However, the range of operation is short. This is an ideal platform when takeoff space is limited or when there is not enough space for the operator to move around

to care due to its vast territory and diverse geographical landscape that creates isolated areas. Of the 39 municipalities, 5, Canelas, Mezquital, Otáez, Tamazula, and Topia, are considered by the SEDESOL Micro-Regions Program as highly marginalized with regard to access to education, living condition, population density, and income (Consejo Nacional de Población (CONAPO), n.d.).

Specifically, this project will focus on acute, subacute, and chronic medical problems in geographical locations with a shortage or absence of healthcare providers and lack of adequate infrastructure to provide immediate medical care when needed.

This pilot project will use UAVs as telemedicine units, which will incorporate basic but technologically advanced digital health systems. For example, these telemedicine drones will incorporate FDA-approved digital health devices including devices able to monitor EKG activity, pulse, blood pressure, temperature, oxygen saturation, and ultrasound (Rhythm Technologies, Inc., n.d.; Sotera Wireless, Inc., n.d.; Zhao et al. 2015). These devices can be incorporated into the drone via small stand-alone devices or a mobile phone. These UAVs will use highly secure networks that will allow patients to connect to healthcare providers immediately in a HIPPA compliant manner with limited broadband.

Overall, this study will evaluate the feasibility and scaling of prompt access to care via drones through the use of digital health, telemedicine, and transportation of necessary health equipment and medication. We hope that this study will provide insight on how to create systems of air bridges with unmanned aircrafts between

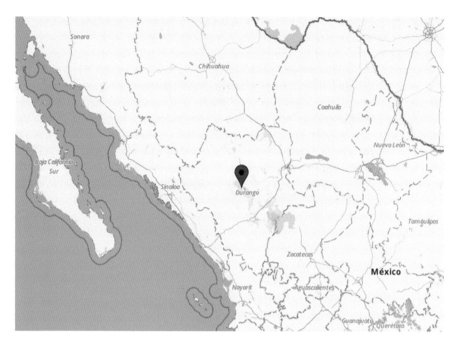

Fig. 11.6 *Map of Durango*. Map showing the location of Durango in Mexico. Map adapted from © OpenStreetMap contributors and this data is available under the Open Database License

marginalized regions and a distribution center offering health equipment and services. Additionally, we hope that this study will provide evidence that drones can be used as effective telemedicine units. If so, we hope that this model will be replicated in the rest of the world.

11.6   Conclusion

If we were to compare drones to the invention and boom of personal computers in the 1980s, at that time computers were expensive, large, and of rustic design. In addition to their operating systems having many errors, few people knew how to use them. People did not imagine that computers would become an integral part of day-to-day life and be able to complete so many diverse and complex tasks. Nevertheless, technology began to develop and mature exponentially. Now, everyone has a computer and it has become an essential tool.

Just like with computers in the 1980s, we have now developed an understanding of drones as an aircraft. However, we have yet to fully develop the use of this technology.

Technology is reaching a point of maturity. This opportunity will allow drones to become viable options for a diverse range of services including health services. Drones can have a large social impact. Drones can be used for natural disasters, search and rescue missions, and transfer units. And if our hypothesis is correct, drones can also serve as telemedicine units. Currently, health services and medical resources in underserved communities are limited to motor transportation and in-person interactions; however, drones have the ability to change communities, access to health all over the world. Drones can make medical services readily available and take road infrastructure out of the equation.

References

Aidronix Drones for good [Internet]. Accessed on April 2, 2017. n.d. http://www.aidronix.com.

Amukele TK, Sokoll LJ, Pepper D, Howard DP, Street J. Can unmanned aerial systems (Drones) be used for the routine transport of chemistry, hematology, and coagulation laboratory specimens? PLoS One. 2015;10:1–15.

Burdakov O, Doherty P, Holmberg K, Kvarnstrom J, Olsson P-M. Relay positioning for unmanned aerial vehicle surveillance. Int J Robot Res. 2010;29:1069–87.

Consejo Nacional de Población (CONAPO). Índice de marginación por entidad federativa y municipio 2010. [Internet]. Accessed on April 2, 2017. n.d. http://www.conapo.gob.mx/work/models/CONAPO/indices_margina/mf2010/CapitulosPDF/1_4.pdf.

DeBusk WM. Unmanned aerial vehicle systems for disaster relief: Tornado alley. AIAA Infotech at Aerospace 2010, Article Number 2010-3506. 2010.

Doherty P, Rudol P. A UAV search and rescue scenario with human body detection and geolocalization. In: Orgun MA, Thornton J, editors. AI 2007: Advances in artificial intelligence, Lecture notes in computer science, vol. 4830. Berlin: Springer; 2007.

Htet ZB. Disaster drones : great potential, few challenges? RSIS Commentaries. Singapore: Nanyang Technological University; 2016.

Lippi G, Mattiuzzi C. Biological samples transportation by drones: ready for prime time? Ann Translat Med. 2016;4:92.

National Institute of Statistics and Geography. Durango, Mexico. [Internet]. Accessed on January 8, 2017. n.d. http://cuentame.inegi.org.mx/monografias/informacion/dur/default.aspx?tema=me&e=10.

Rhythm Technologies, Inc. Zio® XT Patch. [Internet]. Accessed on April 1, 2017. n.d. www.irhythmtech.com.

Scott J, Scott C. Drone delivery models for healthcare. Proceedings of the 50th Hawaii International Conference on System Sciences. 2017, pp. 3297–3304.

Sotera Wireless, Inc. Visi Mobile. [Internet]. Accessed on April 1, 2017. n.d. www.visimobile.com.

Thiels CA, Aho JM, Zietlow SP, Jenkins DH. Use of unmanned aerial vehicles for medical product transport. J Air Med Transp. 2015;34:104–8.

We Robotics. How we create local Flying Labs. Accessed on April 02, 2017. n.d. http://werobotics.org/flying-labs/.

Zhao F, Li M, Tsien JZ. Technology platforms for remote monitoring of vital signs in the new era of telemedicine. Expert Rev Med Devices. 2015;12(4):411–29.

Chapter 12
Digital Health and Obesity: How Technology Could Be the Culprit and Solution for Obesity

Matthew Cooper and John Morton

Abstract Advances in technology over the past century have directly contributed to the growing worldwide obesity epidemic. Streamlined food production, changes in the macronutrient profile of food, and mass marketing of unhealthy food to children have all contributed to an increase in caloric intake. Decreased physical activity and an increase in sedentary behavior both stem from industrialization of the workplace. Conversely technology can help integrate proven behavioral modification models into patients lifestyles and provide patients with biometric data previously unavailable. Web based interventions offer patients access to information and counseling on demand. Relatively new and gaining in popularity, wearables offer patients immediate access to vital signs, biometric data, and various other physiologic and social parameters. However popular they may be their efficacy is unproven and remains to be seen. Integrating technological advances and medical care will provide better treatments for obesity in the future.

Keywords Technology • Obesity • Wearables • Sedentary behavior • Behavior modification

12.1 Introduction

Obesity is a growing problem in The United States and around the globe. Two thirds of Americans are overweight with 35% of these being obese. Worldwide in 2014, 39% of adults aged 18 years or older were overweight and 13% were obese. This amounts to more than 1.9 billion adults worldwide who are overweight (World Health Organization 2016). Of these over 600 million adults were obese (Ogden et al. 2014). These numbers are expected to continue to swell into the future (Kelly et al. 2008).

M. Cooper, M.D. • J. Morton, M.D. (✉)
Stanford University School of Medicine, 291 Campus Drive, Stanford, CA 94305, USA
e-mail: morton@stanford.edu

© Springer International Publishing AG 2018   169
H. Rivas, K. Wac (eds.), *Digital Health*, Health Informatics,
https://doi.org/10.1007/978-3-319-61446-5_12

Obesity is a major area of concern for global health. A well established relationship exists between excess weight and comorbid conditions such as diabetes, increased cancer risk, heart disease, stroke, osteoarthritis, sleep apnea, liver, and pulmonary disease. With such a large portion of the world population being overweight these comorbidities pose a significant stress on health care systems in both developed and developing nations. In the United States, obesity is responsible for approximately 21% of all medical spending (Cawley and Meyerhoefer 2012). Worldwide the economic costs of obesity are estimated at 0.7–2.8% of all health care expenditures (Withrow and Alter 2011).

The dramatic rise in the incidence of obesity worldwide stems from the complex interplay of a variety of factors including genetic, physiologic, environmental, psychological, social, economic, and political. In large part, the recent weight gain of the population can be attributed to behavioral, lifestyle and diet changes made possible through new technology.

The progression of technology and the rise of obesity are linked together. Technological advances in society can be attributed as one of the chief causes of the obesity epidemic around the world. Conversely the future is bright with new and emerging technologies that offer a myriad ways to prevent obesity, enhance care of the obese patient, and manage the disease of obesity.

12.2   Technology as a Cause of Obesity

Although obesity has both genetic and environmental causes, the doubling of the number of obese persons in the United States since 1980 suggests that environmental changes are the likely culprit. Obesity is generally causes by an excess amount of energy consumed (dietary intake) compared to energy expenditure (energy spent via metabolic and physical activity). Technology has affected both the way we consume food as well as the effort required for energy expenditure. Our current "obesogenic" environment facilitates the propagation of obesity by providing virtually unlimited access to inexpensive, energy-dense food, while decreasing the need for prolonged periods of physical activity.

12.2.1   Dietary Modifications

The prevalence of obesity in society today has been greatly facilitated by the unhampered access to inexpensive, energy dense food. This abundance of caloric intake coupled with the decreased need for prolonged periods of physical activity has contributed significantly to the current obesity epidemic.

Over the past 40 years we have seen significant drop in the price of food around the world. This is partially due to expanded industrialisation and automation of food production. However, it just isn't the increased volume of food that has led to an increase in obesity but the type and quality of food produced. It is the cost of energy dense foods high in fat, sugar, and salt has fallen most, while the cost that of healthier options has actually increased in relative terms. This may partly explain why obesity is more common in those on lower incomes (Foresight 2007; Marmot 2005).

Marketers and food production have joined forces to aggressively promote calorie dense, nutrient poor food to all members of society. Consumers are bombarded with a barrage of advertisements via billboards, magazines, television, radio, internet, and cell phones.

(Harris et al. 2009). Robinson found that as little as 30 s of exposure to televised food commercials influenced the food preferences of pre-school aged children (Borzekowski and Robinson 2001).

The average child in the United States for instance, views 15 television food advertisements every day, or nearly 5500 messages per year (Fed Trade Comm (US) 2007). This number will surely continue to rise as advertising permeates more facets of everyday life via advances in technological devices. Focused and personalized advertising is already mainstream and employed by a large number of companies to hone in on customers preferences and desires. Due to social media and vast digital databases, advertisers are able to gather and analyze details about customers demographic and habits to create advertisements that more personalized and effective than in the past.

In the past three decades childhood obesity has more than tripled in the United States. Children are becoming more obese and at younger ages than at any time in history. It is well documented that childhood obesity leads to adult obesity (CDC 2007). According to the AAP children are spending on average 7 h a day on entertainment media including televisions, cell phones, tablets, computers, and other electronic devices (https://www.aap.org/en-us/advocacy-and-policy/aap-health-initiatives/Pages/Media-and-Children.asp).

A recent trial discovered that in young children at or above the 75% BMI that lowering the amount of television watched significantly reduced BMI for young children at or above the 75th BMI percentile. The BMI reductions were due to reduced energy intake and not changes in physical activity (Epstein et al. 2008).

Another technological development that coincides with the start of the rise in obesity in America was the popularization of High Fructose Corn Syrup (HFCS) in the 1970's and 1980's. A systematic review by Malik et al. looking at the correlation between in weight gain in children and consumption of sugar-sweetened beverages. Most, but not all, of the studies, showed a strong positive association between these two factors (Malik et al. 2006). The abundance of corn available due to the automation of corn harvesting and advances in farming technology has led to a surplus of corn. Faced with this surplus farmers and food companies developed new ways to use their crops and one of the results was high fructose corn syrup. In recent years HFCS has found its way into almost every imaginable foodstuff sold in the united states from soft drinks to bread to innumerable processed ready to eat foods.

In addition to helping disseminate less healthy food, technology has made it much easier to obtain food with less and less effort. Starting with vending machines and pizza delivery in the 1980's, the amount of effort and work required to obtain food has dwindled to almost nothing. With the progression of the internet and smartphones, a simple touch of the screen can signal Amazon Prime can deliver a week's worth of groceries in less than an hour. Food delivery companies deliver complete ready to eat meals to your front door. Currently food delivery is still carried out by humans but soon with self driving cars being developed by Google and Uber these deliveries may soon become fully automated. Some companies are even looking a food delivery by drone thus increasing the range and terrain available for delivery.

12.2.2   Sedentary Lifestyle

After increased caloric intake, decreased energy expenditure is the other half of the rise of obesity. For much of history man was required by his circumstances to participate in rigorous physical activity to obtain food and perform work. Time spent performing physical activity has decreased and time spent being sedentary has increased. This began to change after the industrial revolution and continues to evolve today. This change can be attributed to changes in transportation with the global use of automobiles. The move from an agrarian society to an urban one particularly with the increase of time spent sitting at a desk. Finally, leisure activities have become less active due to developments in technology (television, computers, internet, video games etc).

The rise in sedentary behavior (SB) is a large contributor to obesity. Sedentary behavior is defined as as any waking behavior performed while in a sitting or reclining posture that requires very low energy expenditure (Sedentary Behaviour Research Network 2012). Examples of SB are sitting at a desk, driving a car, or watching television). The sedentary lifestyle prevalent in the modern society contributes significantly to the ever increasing prevalence of obesity (Robinson 1999; Levine et al. 2000). It has also been found to be an independent risk factor for cardiovascular-related and all cause mortality that cannot be repaired by an increase in exercise (Wijndaele et al. 2011; Grontved and Hu 2011). Obese patients spend a higher portion on their daily time, nearly 80%, in SB compared to only 57–69% in the general population (Bond et al. 2011; Healy et al. 2008). A review of leisure time activity levels over the past 50 years reveal no decrease in the amount of time set aside solely for exercise (Brownson et al. 2005). Thus the most significant change affecting the decrease in energy expenditure has been the use of technology to decrease the physical labor involved in daily tasks.

For children time spent watching television has had a large effect on obesity. One quarter of US children watch greater than 4 h of television daily and two thirds watch at least 2 h. Studies have suggested that time spent sitting watching television correlated with BMI than the amount of time spent in vigorous activity. As with adults, sedentary behaviors like watching television are associated with decreased caloric expenditure in children as well. As stated earlier children are very suscepti-ble to targeted advertising as well and this likely may encourage excessive caloric intake by snacking while watching television (Andersen et al. 1998).

12.3   Technology as a Solution for Obesity

Comprehensive lifestyle modification programs using behavior based weight loss interventions are well studied in the treatment of obesity. These therapies reinforce health changes in diet and activity and have traditionally been delivered via face to face encounters, group sessions or commercial weight loss programs. Pen and paper self monitoring of diet and activities are integrated with the behavioral based coach-ing (Jensen Michael et al. 2013; Leblanc et al. 2011). These human based therapy sessions are typically used as first line therapy for obese patients because of a long track record of safety and efficacy at helping patients achieve and maintain weight loss. These programs however are often difficult to utilize due to the time and man-power requirements needed to run the programs, lack of referrals from healthcare providers, financial burden to patients, non-coverage by insurance companies, fixed schedule meetings confliction with patients schedules, and patient embarrassment. Technology offers unique solutions to many if not all of these problems. Web based delivery of these programs, mobile health, wearables and even video games are available to help deliver proven behavioral health interventions to obese patients.

12.4   Web Based Intervention

A recent meta analysis (Wieland et al. 2012) reviewed 14 weight loss trials and 4 weight maintenance trials with 4140 participants total. The vast majority of the subjects were female (82%) with and average BMI of 32 and an average age of 46. When compared to control (i.e. minimal intervention) web based weight loss pro-grams led to greater weight loss. However when compared to face to face interven-tions, the web based intervention had significantly less weight loss. Other meta analyses have shown similar results.

One of the criticisms of web based programs is high attrition rates. Without the face to face accountability, patients may be less likely to complete the program. One study looked at a web based intervention in primary care (Cawley and Meyerhoefer 2012). The patients were incentivized in order to abrogate the usually high attrition rate associated with web based intervention. 101 obese patients with hypertension participated in the 12 week randomized control trial. Patients were randomized to either a web-based interactive weight loss approach or usual care where providers managed interventions the help patients lose weight. The study results showed a mean weight of -2.28 ± 3.21 kg (body weight of $-2.6\% \pm 3.3\%$) in the intervention group compared to a mean weight gain of 0.28 ± 1.87 kg (body weight

0.39% ± 2.16%) in the usual care group. Higher number of patient log ins was asso-ciated with the highest amount of weight loss.

12.5 Wearable Technology

Medical practitioners have been using the most up to date electronic devices avail-able to better diagnose, treat, and care for patients. Wearable technology has taken much of the same equipment used for years by medical practitioner and put it in the hands of patients. Today wearables mostly collect patient information and some-times analyze this information to help motivate and inform patients.

As technology moves ahead wearables are expanding the scope of their ability. For the obese patients wearables are an enticing concept to help patients lose weight. Today's wearables are a far cry from the basic pedometers and heart rate monitors of the past. Now they can measure multiple vital signs, activities, sounds, pictures, locations and synthesize and analyze the data in real time. Smart watches can track activity, heart rate, pulse oximetry, and sleep wake cycles. Aside from smart watches there are many other cutting edge devices being developed. An oximeter built into a ring can measure heart rate. Electromyographic sensors embedded into clothing can measure muscle activity. Headbands with non-gelled electroencephalogram elec-trodes can monitor levels of mental attention. Wristbands imbedded with an electro-dermal sensor can measure stress levels. Accelerometers in smartwatches and fitness bands can measure physical activity and sleep wake cycles. Proximity sensors which inform patients of levels of social interaction to promote feelings of well being (Piwek et al. 2016). All these different sensors, meters, and devices are getting smaller and smaller and can be incorporated into usual clothing or accessories. Advances in battery life allow these devices to be worn continuously 24 h a day. Information from these sensors is available in real time to provide patients with immediate, customized goal oriented feedback. Wearable devices are extremely popular with adolescents and children who are increasingly susceptible to obesity and its sequelae.

Wearables have exploded in popularity over the past few years. 15% of American consumers currently use some type of wearable technology such as a smartwatch or fitness band. This number is expected to 110 million by the year 2018 (Juniper Research 2013). Wearables are a promising technological device that may be useful to help analyze and treat obesity. Unfortunately there is very little sound data on wearables and their efficacy as a weight loss tool. The rapid development, constant model updates, evolving features, and inter device compatibility issues have ham-pered any thorough long term studies from being performed. In addition, patients may see wearables as a cure all and then stop using them when they do not see results. A recent survey showed that 32% of users stopped wearing their device after just 6 months and half had stopped wearing at 1 year (Ledger et al. 2014).

Jakicic et al. recently published one of the first studies to evaluate the effect of wearable technology on weight loss with substantial follow up (Jakicic et al. 2016).

They took 471 adult participants aged 18–35 with a BMI between 25 and 40 and randomized them to a standard behavioral weight loss intervention versus a technology enhanced weight loss intervention in a randomized clinical trial. Primary outcome was weight loss at 24 months with additional outcomes of body composition, fitness, physical activity and dietary intake. Patients in the technology arm were provided with and encouraged to use a FIT core arm band with a web interface which provided information on physical activity and could also be used to track dietary input. 74.5% of patients completed the study. After 24 months weight change differed significantly between the groups with the technology aided group losing less weight (difference, 2.4 kg '95% CI 1.0–3.7]; $P = 0.002$) Although both groups had significant improvements in body composition, fitness, physical activity and diet there were no significant differences between the groups. This is one of the largest studies to evaluate the effectiveness of wearable devices in the augmentation of weight loss. This study did not find that the addition of wearables improved weight loss any more than standard behavioral therapy. Limitations were that the study was restricted to young adults. The device was worn on the upper arm rather than the wrist which may have affected its ability to accurately collect data. Though this study did not find an appreciable difference in weight loss when a wearable was added to the mix additional research with possibly different more advanced or accurate devices in a more diverse demographic group would provide more definitive information.

Other possible reasons for the lack of efficacy of wearables is they primarily track activity or exercise. An individual must burn 3500 calories in order to lose a single pound of fat. Diet is a more important factor in getting patients to lose weight than exercise. It is also possible that the detailed information on patients activity levels gives them a false sense that they have accomplished their workout goal for the day and can therefore indulge in less healthy eating habits. This concept of moral licensing (see paragraph below) is well described and is very applicable in this situation. Whether or not wearables are just a passing fad to be forgotten in the next couple of years or the next health revolution promised by manufacturers remains to be seen.

12.6 Moral Licensing

Also known as self-licensing is a term used in social science to describe the subconscious tendency of individuals to indulge in something after doing something positive first (Merritt et al. 2010). In short, when we do something good for our health such as exercising we have a subconscious tendency to do something unhealthy because we feel justified by our exercise. This phenomenon has been well described in politics, consumer purchases, political opinions, charitable giving, hiring practices, energy policy and home energy use, race relations, health-related decision-making, risky sexual behavior, alcohol consumption, and even dietary supplement use (Khan and Dhar 2006).

12.7 Video Games

The problem of childhood obesity was discussed earlier. Currently only 29% of high school seniors are reaching prescribed goals for physical fitness and activity (CDC 2012). Many modern video games are equipped with sensors and controllers that allow patients to play by moving their bodies or even exercising.

Pokemon Go is a augmented reality based mobile phone game in which players advance in the game by walking or exercising. Its immense popularity, over 65 million downloads in its first week of availability has raised questions about its benefit for obese patients (Serino et al. 2016). A game such as this is primarily directed towards children and adolescents who are at high risk of being overweight or obese. Though no clinical data exists on whether or not playing Pokemon Go can actually lead to weight loss, its popularity alone and its unique gameplay involving physical activity raises good questions about this viability of these sorts of future interventions for obese patients.

12.8 Future

Technology offers many attractive new methods to help patients lose weight as well as augmentation of tried and true weight loss methods. Though many of the early studies show mixed results for web based, mobile and wearable interventions it is possible that there may be synergy between them when used together. We are on the forefront of this current wave of technology. As patients become more familiar with these new technologies and they become better integrated with the healthcare system we will likely see better results in the future.

12.9 Summary

Technology is both a cause and a solution to the obesity epidemic. Technology driven changes in food production, advertising, makeup and delivery have all contributed to the increased prevalence of obesity. On the other hand technology offers many unique solutions to the problem of obesity and other chronic diseases. Though the use of technology to treat obesity is still in its infancy it shows great promise.

12.10 Conclusion

Obesity is clearly a twenty-first century problem that will require twenty-first century solutions. It is clear that a side effect of many of the technologies that improve and streamline our lives have had the unfortunate side effect of increasing the prevalence of obesity. As technology and medicine work together new developments and devices will be discovered to treat and manage obesity and likely other chronic diseases.

References

Andersen RE, Crespo CJ, Barlett SJ, et al. Relationship of physical activity and television watching with body weight and level of fatness among children. J Am Med Assoc. 1998;279(12):938–42.

Bond DS, Unick JL, Jakicic JM, et al. Objective assessment of time spent being sedentary in bariatric surgery candidates. Obes Surg. 2011;21:811–4.

Borzekowski DL, Robinson TN. The 30-second effect: an experiment revealing the impact of television commercials on food preferences of preschoolers. J Am Diet Assoc. 2001;101:42–6.

Brownson RC, Boehmer TK, Luke DA. Declining rates of physical activity in the United States: what are the contributors? Annu Rev Public Health. 2005;26:421–43.

Cawley J, Meyerhoefer C. The medical care costs of obesity: an instrumental variables approach. J Health Econ. 2012;31:219–30.

CDC. Youth risk behavior surveillance—United States, 2011. MMWR. 2012;61(SS-4).

Cent. Dis. Control, Natl. Cent. Health Stat. 2007. Prevalence of overweight among children and adolescents: United States, 2003–2004. http://www.cdc.gov.

Epstein LH, Roemmich JN, Robinson JL, Paluch RA, Winiewicz DD, et al. A randomized trial of the effects of reducing television viewing and computer use on body mass index in young children. Arch Pediatr Adolesc Med. 2008;162:239–45.

Fed Trade Comm (US). 2007. Children's exposure to TV advertising in 1977 and 2004. Bur Econ Staff Rep.

Foresight. Tackling obesities: future choices—project report. 2007. www.foresight.gov.uk/OurWork/ActiveProjects/Obesity/KeyInfo/Index.asp.

Grontved A, Hu FB. Television viewing and risk of type 2 diabetes, cardiovascular disease, and all-cause mortality: a meta analysis. JAMA. 2011;305:2448–55.

Harris JL, Pomeranz JL, Lobstein T, Brownell KD. A crisis in the marketplace: how food marketing contributes to childhood obesity and what can be done. Annu Rev Public Health. 2009;30:211–25.

Healy GN, Wijndaele K, Dunstan DW, et al. Objectively measured sedentary time, physical activity and metabolic risk: the Australian diabetes, obesity and lifestyle study (AusDiab). Diabetes Care. 2008;31:369–71.

https://www.aap.org/en-us/advocacy-and-policy/aap-health-initiatives/Pages/Media-and-Children.asp.

Jakicic JM, Davis KK, Rogers RJ, King WC, Marcus MD, Helsel D, Rickman AD, Wahed AS, Belle SH. Effect of wearable technology combined with a lifestyle intervention on long-term weight loss: the IDEA randomized clinical trial. JAMA. 2016;316(11):1161–71. doi:10.1001/jama.2016.12858.

Jensen Michael D, Ryan Donna H, Apovian Caroline M, Ard Jamy D, Comuzzie Anthony G, Donato Karen A, Hu Frank B, Hubbard Van S, Jakicic John M, Kushner Robert F, Loria Catherine M, Millen Barbara E, Nonas Cathy A, Pi-Sunyer F Xavier, Stevens June, Stevens Victor J, Wadden Thomas A, Wolfe Bruce M, Yanovski Susan Z. AHA/ACC/TOS guideline for the management of overweight and obesity in adults: a report of the American College of Cardiology/American Heart Association Task Force on Practice Guidelines and The Obesity Society. Circulation. 2013;135.

Juniper Research. 2013. Smart wearable devices. Fitness, healthcare, entertainment & enterprise 2013–2018.

Kelly T, Yang W, Chen C, Reynolds K, He J. Global burden of obesity in 2005 and projections to 2030. Int J Obes. 2008;32:1431–7. doi:10.1038/ijo.2008.102.

Khan U, Dhar R. Licensing effect in consumer choice. J Mark Res. 2006;43(2):259–66.

Leblanc E, O'Connor E, Whitlock E, Patnode CD, Kapka T. Effectiveness of primary care-relevant treatments for obesity in adults: a systematic evidence review for the U.S. Preventive Services Task Force. Ann Intern Med. 2011;155(7):434–47.

Ledger D, Partners E, Scientist B, Manager P. Inside wearables. How the science of human behavior change. Endevour Partners. 2014.

Levine JA, Schleusner SJ, Jensen MD. Energy expenditure of nonexercise activity. Am J Clin Nutr. 2000;72:1451.

Malik VS, Schulze MB, Hu FB. Intake of sugar-sweetened beverages and weight gain: a systematic review. Am J Clin Nutr. 2006;84(2):274–88.

Marmot M. Social determinants of health inequalities. Lancet. 2005;365:1099–104.

Merritt AC, Effron DA, Monin B. Moral self-licensing: when being good frees us to be bad. Soc Personal Psychol Compass. 2010;4(5):344–57.

Ogden CL, Carrol MD, Kit BK, Flegal KM. Prevalence of childhood and adult obesity in the United States, 2011-2012. JAMA. 2014;31:806–14.

Piwek L, Ellis DA, Andrews S, Joinson A. The rise of consumer health wearables: promises and barriers. PLoS Med. 2016;13(2):e1001953.

Robinson TN. Reducing children's television viewing to prevent obesity: a randomized controlled trial. JAMA. 1999;282:1561.

Sedentary Behaviour Research Network. Letter to the editor: standardized use of the terms "sedentary" and "sedentary behaviours". Appl Physiol Nutr Metab. 2012;37(3):540–2.

Serino M, Cordrey K, McLaughlin L, Milanaik RL. Pokémon go and augmented virtual reality games: a cautionary commentary for parents and pediatricians. Curr Opin Pediatr. 2016;28(5):673–7. PubMed

Wieland L, Falzon L, Sciamanna C, Trudeau K, Brodney F, Davidson K. Interactive computer-based interventions for weight loss or weight maintenance in overweight or obese people (Review). Cochrane Database Sys Rev. 2012;15:8.

Wijndaele K, Brage S, Besson H, et al. Television viewing time independently predicts all-cause and cardiovascular mortality: the EPIC Norfolk study. Int J Epidemiol. 2011;40:150–9.

Withrow D, Alter DA. The economic burden of obesity worldwide: a systematic review of the direct costs of obesity. Obes Rev. 2011;12:131–41. doi:10.1111/j.1467-789X.2009.00712.x.

World Health Organization. 2016. Fact Sheet No 311 [2016–06–21]. Obesity and overweight.

Chapter 13
Engaging a Digital Health Behavior Audience: A Case Study

David Bychkov and Sean D. Young

Abstract The majority of public health challenges, including infectious diseases like HIV as well as drug addiction, can be prevented through behavioral modification. New technologies may help to address these challenges and improve behavior change interventions. Much of the research in this area has been corporate-sponsored (i.e., external to the field of public health). For example, advertisers have shown tremendous progress in persuading consumers to act upon triggers embedded within technology platforms, specifically smartphone apps and websites. Consumer market research firms have studied and advocated for a variety of tactics to help their clients convert ad viewers into product buyers. When consumer behavior fails to meet market research expectations, advertisers are quick to adapt their own approaches and messages. Indeed, corporations have been armed with significant investment capital and profits to fuel this body of research for the past 50 years. Public health researchers and organizations, on the other hand, have fewer resources and therefore need to focus on research and behavior change "best practices" that are highly cost-effective and scalable. In this chapter, we explore two potential methods of using social media sites to engage people and seek to use data from an academic Twitter handle to study whether they can be successfully applied to engage an audience in public health research. The two methods used are: (1) combining Twitter text with pictures to garner more engagement, and (2) inclusion of hashtags with text that is relevant and timely.

Keywords Social media • Twitter • Persuasion • Public health • Consumerism • Behavioral modification

D. Bychkov, Ph.D. (✉)
InHealth, Johns Hopkins University, Baltimore, MD 21218, USA

S.D. Young, Ph.D., M.S. (✉)
Department of Family Medicine, Center for Digital Behavior, University of California
Institute for Prediction Technology, University of California, Los Angeles,
10880 Wilshire Blvd., Ste. 1800, Los Angeles, CA 90024, USA
e-mail: sdyoung@mednet.ucla.edu

© Springer International Publishing AG 2018
H. Rivas, K. Wac (eds.), *Digital Health*, Health Informatics,
https://doi.org/10.1007/978-3-319-61446-5_13

179

13.1   Persuasion Technology and Behavioral Change in Digital Health

13.1.1   Introduction: How Do Advertisers Impact Health Behavior?

The United States has made tremendous advancements in medical research and spends billions of dollars each year on public health communications, and yet massive challenges remain (World Health Organization 2002). According to the U.S. Centers for Disease Control and Prevention (CDC), America's top public health dangers are alcohol-related harm, food safety, healthcare-associated infections, heart disease and stroke, HIV infection, motor vehicle injury, nutrition, physical activity and obesity, prescription drug overdose, teen pregnancy, and tobacco use (CDC 2016). On a global basis, health behaviors related to each of these issues affect hundreds of millions of people and are projected to cost trillions of dollars in treatments for chronic disease, addiction treatment, counseling, incarceration, and lost productivity (Anderko et al. 2012; WHO 2016). In response, government agencies have launched prevention campaigns, used advertising to increase awareness, and developed new technologies to modify behavior.

Some of these high risk, unhealthy, or addictive behaviors were cultivated by technology users. Television advertising, for example, has been singled out for its role in convincing minors to eat junk food, consume sugary drinks, drink alcohol, and smoke cigarettes (Strasburger et al. 2009). The massive expansion of personal computer, television, and video game sales has been implicated as a factor in the explosive growth of obesity in America (French et al. 2001). Corporations are clearly successful at using advertising technology platforms to persuade the public to make poor health decisions. Unlike public health researchers, corporations are able to devote significant resources and manpower to collecting data on which tools and platforms are most likely to persuade audiences to try their products.

Social media websites gather a large amount of user information, which allows them to target audiences in a variety of ways. For example, Twitter has proven to be an especially effective tool for persuading people to visit e-cigarette websites (Grana et al. 2014; Huang et al. 2014). Unlike Facebook or other social media platforms, Twitter does little to prevent minors from gaining access to e-cigarette marketing messages (Advertising Policies 2016). At the same time, advertisers gain rich insight from their audiences, including which tweets gained the most views ("impressions"), which tweets convinced people to look at their profile ("profile clicks"), which tweets were able to persuade viewers to click on embedded websites ("URL clicks"), and how many were able to get them to maximize their view of the tweet itself ("detail expands") (Twitter Help Center 2016).

According to one study by Twitter, these engagement metrics are directly linked to the presence within each tweet of photographs, hashtags, links, videos, and/or statistics (Twitter Blogs 2016). Hashtags combined with plain text provide a 16% boost, while graphics can increase engagement by 28–35%. Although Twitter states that their best practices are derived from analyzing millions of tweets related to the fields of television, music, politics, and sports, there are little peer-reviewed data to confirm such results can be achieved by public health researchers. Thanks to Twitter's open access tools, we were able to develop an academic social media account (@SeanYoungPhD) to promote behavior change awareness and test both hashtags and graphics with text. We therefore sought to look back at the analytics of this account and, based on results, create initial hypotheses for best practices that public health researchers can use for applying social media to get people interested in public health research.

13.2 Method: Deploying Tweets from a Public Health Researcher Account

From April 11, 2016, to July 18, 2016, we published 272 tweets from an academic healthcare researcher's Twitter account (@SeanYoungPhD), of which 44 contained graphics. The profile featured website links for the UCLA Center for Digital Behavior (digitalbehavior.ucla.edu; blackboxphd.com) and the University of California Institute for Prediction Technology (predictiontechnology.ucla.edu), as did the tweets. Tweets that included graphics featured stylized versions of the text (Fig. 13.1); not all of the tweets that included graphics featured photographs or citation of the text portion of the tweet. We also created tweets with graphics where the

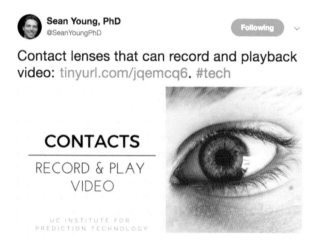

Fig. 13.1 @SeanYoungPhD tweet at 1:51 P.M. on May 2, 2016. The tweet features text, a URL, a hashtag, a photo, and stylized version of the text

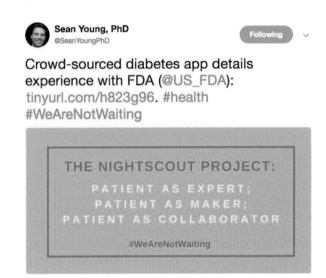

Fig. 13.2 @SeanYoungPhD tweet from 6:25 A.M. on April 26, 2016. The tweet features text, a mention of the U.S. Food and Drug Administration's Twitter handle, a URL, two hashtags, and a graphic of stylized text that refers to the second hashtag

image featured stylized text referring to the content implied by the link we were promoting (Fig. 13.2).

All of the tweets featured several key elements intended to make a positive first impression with audiences and encourage them to click. Profile "approachability" plays a role in user engagement with tweets (Vernon et al. 2014), thus the @SeanYoungPhD account features a close-up photograph, as opposed to a medium or long shot. We refrained from using scientific terminology, institutional verbiage, or acronyms that would require prior knowledge of public health issues to comprehend the messages. In order to maximize response to our campaign, we decided to produce content that was consistent with the keywords most frequently mentioned in the user profiles of @SeanYoungPhD's existing followers. According to Moz.com's free FollowerWonk tool, the keywords most associated with @SeanYoungPhD's followers' profiles as of April 11, 2016, included: "health," "love," and "social" (Fig. 13.3).

We also deployed tweets without graphics in order to determine whether and when it would be best to use images compared to text alone. Tweets without images featured content and hashtags, so that the public could easily find more information on a trending topic. During the study, we released at least one tweet between Monday to Friday between 6:00 A.M. to 9:00 A.M.; 11:00 A.M. to 1:00 P.M.; and 3:00 P.M. to 6:00 P.M. Eastern Standard Time. According to Moz.com's

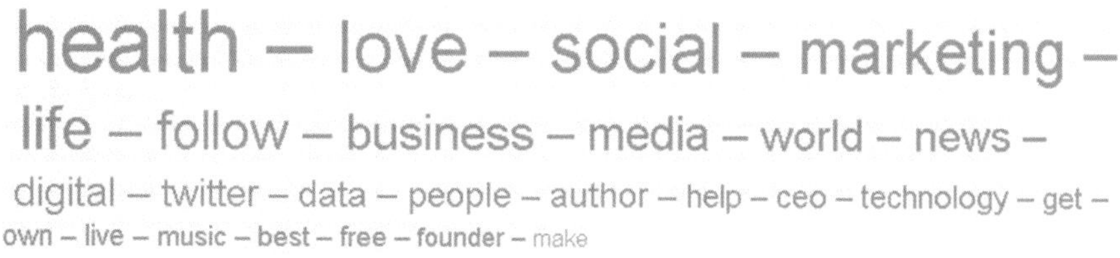

health – love – social – marketing –
life – follow – business – media – world – news –
digital – twitter – data – people – author – help – ceo – technology – get –
own – live – music – best – free – founder – make

Fig. 13.3 Moz.com FollowerWonk word cloud of the most common keywords associated with @ SeanYoungPhD's followers (April 11, 2016)

FollowerWonk tool, these were the hours of the day when @SeanYoungPhD's followers were most active on Twitter.

13.3 Results: Engagement with an Academic Twitter Account

Between April 11, 2016, and July 18, 2016, there were 3449 total engagements with @SeanYoungPhD. The account's 272 tweets earned a total of 874,201 impressions. Tweets with graphics ($n = 44$) earned 180,395 impressions, which resulted in a mean of 4099 impressions per tweet. Tweets without graphics ($n = 228$) earned 693,806 impressions and, therefore, a mean of 3043 impressions per tweet. Tweets with graphics received a total of 23 profile clicks (a mean of 0.52 profile clicks per tweet) while plain text tweets received 113 profile clicks (a mean of 0.50 profile clicks per tweet). The 44 tweets that contained graphics and embedded URLs garnered a total of 81 URL clicks. This resulted in a mean of 1.84 URL clicks per tweet, while the other 230 tweets with plain text and URLs received 179 URL clicks, which results in a mean average of 0.79 URL clicks per tweet. Tweets with graphics received a total of 79 detail expands (an average of 1.80 detail expands per tweet), while plain text tweets received a total of 126 detail expands (an average of 0.55 detail expands per tweet) (Table 13.1).

Tweets were also analyzed by rank. Accordingly, there were three tweets that achieved the highest rankings in different areas related to persuasion. For example, a tweet that discussed contact lenses and featured an image tied for number in detail expands and ranked number one in URL clicks. Another tweet with a graphic related to diabetes ranked a distant second place in URL clicks but achieved nearly the same number of impressions as the contact lens tweet. A third tweet, related to the Boelter Hall campus shooting at UCLA on June 1, 2016, featured no graphics but ranked first in terms of detail expands, impressions, and profile views (Table 13.2).

Table 13.1 @SeanYoungPhD tweets with and without graphics (April 11, 2016–July 18, 2016)

@SeanYoungPhD	Impressions	Mean impressions	Profile clicks	Mean profile clicks	URL clicks	Mean URL clicks	Detail expands	Mean detail expands
272 total tweets	874,201	3213.97	136	0.49	260	0.93	205	0.73
44 tweets (with graphics)	180,395	4099	23	0.52	81	1.84	79	1.80
228 tweets (without graphics)	693,806	3043	113	0.50	179	0.79	126	0.55

Table 13.2 @SeanYoungPhD's most persuasive tweets (April 11, 2016–July 18, 2016)

Tweet	Graphics	Impressions	Impression rank	Profile views	Profile views rank	Detail expands	Detail expands rank	URL clicks	URL click rank
Contact lenses that can record and playback video: https://t.Co/6QiTzlwezw. #tech https://t.Co/M26ch63xx1.	Yes	5473	16th	7	2nd	55	1st	22	1st
Crowd-sourced diabetes app details experience with FDA (@US_FDA): https://t.Co/W7TSfegLYS. #health #WeAreNotWaiting https://t.Co/OCPPdBWlg9	Yes	5515	14th	0	N/A	0	N/A	9	2nd
Our #ucla lab is safe. We have students and researchers in bolter where the shooter was	None	6623	2nd	55	1st	55	1st	0	N/A

13.4 Discussion: Moving from Getting Attention to Behavior Modification in Digital Health

Our results uncovered two techniques that public health researchers can use to persuade audiences to engage with their messages on Twitter: usage of graphics, and hashtags along with timely relevant content. Appending graphics to tweets is likely to increase the overall quantity of clicks, impressions, and profile views earned by academic tweets during a social media campaign. This is consistent with the history of visual communication research, which has proven that messages with color, dynamic form, depth, and movement elicit stronger emotional responses, are more likely to be remembered later, and command more attention than static, plain-text message (Lester 2013). Market research studies show that consumer choices are driven by product colors (Grossman and Wisenblit 1999). Neurobiological studies confirms that stimuli with dynamic elements are pleasing and stimuli that are static may be agitating (Zeki 1992).

Communicating to Twitter users, however, is not the same as persuading. During our study, we had to create original messages that would generate interest for @SeanYoungPhD's followers. Although the fact that the top keyword associated with @SeanYoungPhD's user profiles ("health") demonstrated interest in our research and mission, we decided to ensure that the images and text posted to the account reflected the wider range of words as well. For example, we posted health tips like how to increase exercise motivation. We also created tweets that featured news on scientific breakthroughs, such as "A better way to predict #diabetes: https://t.co/dgGAHCGDYY." Tailoring tweets to user profiles is consistent with persuasion theory, whereby messages are employed to convince audiences to adopt a point of view or buy a new product (Lester 2013).

The challenge with tailored health communications is to create the most persuasive content and deliver it at the optimal moment for behavior change (Rimer and Kreuter 2006). Twitter's main mechanism for sorting and distributing tweets is the hashtag. This allows users to view what topics are trending on Twitter based on how many people append their tweets with a particular hashtag. Users can also perform advanced searches by using hashtag queries. For this reason, we decided that our hashtags would in some cases be based on the Moz.com FollowerWonk word cloud. For example, we used the word "health" 55 times and "business" 7 times as hashtags among our tweets. In other cases, hashtags were based on the content itself.

Two of our most persuasive tweets contained graphics. The tweet discussing contact lenses showed an eye with stylized text (Fig. 13.1) and the tweet discussing diabetes featured a simple graphic with stylized text (Fig. 13.2). While both of these tweets earned a nearly identical number of impressions, the contact lens tweet earned more than double the number of URL clicks. In addition, the contact lens tweet earned 55 detail expands whereas the diabetes tweet earned none (Table 13.2). Users clicked on the tweet for several possible reasons: (1) to see the photograph contained in the graphic more clearly, (2) to more easily read the stylized text contained in the graphic, or (3) to see publicly available engagement data. All of these types of inspection by an end user meant that we had persuaded the user to commit time and attention to our message at little to no cost.

One of our most persuasive tweets took place during a campus shooting at UCLA. The tweet was a plain text message with one hashtag ("Our #UCLA lab is safe. We have students and researchers in Bolter where the shooter was"). This tweet earned the highest number of profile views. While other tweets persuaded users to click on external URLs, this message compelled our audience to want to learn more about our point of view and mission. The Boelter Hall-related tweet demonstrates the potential of proper hashtag selection and tweet timing to earn engagement. As the @SeanYoungPhD profile is followed by other UCLA Twitter users, it is not surprising that this tweet generated the highest number of profile views. Finally, the text itself ("shooter") was directly relevant to its hashtag.

The effectiveness of graphics and hashtags for public health tweets presents a wide range of public health implications. Currently, influenza is tracked through Twitter. If this same platform can be better used for tailored health communications, social media campaigns can be developed at an extraordinarily low cost to promote disease prevention. At the same time, greater research is needed to understand how these same techniques can exacerbate public health obstacles (e.g., tweets with graphics or hashtags by celebrities in the anti-vaccination movement that deride flu shots may be more effective than text tweets released by government agencies during flu season).

Our study was limited by a lack of direct communication Twitter users who clicked URLs posted on @SeanYoungPhD, visited the profile, or viewed its tweets. Without the ability to interview users independently, it is impossible to gauge their genuine interest and understanding of the social psychology issues promoted by our Twitter account. In a future study, we would like to collect offline information from @SeanYoungPhD followers to compare against their online engagements with our messages. This study was also limited in that it did not use a formal design such as a randomized controlled trial; its primary function was as a pilot study to review marketing efforts intended to engage a public health audience and to explore ideas for future research about how to engage social media users in public health marketing. We hope that the exploratory nature of this study will provide new insights for researchers and healthcare organizations interested in using social media to engage the public in positive health behavior changes.

13.5 Conclusion

Public health organizations and researchers can use social media tools such as Twitter to deliver public health messages and engage followers. Well-timed posts that include graphics, hashtags, URLs, and timely information are the most likely factors to attract engagement. Persuading Twitter audiences to act on the information that is communicated to them requires usage of a variety of analytics tools, in addition to those free ones provided by the platform itself. The results we achieved during our four-month campaign were possible thanks to data that Moz.com provided on our followers, such as their user profile keywords and time spent on Twitter.

References

Advertising Policies [Internet]. [cited 2016 Aug 31.] Available from: https://www.facebook.com/policies/ads/.
Anderko L, Roffenbender JS, Goetzel RZ, Howard J, Millard F, Wildenhaus K, et al. Promoting prevention through the affordable care act: workplace wellness. Prev Chronic Dis [Internet]. 2012. [cited 2016 Aug 31];9. Available from: http://www.cdc.gov/pcd/issues/2012/12_0092.htm.
CDC Prevention Status Reports (PSR)—National Summary—STLT gateway [Internet]. [cited 2016 Aug 30]. https://www.cdc.gov/psr/national-summary.html.
French SA, Story M, Jeffery RW. Environmental influences on eating and physical activity. Annu Rev Public Health. 2001;22(1):309–35.
Grana R, Benowitz N, Glantz SA. E-Cigarettes. Circulation 2014;129(19):1972–1986.
Grossman RP, Wisenblit JZ. What we know about consumers' color choices. J Mark Pract Appl Mark Sci. 1999;5(3):78–88.
Huang J, Kornfield R, Szczypka G, Emery SL. A cross-sectional examination of marketing of electronic cigarettes on Twitter. Tob Control. 2014;23(suppl 3):iii26–30.
Lester PM. Visual communication: images with messages. In: Cengage learning; 2013. 484.
Rimer BK, Kreuter MW. Advancing tailored health communication: a persuasion and message effects perspective. J Commun. 2006;56:S184–201.
Strasburger VC, Wilson BJ, Jordan AB. Children, adolescents, and the media: SAGE; Thousand Oaks, CA. 2009. 641.
Tweet activity dashboard [Internet]. Twitter Help Center. [cited 2016 Aug 31]. https://support.twitter.com/articles/20171990.
Vernon RJW, Sutherland CAM, Young AW, Hartley T. Modeling first impressions from highly variable facial images. Proc Natl Acad Sci U S A. 2014;111(32):E3353–61.
What fuels a Tweet's engagement? [Internet]. Twitter Blogs. [cited 2016 Aug 30]. https://blog.twitter.com/2014/what-fuels-a-tweets-engagement.
WHO|Tobacco [Internet]. WHO. [cited 2016 Aug 30]. http://www.who.int/mediacentre/factsheets/fs339/en/.
World Health Organization. The world health report 2002: reducing risks, promoting healthy life. Geneva: World Health Organization; 2002. 278.
Zeki S. The visual image in mind and brain. Sci Am. 1992;267(3):69–76.

Chapter 14
How Digital Health Will Deliver Precision Medicine

Pishoy Gouda and Steve Steinhubl

Abstract Digital health can be briefly described as the intersect between smartphone-enabled mobile computational and connectivity capabilities, but also encompass genomics, information systems, wireless sensors, cloud computing and machine learning with modern healthcare. Globally, we are seeing an increase in the desire for patients to play an active role in their healthcare management. Combined, digital technology and patient engagement, advances the possibility of providing personalised medicine. This entails tailoring the medical experience to an individual patient, based on their genetics, molecular, physiologic and cellular analysis in addition to their socio-demographics and personal history. Advancements in this field have seen digital health being incorporated into a variety of aspects of healthcare: including diagnosis, management and follow-up of patients. However, many challenges still exist preventing their disseminated use, including security concerns as well a lack of evidence base demonstrating both clinical and cost effectiveness.

Keywords Digital health • Digital medicine • Personalised medicine • Genomics • Biotechnology

14.1 Scenario

You are seeing a 55-year-old male coming into your clinic with newly diagnosed atrial fibrillation requesting to be started on a DOAC (Direct oral anticoagulant). You go over the risks and benefit of the agents, stating an average bleeding risk of ~ 2% each year. In most patients, the prevention of ischemic stroke outweighs the risk of bleeding. Unfortunately, this is not always the case and occasionally a

P. Gouda, MB BCh BAO, MSc (✉)
Division of Internal Medicine, Foothills Medical Centre, University of Calgary,
Room 933, 1403 - 29 Street NW, North Tower, Calgary, Canada, AB T2N 2T9
e-mail: pishoy.gouda1@ucalgary.ca

S. Steinhubl, M.D.
Scripps Translational Science Institute, La Jolla, CA, USA

© Springer International Publishing AG 2018
H. Rivas, K. Wac (eds.), *Digital Health*, Health Informatics,
https://doi.org/10.1007/978-3-319-61446-5_14

patient unexpectedly experiences a major bleeding event when treated with a DOAC or never has a thromboembolic stroke despite not being treated with one. What if you had a tool that could predict which of your patients were essentially guaranteed to experience a major bleeding or a thromboembolic event? Would that change your clinical practice?

14.2   What Is Precision Medicine?

Precision medicine refers to the process of tailoring the medical experience to an individual patient, taking into account a combination of their genetics, molecular, physiologic and cellular analysis in addition to their socio-demographics and personal history. This is not only pertinent to deciding treatment options, but also has an important role in prevention, establishing diagnosis and predicting outcomes. With the rising costs of healthcare, funding mass population screening for diseases that most patients will never develop and prescribing costly medications that may have no clinical benefits for an individual patient is no longer feasible. Improving precision medicine offers a solution, where we can tailor a patient's therapy using their unique genomic and physiological characteristics.

14.3   What Is Digital Medicine?

Digital medicine is relatively new term first described in the early 2000's by Shaffer et al. (Shaffer et al. 2002). The term covers the large intersect between smartphone-enabled mobile computational and connectivity capabilities, but also encompass genomics, information systems, wireless sensors, cloud computing and machine learning (Topol et al. 2015; Topol 2010; Steinhubl et al. 2015). Together these technologies represent the future of medicine, where they can be incorporated into health management systems, using patient-generated data to inform clinical decisions.

14.4   How Digital Health Can Augment Precision Medicine?

With the FDA approving the very first set of mobile medical applications in 2015 (US Food and Drug Administration 2016) and with over 4.5 billion USD being pumped into the industry that year, it is becoming apparent that digital health will become part of clinical practice over the next decade. However, how digital health will permeate into the healthcare system remains to be seen. These technologies have the potential to enhance virtually every aspect of healthcare including: prevention, diagnosing, tailoring treatment, symptom monitoring and improving medication adherence. Below we have outlines these various components, highlighting the potential uses and evidence that already exist for digital health in each one.

14.4.1 Prevention

Chronic diseases undisputedly place the largest burden on the healthcare system worldwide, and is estimated to contribute to >40 million death per year (Strong et al. 2005). However, our current healthcare model is ill equipped to manage this epidemic of chronic disease, which places an emphasis on treating patients in the acute phase of their illness. Chronic diseases by definition are a longitudinal process that requires an equally "chronic" solution. Management of these conditions require frequent, personalised evaluations guided by repeated clinical data collection (Kvedar et al. 2016). Such interventions are time consuming for both patients and clinicians and as a result, place a significant financial burden on the healthcare system. Digital medicines may provide the key to decreasing the incidences of chronic disease and resultant complications.

One example of this is the battle against the diabetic epidemic; several companies have harnessed digital medicine to provide tailored treatments and education to individual patients. BlueStar is an FDA approved app that teaches individuals with diabetes about how their blood sugar varies during the day and optimal testing time, that was able to demonstrate a 1.2% in HbA1C compared to the standard of care (Quinn et al. 2011). Similarly, Prevent is an online lifestyle modification tool that provides education and collects data on patients that also demonstrated a reduction in HbA1C as well as BMI (Sepah et al. 2015). However, Prevent is currently not FDA approved and targets employers who seek to decrease the healthcare costs of their employees.

Hypertension is another area where digital medicine promises to make a substantial impact on the prevention of subsequent disease progression and complications. Using novel technology of photoplethysmography, sensors are able to measure blood pressures by detecting differences in light absorption (Steinhubl et al. 2016). This technology provides a much less obtrusive method of measuring blood pressure than the current standard inflating cuff. In the near future it is feasible to imagine that this technology will collect continuously without any effort or awareness from the patient. This data can be further fed into a treatment algorithm and either recommend treatment changes to the clinical team or even directly to the patient through a virtual consultation.

14.4.2 Diagnosing

In the past decade, the scientific community has made extraordinary advances in the world of genomics, identifying genetic pathways for more than 80 common disease (Topol 2010; Visscher and Montgomery 2009). While whole genome sequencing has demonstrated that it can provide clinically actionable information on the individual patient level (Pierce and Ahsan 2010; Lumley and Rice 2010), large scale studies have yet to demonstrate long term outcomes of such interventions on a large scale. As a result, while the field of genomics has made considerable its routine implementation for the diagnosis of disease should be met with caution (Manolio 2010).

While genomics will play a key role in precision diagnostics, digital medicine technologies can aid in the ease and timeliness of diagnosis for many acute illnesses. Digital medicine has the potential of vastly improving our ability to conduct point of care testing for a wide range of infection diseases, streamlining management in an exceedingly complex healthcare system (Pai et al. 2012). Cellscope is a mobile smartphone attachment that employs fibre optic illumination technology that may allow for home diagnosis of inner ear infections in children (Rappaport et al. 2015), one of the most common reasons for children presenting to a healthcare provider. Other promising venues for implementing digital medicine include: point of care tests for the diagnosis of urinary tract infections (Mach et al. 2011) and upper respiratory tract infections (Lai et al. 2002). In the future, these technologies will allow us to identify the genomic signature of specific pathogens and their antibiotic susceptibility.

Other demonstrable uses and future uses include the diagnosis of cardiac arrhythmias (Lowres et al. 2014), detection of seizures (Heldberg et al. 2016), sleep apnea (Oliver and Flores-Mangas 2016) and non-invasive diagnosis of many forms of cancer (Bajtarevic et al. 2009).

14.4.3   Tailoring Treatment Decisions

It is clear that genomic variations influence the absorption and metabolism of almost all pharmaceutical agents. While there is great promise in pharmacogenetic testing its clinical applicability has yet to be convincingly demonstrated. One of the better-chronicled failures of digital medicine is the use of CYP450 testing to tailor use of selective serotonin reuptake inhibitors in patients with depression. In theory, identifying patients with particular variants of CYP450 may be able to predict what dose of SSRI the patient should receive, based on whether metabolizing strength of their CYP450 variant. This led to mass retail availability of testing for CYP450, with several tests even receiving FDA clearance. This is despite the recommendation from the Evaluation of Genomic Applications in Practice and Prevention (EGAPP) Working Group that CYP450 testing not be routinely used stating a lack of evidence to support its use (Evaluation of Genomic Applications in Practice and Prevention (EGAPP) Working Group 2007).

That being said, CYP450 variants have been able to provide some potentially valuable insight in other settings, such as determining which patients will be responsive to clopidogrel, an antiplatelet agent used in acute coronary syndrome (Hulot et al. 2006), with large scale trials currently underway (Pulley et al. 2012). Despite being a promising venue, the American Heart Association does not currently recommend routine testing due to the lack of evidence that use of this technology leads to improved clinical outcomes, which poses the largest challenge to the implementation of this class of technology (Lanham and Oestreich 2010).

Interestingly, even when there is evidence to support the implementation of genetic guided pharmacotherapy, there is limited uptake in the clinical realm. One such example is the use genotype-guided warfarin therapy in patients requiring anticoagulation. Several large studies have already demonstrated the feasibility and efficacy of the use of this technology in this setting (International Warfarin Pharmacogenetics Consortium 2009; Anderson et al. 2007). Despite this evidence, recommendations from governing bodies only go so far as to state that this technology may be used. The major limitations to the adoption of this technology, when evidence supports its use, seem to be a lack of demonstrable clinical outcomes benefit, cost effectiveness as well as logistics of obtaining timely genotype data.

14.4.4   Medication Adherence

Key difficulties in the management of chronic disease include: determining whether the observed lack of treatment effect is the result of pharmacological unresponsiveness or inadequate adherence, difficulties accessing specialists and insufficient patient data to optimize treatment.

An early informal study of eight hypertensive patients explored the use of digital feedback system to monitor blood pressure medication effect and adherence, where ingestible sensors were taken with their regular medication and sensed by a wearable device (Godbehere and Wareing 2014). This proof of concept study was able to provide clinicians with data that allowed them to increase or decrease medication dosages discuss non-adherence and identify unresponsiveness to therapy.

Several other formal studies have demonstrated that digital blood pressure medicines, incorporating active medical ingredients with digestible sensors, is acceptable to patients, can accurately reflect adherence and can improve the efficacy of therapy (DiCarlo et al. 2016; Noble et al. 2015; Naik et al. 2015).

However, not all digital medicines have to be complex to improve medication adherence. Over a dozen clinical trials, in variety of disease settings, have demonstrated that a simple text messaging program can double medication adherence (Thakkar et al. 2016). When you take into consideration the implications of such a difference this can make in terms of reducing disease progression and complications, it is evident that providing personalised adherence programs through mobile technologies will soon be the norm.

14.4.5 Disease Symptoms and Sign Monitoring

A known challenge in the management of Parkinson's disease is that the clinical assessment only provides the clinician a snapshot of the disease state. Many signs are difficult to elicit on command such as the infamous freezing of gait, a sensation of being "glued to the floor" despite making a conscious effort to move. In an effort to help collect this vital data, a variety of wearable technologies have been developed employing accelerometers, gyroscopes, and magnetometer technologies (Maetzler et al. 2013). These wearables provide the opportunity to collect continuous data, in-between clinic visits, allowing clinicians to make treatment decisions based on symptom trends.

In addition, this digital technology provides a unique opportunity to quantitatively assess physical symptoms such as gait deficits and tremor that have been previously relied on clinically subjective scales.

While there is a general consensus that digital technologies has the opportunity to improve the diagnosis and monitoring of Parkinson's disease on an individual level, there are no studies that demonstrate long term treatment benefits (Espay et al. 2016).

Asthma is another challenging condition, which requires patients to routinely measure their peak flow measurements. Simple smartphone based applications have demonstrated that digital monitoring of asthmatic symptoms is feasible, acceptable to patients and improves compliance (Holtz and Whitten 2009; Ryan et al. 2005). Despite this, there is a paucity of evidence to support that this technology provides meaningful clinical benefit (Nickels and Dimov 2012).

14.5   Challenges in the Implementation of Digital Health

Despite the promising evidence that we have highlighted, there are a variety of barriers that must be overcome before digital health becomes integrated into our healthcare system. First, we must expand our evidence base for supporting the implementation of these technologies. This includes demonstrating that the intervention is feasible and acceptable to the patient population. Clinical trials also are also desperately needed to demonstrate non-inferiority, or better yet, superiority to the current gold standards, but also need to demonstrate cost-effectiveness and the ability to change current medical practice. The current fee-for-service reimbursement structure remains a major impediment to incentivizing changes in clinical practice that decrease office visits. Another concern is the security surrounding electronic devices and cloud based data storage. The industry must demonstrate that data can be transmitted and stored in a manner that is in compliance with the Health Insurance Portability and Accountability Act.

Only when these substantial challenges are addressed will we begin to see recommendations from governing bodies to support digital health and accelerated uptake by medical providers and consumers.

References

Anderson JL, Horne BD, Stevens SM, Grove AS, Barton S, Nicholas ZP, et al. Randomized trial of genotype-guided versus standard warfarin dosing in patients initiating oral anticoagulation. Circulation. 2007;116(22):2563–70.

Bajtarevic A, Ager C, Pienz M, Klieber M, Schwarz K, Ligor M, et al. Noninvasive detection of lung cancer by analysis of exhaled breath. BMC Cancer. 2009;9(1):164–16.

DiCarlo LA, Weinstein RL, Morimoto CB, Savage GM, Moon GL, Au-Yeung K, et al. Patient-centered home care using digital medicine and telemetric data for hypertension: feasibility and acceptability of objective ambulatory assessment. J Clin Hypertens (Greenwich). 2016;18:n/a.

Espay AJ, Bonato P, Nahab FB, Maetzler W, Dean JM, Klucken J, et al. Technology in Parkinson's disease: challenges and opportunities. Mov Disord. 2016;31(9):1272–82. doi:10.1002/mds.26642.

Evaluation of Genomic Applications in Practice and Prevention (EGAPP) Working Group. Recommendations from the EGAPP working group: testing for cytochrome P450 polymorphisms in adults with nonpsychotic depression treated with selective serotonin reuptake inhibitors. Genet Med. 2007:819–25.

Godbehere P, Wareing P. Hypertension assessment and management: role for digital medicine. J Clin Hypertens. 2014;16(3):235.

Heldberg BE, Kautz T, Leutheuser H, Hopfengartner R, Kasper BS, Eskofier BM. Using wearable sensors for semiology-independent seizure detection - towards ambulatory monitoring of epilepsy. Conf Proc IEEE Eng Med Biol Soc. 2016;2015:593–6.

Holtz B, Whitten P. Managing asthma with mobile phones: a feasibility study. Telemed J E-Health. 2009;15(9):907–9.

Hulot J-S, Bura A, Villard E, Azizi M, Remones V, Goyenvalle C, et al. Cytochrome P450 2C19 loss-of-function polymorphism is a major determinant of clopidogrel responsiveness in healthy subjects. Blood. 2006;108(7):2244–7.

International Warfarin Pharmacogenetics Consortium. Estimation of the warfarin dose with clinical and pharmacogenetic data. N Engl J Med. 2009;360(8):753–64.

Kvedar JC, Fogel AL, Elenko E, Zohar D. Digital medicine's march on chronic disease. Nat Biotechnol. 2016;34(3):239–46.

Lai SY, Deffenderfer OF, Hanson W, Phillips MP, Thaler ER. Identification of upper respiratory bacterial pathogens with the electronic nose. Laryngoscope. John Wiley & Sons Inc. 2002;112(6):975–9.

Lanham KJ, Oestreich JH, Dunn SP. Impact of genetic polymorphisms on clinical response to antithrombotics. Pharmacogenomics Pers Med. 2010;3:87–99.

Lowres N, Neubeck L, Salkeld G, Krass I, McLachlan AJ, Redfern J, et al. Feasibility and cost-effectiveness of stroke prevention through community screening for atrial fibrillation using iPhone ECG in pharmacies. Thromb Haemost. 2014;111(6):1167–76.

Lumley T, Rice K. Potential for revealing individual-level information in genome-wide association studies. JAMA. 2010;303(7):659–60.

Mach KE, Wong PK, Liao JC. Biosensor diagnosis of urinary tract infections: a path to better treatment? Trends Pharmacol Sci. 2011;32(6):330–6.

Maetzler W, Domingos J, Srulijes K, Ferreira JJ, Bloem BR. Quantitative wearable sensors for objective assessment of Parkinson's disease. Mov Disord. 2013;28(12):1628–37.

Manolio TA. Genome wide association studies and assessment of the risk of disease. N Engl J Med. 2010;363(2):166–76.

Naik R, Macey N, West RJ. An ingestible sensor and wearable patch tracking adherence and activity patterns identified underlying factors leading to persistent hypertension: a real-world registry study. 2015.

Nickels A, Dimov V. Innovations in technology: social media and mobile technology in the care of adolescents with asthma. Curr Allergy Asthma Rep. 2012;12(6):607–12.

Noble K, Xiang P, Kim Y, Leadley S, Dicarlo L. Medication adherence and activity patterns measured by sensor technologies guided hypertension management in the community pharmacy. Pharmacotherapy: The Journal Of Human Pharmacology and Drug Therapy. 2015; 35(11):e180.

Oliver N, Flores-Mangas F. HealthGear: a real-time wearable system for monitoring and analyzing physiological signals. InWearable and Implantable Body Sensor Networks, 2006. BSN 2006. International Workshop on 2006; p. 4. IEEE.

Pai NP, Vadnais C, Denkinger C, Engel N, Pai M. Point-of-care testing for infectious diseases: diversity, complexity, and barriers in low- and middle-income countries. PLoS Med. 2012;9(9):e1001306–7.

Pierce BL, Ahsan H. Clinical assessment incorporating a personal genome. Lancet. 2010;376(9744):869–70.

Pulley JM, Denny JC, Peterson JF, Bernard GR, Vnencak-Jones CL, Ramirez AH, et al. Operational implementation of prospective genotyping for personalized medicine: the design of the Vanderbilt PREDICT project. Clin Pharmacol Ther. 2012;92(1):87–95.

Quinn CC, Shardell MD, Terrin ML, Barr EA. Cluster-randomized trial of a mobile phone personalized behavioral intervention for blood glucose control. Diabetes Care. 2011;34:1934–42.

Rappaport KM, McCracken CC, Beniflah J, Little WK, Fletcher DA, Lam WA, et al. Assessment of a smartphone otoscope device for the diagnosis and management of otitis media. Clin Pediatr (Phila). 2015;7:1–11.

Ryan D, Cobern W, Wheeler J, Price D, Tarassenko L. Mobile phone technology in the management of asthma. J Telemed Telecare. 2005;11 Suppl 1(5):43–6. SAGE Publications

Sepah SC, Jiang L, Peters AL. Long-term outcomes of a web-based diabetes prevention program: 2-year results of a single-arm longitudinal study. J Med Internet Res. 2015;17(4):e92–8.

Shaffer DW, Kigin CM, Kaput JJ, Gazelle GS. What is digital medicine? Stud Health Technol Inform. 2002;80:195–204.

Steinhubl SR, Muse ED, Topol EJ. The emerging field of mobile health. Sci Transl Med. 2015;7(283):283rv3.

Steinhubl SR, Muse ED, Barrett PM, Topol EJ. Off the cuff: rebooting blood pressure treatment. Lancet. 2016;388:749.

Strong K, Mathers C, Leeder S, Beaglehole R. Preventing chronic diseases: how many lives can we save? Lancet. 2005;366(9496):1578–82.

Thakkar J, Kurup R, Laba T-L, Santo K, Thiagalingam A, Rodgers A, et al. Mobile telephone text messaging for medication adherence in chronic disease. JAMA Intern Med. 2016;176(3):340–10.

Topol EJ. Transforming medicine via digital innovation. Sci Transl Med. 2010;2(16):16cm4.

Topol EJ, Steinhubl SR, Torkamani A. Digital medical tools and sensors. JAMA. 2015;313(4):353–5.

US Food and Drug Administration. FDA permits marketing of first system of mobile medical apps for continuous glucose monitoring [Internet]. 2016. [cited 8 Jul 2016]. http://www.fda.gov/NewsEvents/Newsroom/PressAnnouncements/ucm431385.htm.

Visscher PM, Montgomery GW. Genome-wide association studies and human disease: from trickle to flood. JAMA. 2009;302(18):2028–9.

Chapter 15
The Digital and *In Silico* Therapeutics Revolution

Carolina Garcia Rizo

Abstract Digital therapeutics, i.e., adding digital components to traditional thera-peutics, can improve or even prevent diseases through behavioral change in cases where traditional drugs have not succeeded. The inclusion of digital components provides significant value not only to the therapeutics by improving their effective-ness, but also to the drug development process by reducing costs and increasing efficiency. The combination of digital therapeutics and diagnostics empowers the provider to deliver personalized medicine by better diagnosing and managing the patient, potentially enabling early disease detection. The implementation of compu-tational, or "*in silico*" tools in therapeutics and diagnostics, such as deep learning algorithms, is taking the digitalization improvements to its next level, fueling the healthcare revolution from curing diseases to preventing them.

Keywords Digital therapeutics • *In silico* therapeutics • Behavior change • *In silico* diagnostics • *In silico* clinical trials • Deep learning • *In silico* Genomics

15.1 Introduction

In the first chapter of this book, Dr. Rivas, Prof. at Stanford University, explained why digital health is a logical progression in healthcare. A key component of that explanation was the understanding of the different stakeholders in the digital health ecosystem. There is no need to emphasize that each of their different stakeholders has to be understood and considered as they are all interconnected and, therefore, each influences and affects the others. Within the topics discussed throughout this book, various stakeholders in digital health and their relationships are described.

Pharmaceutical companies are key stakeholders in the healthcare ecosystem as they are responsible for developing the "product" to improve and hopefully cure

C.G. Rizo, Ph.D., M.B.A.
Roche Molecular Systems, San Francisco, CA, USA
e-mail: carolina_rizo@sloan.mit.edu

© Springer International Publishing AG 2018   197
H. Rivas, K. Wac (eds.), *Digital Health*, Health Informatics,
https://doi.org/10.1007/978-3-319-61446-5_15

diseases. Under the control of countries' regulatory agencies, prescribed by the providers and reimbursed by the payers, the therapeutics developed by pharmaceutical companies have played a key role in the traditional healthcare ecosystem and will play an even bigger role in the digital health ecosystem by adding digital tools and delivering digital therapeutics.

In this chapter, the focus is on digital therapeutics and diagnostics. We will explore the meaning of this concept and discuss the value of digital components to traditional, therapeutics, diagnostics, and to their development. We will also explore the potential added value to traditional therapeutics and diagnostics of not only digital, but also "in silico" (computational) technologies.

15.2 The Foundation and Value of Digital Therapeutics

While talking about innovation and "digitalization" (i.e., adding digital tools to the existing practices) (De Clerck 2016) we should never forget the most pressing questions: What is the reason behind what we do?, why do we add digital components to therapeutics?, why do we need digital therapeutics?, what is the foundation of digital therapeutics and what are we trying to achieve?

Given the state of stakeholders of the healthcare ecosystem, our assumption is that only when the patient is placed at the center of the healthcare ecosystem, we can have a clear vision of what is important and what is the final objective of our work.

The objective in healthcare is to assure the highest effectiveness of patient treatment to achieve the best outcome. The pharmaceutical companies' role is developing safe and effective compounds make it possible to achieve this goal.

Traditionally, diseases have been treated with drugs that have varying effectiveness. Indeed, in some diseases traditional drugs may have limited or no positive effect, but could have negative side effects that cause more harm than benefits. This is the case of medical conditions with a behavioral component, such as type II diabetes, lung cancer caused by smoking, and heart disease where traditional therapeutics often have not succeeded. In these cases, if patients would be able to change their behaviors by eating healthier, quitting smoking, and exercising more, they would improve their health status and those at high-risk of these diseases could prevent their onset. By adding a digital component to traditional therapeutics, these patients may be able to change their behavior and, thereby, improve their health status, providing evidence of the value of digital therapeutics.

Joseph C. Kvedar, MD, vice president of Partners HealthCare's Connected Health unit, conveys a thorough description of digital therapeutics, in an article published by Harvard Business Review (Fogel and Kvedar 2016), as *"technology-based solutions that have a clinical impact on disease comparable to that of a drug. They primarily use consumer-grade technology, such as mobile devices, wearable sensors, big data analytics, and behavioral science and can be delivered through web browsers, apps, or in conjunction with medical devices. They can also be deployed in real-time and at scale, which is critical for intervention in chronic diseases*" (Fogel and Kvedar 2016).

In an interview regarding the founding of digital therapeutics (https://a16z.com/2016/10/25/bio-cs-machinelearning-medicine/), Vijay Pande, partner of the Silicon Valley-based VC firm Andreessen Horowitz, states: "*The foundation of digital therapeutics lies in diseases like type II diabetes, anxiety, depression, PTSD…, where traditionally efforts were coming only from traditional pharma, but actually they are different from other diseases since the main issue is behavior-related. Therefore, they should be approached not by using "the traditional pill," but using behavioral solutions, which is a better solution from the point of view of toxicity and efficacy. Traditionally, there were behavioral therapies, but they don't scale. Digital solutions help them to scale*" (https://a16z.com/2016/10/25/bio-cs-machinelearning-medicine/).

If one considers that medical conditions like heart disease, type II diabetes and lung cancer could be prevented by behavioral change, moreover they are responsible for 70% of Americans' premature death (https://www.cdc.gov/healthcommunication/toolstemplates/entertainmented/tips/preventivehealth.html) and account for 75% of health spending in the US (https://www.cdc.gov/healthcommunication/toolstemplates/entertainmented/tips/preventivehealth.html), then it is easy to understand the huge impact that digital therapeutics might have on the American society.

It is recognized that chronic diseases and behavior-based diseases also have a huge impact worldwide (http://www.who.int/nutrition/topics/2_background/en/). Nevertheless, for the sake of simplicity and space and time constraints, this chapter only references the US healthcare ecosystem, but can be extended also to other countries, albeit with regional differences in concepts, solutions, and strategies.

The huge negative impact on society that these diseases bring can be reduced through advancements in digital therapeutics, an industry now hailed by mHealth Intelligence as the "next big thing" in digital health (Wicklund 2016). Digital therapeutics is projected to become a $6 billion industry in 5–8 years based on a research report by Goldman Sachs and supplementary Psilos research, which predicts digital therapeutics to become the biggest component of digital health (Krupa et al. 2016).

For this reason, Joseph Riley, managing partner at Psilos Group, says, "the potential [of the digital therapeutics industry] is tremendous", outlining six factors that dictate the rise in digital therapeutics (Wicklund 2016; Krupa et al. 2016):

- Increasing healthcare costs
- The shift toward value-based care and reimbursement models
- Employers looking to improve their workforce through health management
- The consumerization of healthcare
- The prevalence of smartphones and the "quantified self" movement
- Strong support from investors, especially venture funds.

These factors have created an ecosystem where a new type of start-up has been developing. For example, the pioneer Omada Health (https://www.omadahealth.com/) has demonstrated that traditional therapeutics are not always the solution and that digital technologies are able to complement traditional therapies, thus creating this new digital therapeutics industry (Wicklund 2016).

15.3   Start-Ups Fueling the Digital Therapeutics Revolution

Omada Health (https://www.omadahealth.com/), the San Francisco (US) based start-up, is a pioneer company in the field of digital therapeutics, as we mentioned before, and its initial focus was, and still is type II diabetes.

Its marketing materials, though, suggest specific target on the four most costly and dangerous chronic conditions that lead to type II diabetes and other diseases: high blood sugar, high blood pressure, high blood fats, and obesity (https://www.omadahealth.com/).

In an article about the future of business and tech in addressing the growing number of diabetes cases, Dr. Anne Peters, director of the USC Clinical Diabetes Program, states: *"Type II diabetes happens when the body doesn't respond to insulin or doesn't produce enough insulin. It is the most prevalent type of diabetes and can be treated by exercising, eating healthier, and taking medications. In the United States, there are more than 29 million with diabetes and approximately 27 million have type II diabetes"* (http://www.joslin.org/info/common_questions_about_type_2_diabetes.html; Codemo 2016).

Omada Health (https://www.omadahealth.com/) created a program called "Prevent" (Fontil et al. 2016), where participants who are at risk of developing diabetes enroll in a 16-week-program. The program objective is to improve their behavior so they eat healthy and exercise in order to avoid developing diabetes. The participants are divided in groups of 10–12 based on age, body mass (BMI), and residence. They are assigned a "health coach" who monitors their progress and offers extra support. The participants will continue receiving support after they complete their program.

Omada Health (https://www.omadahealth.com/) is not just a digital system, but a true digital therapeutic, which product value have been proven through clinical data generation, that has cost the company significant time and money, but has allowed them to collect a per-member-per-month (PMPM) fee from self-insured employers and, importantly, from insurance companies. Omada Health also provides adherence feedback to payers, identifies the appropriately motivated patients, and provides tracking measures. This is very valuable to payers and is an example of the value that digital components add to traditional therapeutics that does not capture patient adherence or patient differentiation. Health Ventures mentions in its article about digital therapeutics: *"with prospective randomized data and a way to verify adherence, Omada could move to a much higher PMPM for the perfect patients. Essentially, the "personalized medicine" promise, but digitally"* (Healthy Ventures 2016).

There are other digital therapeutics companies like Omada that have developed mobile platforms for people with chronic conditions like diabetes, for example, HealthMine (http://www.healthmine.com), Canary Health (https://www.canary-health.com), Telcare (https://telcare.com), and WellDoc (https://www.welldoc.com/).

Chrono Therapeutics (https://chronothera.com/), a Bay Area based start-up, is another digital therapeutics company that improves the drug delivery process thanks to its digital components. It has a motivational app to deal with the psychological aspects of smoking addiction that is paired with a programmed patch that delivers tailored doses of nicotine (Tansey 2016). Chrono is currently in a phase 2 clinical trial for its nicotine patch and has a pending submission to the FDA (https://chrono-thera.com/flagship-product/). This clinical trial will probe the higher efficiency of a "personalized wearable patch" that is better able to deliver nicotine when the body is craving for it, than traditional therapeutics such as Chantix from Pfizer, nicotine patches, or anti-smoking behavioral coaching alone.

Jenny Hapgood, Chronos Vice President of product and marketing, in an interview for Xconomy (Tansey 2016), mentioned that *"Another plan on the horizon is to adapt the Chrono system for other disorders where there would be an advantage in being able to precisely control a drug dosage over the course of a day or a long course of treatment. Two possibilities are Parkinson's disease, where dose timing might help minimize the tremors that can be a side effect of the current drug used for the illness, and addiction to prescription opioids, where metered drug delivery might be better than dispensing a full bottle of pills to patients and relying on their will-power to limit their daily intake and taper it off over time."*

Another interesting start-up is Akili (http://www.akiliinteractive.com/), which utilizes technology developed at the University of California, San Francisco (UCSF), but is located in Boston where was co-created with Pure-Tech Ventures. Among its investors include the venture arm of Amgen and the one of Merck KGaA from Germany (http://www.londonstockexchange.com/exchange/news/market-news/market-news-detail/PRTC/12898803.html). Akili is developing a gaming platform for people with cognitive disorders.

"The idea behind Akili is that a doctor would prescribe this treatment and the patient would get a prescription code, download it, and play the game for a certain amount of time," explains Daphne Zohar, co-founder and CEO of PureTech in a report about digital therapeutics published by the New York City-based digital healthcare venture capital and growth equity investor firm, Psilos (Wicklund 2016). *"It is really a treatment, we believe, with drug-like efficacy, but without the drug. That is actually a theme across a number of things we are doing."*

"The drug industry has done a lot to influence the brain through drugs, but it's so complex," Daphne Zohar says in an article in Xconomy (Timmerman 2012). *"What's interesting about these approaches is that you can get real human data about indications you're going after, without drugs."*

Akili (http://www.akiliinteractive.com/) would belong to this class of Digital therapeutics, where the "digital tool or offer" even substitute the "traditional drugs". This is described as "Medication Substitution" by Peter Hames, the CEO of Big Health (https://www.bighealth.com/), in a recent MIT Technology Review article (Farr 2017). In this article, this concept is compared with "Medication augmentation" where the "digital tool" adds value, like would be the case of Cronos therapeutics (https://chronothera.com/flagship-product/), previously mentioned.

An example of "Medication Substitution" is also this San Francisco and London based start-up, Big Health (https://www.bighealth.com/), that offers an online therapy program, called "sleepio" for people suffering insomnia. This program is supposed to replace the traditional drugs with visualization exercises.

Steve Kraus, an investor at Bessemer Venture Partners, corroborated, in the mentioned MIT Review article (Farr 2017) the importance of digital therapeutics, which sweet spot, he believes, is when used "in combination" with drugs to make them work better, thus "Medication augmentation" (Farr 2017).

Digital therapeutics add value to traditional drugs, and in some cases, they are even able to substitute them, however, what is key for the success of any digital therapeutics start-up is showing evidence-based value. By showing validation, digital therapeutics will be considered seriously by the consumers, will be prescribed by the providers and will be reimbursed by the payers.

This is why some of these (digital therapeutics start-ups) are following the traditional pharma route by conducting clinical trials (Mack 2017). Some of them, like WellDoc (https://www.welldoc.com), a start-up based in Columbia, MD, followed the traditional pharma development route and got FDA approval in January 2017 (https://www.accessdata.fda.gov/scripts/cdrh/cfdocs/cfpmn/pmn. cfm?ID=K162225) for its offer of a non- prescription version of its BlueStar® digital therapeutics, which consists in a phone app for managing type 2 diabetes (Mack 2017). Previosuly, in June 2013, WellDoc Launched BlueStar®, First FDA-Cleared, Mobile Prescription Therapy for Type 2 Diabetes with Insurance Reimbursement.

WellDoc recently raised $29.5M in a series B funding, led by Samsung Ventures and Merck Global Health Innovation (GHI) Fund and with participation of Johnson & Johnson Innovation –JJDC Inc. (Globenewswire 2015; Sherman 2017).

This is just the beginning of the power that digital components offer to traditional therapeutics: apps that monitor basic patient variables like cardiac function, glucose level, stress, etc. and systems or platforms that enable greater patient control over their health by anticipating health conditions and modifying patients' behavior. Digital technology enables the health variables monitoring in real-time and, thereby, track the patient's progress continuously. As pharmaceutical companies leverage more digital opportunities, more data will become available that can be mined to enhance the therapeutic–patient relationship with the objective to increase the effectiveness and, therefore, the value of the drug, while improving the patient's health.

15.4   The Value Added of Digital and *In Silico* Components to the Traditional Drug Development Process

Digital components can add value to therapeutics in two main ways: (1) by improving the effectiveness of a "traditional drug", as we have seen already, and (2) by improving the process of developing therapeutics.

Therapeutics development requires a huge amount of capital and carries high risk as well (Paul et al. 2010). Research has shown that R&D productivity remains the biggest challenge for the pharmaceutical industry (Paul et al. 2010). Therefore, making the drug development process more efficient by reducing cost and risk brings enormous value to pharmaceutical companies.

Pharmaceutical development companies spend between $4 and $6 billion each year in unnecessary clinical trial expenses (http://csdd.tufts.edu/news/complete_story/pr_tufts_csdd_2014_cost_study). Roughly 25% of clinical trials are inefficient and extremely expensive (http://csdd.tufts.edu/news/complete_story/pr_tufts_csdd_2014_cost_study). A big portion of this inefficiency is due to collecting irrelevant data. As an example, 23% of Phase III clinical trials collect peripheral, unneeded data.

The efficiency of clinical trials could be improved by implementing digital components currently on the market. Such components might be used to improve recruitment, monitor adverse events, and confirm participants' compliance with the protocol (Garcez 2016). One start-up tackling the inefficiency of clinical trials is the Los Angeles based Science 37 (https://www.science37.com/), that assists with clinical trial recruitment and remote monitoring using digital tools.

Digital tools such as sensors, connected devices and apps, can also be very valuable for monitoring the effect of the drug in the patient while collecting real-time data as evidence of clinical improvement. Using digital tools during clinical trials can increase patient engagement and compliance and can even allow participants to follow a regular life, with minor changes in habits. Therefore, using digital therapeutics during clinical trials would be beneficial for traditional pharmaceutical companies which could save time and money and use these data to support applications for FDA approval.

Another area of the "traditional pharma"' research and development (R&D) process, where entrepreneurs see a great benefit when using computational tools is in the early discovery phase. The efficiency of this phase can improve by using "*in silico*" tools to find appropriate drug candidates to match specific conditions (Sliwoski et al. 2014; Tollman et al. 2011; Scannell et al. 2012; Vanhaelen et al. 2017). Among these start-ups trying to find *in silico* drug candidates to bring them later on to clinical trials are TwoXAR (http://www.twoxar.com), Atomwise (http://www.atomwise.com), Numedii (http://numedii.com), and Berg Health (https://berghealth.com), just to mention some.

TwoXAR (http://www.twoxar.com) was created by MIT and Stanford graduates and began its incubation at StartX, a start-up incubator at Stanford. The company has successfully identified potential drug candidates for treating Parkinson's disease. In an interview in Datanami (Woodie 2015), TwoXAR co-founder Andrew A. Radin said, "*We loaded a bunch of data on Parkinson's disease into the system, pressed the go button, a few minutes later we had a list of drugs that were listed as highly efficacious*." (Woodie 2015).

Atomwise (http://www.atomwise.com), a San Francisco-based start-up, describes themselves as "an artificial intelligence-based company for drug discovery" (http://www.atomwise.com). Dr. Heifets, Atomwise's CEO, mentioned in an interview (Martin 2016): "*we have successfully found two potential drug candidates to tackle Ebola*".

Numedii (http://numedii.com), a Silicon Valley-based start-up has formed partnerships with three pharma companies including Astellas and Allergan. Berg Health (https://berghealth.com; https://www.economist.com/news/science-and-technology/21713828-

silicon-valley-has-squidgy-worlds-biology-and-disease-its-sights-will) a Massachusetts-based start-up, discovered a potential drug candidate to treat pancreatic cancer and it is already in phase II clinical trial for a drug compound (https://berghealth.com/berg-initiates-phase-ii-combination-trial-of-bpm-31510-and-gemcitabine-in-patients-with-pancreatic-cancer/).

These companies all apply artificial intelligence to the earliest stages of drug discovery (i.e., finding possible drug candidates). This might well be the beginning of a continuous *in silico* drug development process and even *in silico* clinical trials (Viceconti et al. 2016; Viceconti et al. 2016). When modeling wet-lab experiments *in silico*, more experiments can be performed, because the costly and time-consuming lab experiments are simulated in the computer. *In silico* models, therefore, lead to faster and cheaper drug development, improving the efficiency of drug development process.

Traditional pharmaceutical companies have seen the cost of their R&D efforts increase (valuatePharma® 2015) and their discovery pipelines become drier. However, these "*in silico*" therapeutics start-ups are bringing new potential drug candidates to market; The "digital" therapeutics ones are improving clinical trials efficiency by reducing cost and time, and obtaining real-world evidence data on disease reduction. In some cases, like Omada Health, digital therapeutics are even receiving insurance reimbursement. Therefore, some traditional pharmaceutical companies have started to tap into digital and even "*in silico*" opportunities by creating digital accelerators, like is the case of Takeda (Bulik 2016), or by partnering with digital start-ups. An example of the latter is the partnership between Glaxo Smith Klein (GSK) and the San Francisco-based start-up Propeller (https://www.propellerhealth.com/2015/12/01/propeller-health-announces-development-agreement-and-rd-collaboration-with-gsk-to-develop-a-digital-sensor-for-the-ellipta-inhaler/). They announced (https://www.propellerhealth.com/2015/12/01/propeller-health-announces-development-agreement-and-rd-collaboration-with-gsk-to-develop-a-digital-sensor-for-the-ellipta-inhaler/) a development agreement and R&D collaboration to create a digital sensor for GSK's dry powder inhaler, Ellipta®; and exactly 1 year later, on November 2016, Propeller's digital respiratory disease management system with Ellipta received FDA approval (Al Idrus 2016).

As digital therapeutics further demonstrate their clinical utility and validity, more successful partnerships between traditional and digital therapeutics should be established. This will prove the viability of digital therapeutics as an industry. Digital therapeutics start-ups can benefit from relationships with traditional pharma by seeking not only the financial, but also the operational support from traditional pharma, such as clinical trials and regulatory expertise, and partnerships and contacts established with different healthcare stakeholders from providers to payers, and their worldwide outreach. Traditional pharmaceutical companies have a long history of having established partnerships with most of the stakeholders of the healthcare ecosystem globally.

Traditional pharmaceutical will benefit from these digital therapeutics and *in silico* drug discovery start-ups because they can tap into digital and computational offers that can improve the effectiveness of the traditional pill and increase the efficiency and decrease the cost and risk of the traditional drug discovery and development process. By doing so, pharma companies can identify new business opportunities that increase their market share, competitiveness and consequently profitability.

15.5   Digital Therapeutics and Diagnostics' Next Level: *In Silico* Therapeutics and Diagnostics

Chronic diseases, like type II diabetes, heart disease, and lung cancer due to smoking could be improved and even prevented if patients with chronic or high-risk diseases would eat healthier, exercise regularly, and avoid smoking. For some types of cancer, such as breast cancer, regular screenings allow early detection (http://www. apa.org/pubs/journals/releases/amp-a0037357.pdf;   https://www.cancer.org/ research/cancer-facts-statistics/cancer-prevention-early-detection.html;   https:// www.cancer.org/treatment/survivorship-during-and-after-treatment/when-cancer-doesnt-go-away.html). Early detection of several diseases through screening programs improves the effectiveness and outcome of treatment (Etzioni et al. 2003).

Adding "digital components" to traditional therapeutics (i.e., digital therapeutics) have been proven successful in helping change patient behavior, influencing patients to perform those activities that will prevent and/or delay their chronic disease evolution. Digital therapeutics, therefore, are very valuable for healthcare systems as they improve patient care, prevent disease and, thus, reduce healthcare cost. Early and regular screening, for example, in the case of breast cancer, also helps detect early disease so that the patient can respond better to the early treatment.

Digital therapeutics are also very valuable by monitoring the effect of the drug in the patient while collecting real-time data as evidence of clinical improvement. This can improve patient adherence and behavior change. Diagnostics are also able to "accompany" the drug, monitoring its effect in the patient, assuring its effectiveness. This is what is called "companion diagnostics" (https://www.fda.gov/MedicalDevices/ ProductsandMedicalProcedures/InVitroDiagnostics/ucm407297.htm).

Therefore, when talking about digital therapeutics, we should also mention the role of diagnostics, as enabler of its value added. Robert Mittendorf, partner at Norwest Ventures, already included diagnostics (Salemi 2016) when describing "Digital Therapeutics and Diagnostics" at the 2016 Digital Healthcare Innovation Summit in in Boston (http://healthegy.com/digital-healthcare-innovation-summit-2016/presentations/), suggesting that *"these companies (digital therapeutics and diagnostics) apply information technology, mobile devices, wearables, and other interactive technologies in clinical protocols and insights to help change behavior in the treatment of a clinical condition"*.

Diagnostics are means and measures used to evaluate a state of the patient's health towards a disease diagnosis. Once a diagnosis is established, the appropriate treatment is applied. We then can monitor the patient to ensure that the drug is having a positive effect (i.e., clinical improvement). As mentioned before, this use of diagnostics is called "companion diagnostics (CDx), (https://www.fda.gov/

MedicalDevices/ProductsandMedicalProcedures/InVitroDiagnostics/ucm407297.
htm)" which indicates that these CDx specifically "accompany" the drug to monitor
its safety and effectiveness. Companion diagnostics are frequently developed to
monitor oncology patients during treatment; however, they are being increasingly
developed in other disease areas like cardiovascular, neurological, and metabolic
disorders, among others (Mckinsey and Company 2016).

Pharmaceutical companies use these companion diagnostics during clinical trials
to stratify participating patients and monitor them, assuring the beneficial effect of
the drug in the patient and identifying those that are not (or no longer) benefiting
from the drug. An example of companion diagnostics would be the Roche cobas®
EGFR Mutation Test v2 (GenomeWeb 2015) that is able to identify those NSCLC
(non-small cell lung cancer) patients with EGFR exon 19 deletions or L858R mutations that are candidates for the EGFR-targeted therapy Tarceva® (erlotinib), in first-
line treatment. On the other hand, patients who have the EGFR resistance mutation
T790M are candidates for AstraZeneca's TAGRISSO™ in subsequent lines of treatment (https://molecular.roche.com/news/fda-grants-roche-label-extension-for-the-
cobas-egfr-mutation-test-v2-for-use-with-plasma-as-a-companion-diagnostic-for-
tagrisso/). Companion diagnostics enable personalized medicine because, based on
the characteristics of the patient, the appropriate therapeutic will be administered
(Mckinsey and Company 2016).

Diagnostics enable the provider, in this case the doctor, to treat the patient more
precisely. The more clinically relevant data that can be gathered about the disease
and the patient, the sooner and better the medical doctor can achieve a more accurate diagnosis and, therefore, prescribe the most appropriate treatment. These data
can be gathered by using "digital tools", which added to "traditional diagnostics"
would translate into "digital diagnostics".

This concept of "digital diagnostics" is not yet broadly adopted; however, it
could become an important one in the future. Before discussing the role of digital
diagnostics for the patient, for the pharmaceutical companies, and the healthcare
system in general, we will review the diagnostics industry.

The diagnostics industry has evolved rapidly in recent years (Mckinsey and
Company 2016; http://www.decibio.com/market-report/clinical-dianostics/ivd):
new players, new technologies, and a larger offering of tests are enabling broader
diagnosis of diseases. The specificity and sensitivity of diagnostic tests as well as
the automation of instruments has been improving drastically. The development of
robust point-of-care systems is allowing a faster turnaround of patient samples. All
these improvements, therefore, enable faster diagnosis and treatments.

Genomics has been one of the diagnostics areas with the biggest improvements.
Since the completion of the Human Genome project in 2003 (http://www.compan-
iondiagnostics2016.com/wp-content/uploads/2016/04/McKinseyCo_
Personalized-Medicine_2013_0214-v2.pdf; https://www.genome.gov/10001772/
all-about-the-human-genome-project-hgp/), the extraordinary progress in sequencing technology has allowed a decrease in cost per mega base and an increase in the
number and variety of sequenced genomes (Goodwin 2016). The improvement in
genomics technology and scientific and medical discoveries has enabled liquid

biopsy to start becoming a reality today in cancer diagnostics (https://molecular.roche.com/news/fda-grants-roche-label-extension-for-the-cobas-egfr-mutation-test-v2-for-use-with-plasma-as-a-companion-diagnostic-for-tagrisso/). The first FDA-approved liquid biopsy test (https://www.fda.gov/NewsEvents/Newsroom/PressAnnouncements/ucm504488.htm) was the PCR (Polymerase Chain Reaction)-based test developed by Roche, called cobas® EGFR Mutation Test v2 (Mckinsey and Company 2016).

No NGS (Next-Generation Sequencing) based liquid biopsy test has yet been approved by the FDA, but several companies are working towards this goal (https://www.fda.gov/NewsEvents/Newsroom/PressAnnouncements/ucm504488.htm; Carlson 2016; Pagliarulo 2017).

Given the noninvasive character of these types of tests, the patient can be monitored more frequently than with tissue biopsy, which oftentimes requires hospital intervention (Insight Pharma Reports 2017). Liquid biopsy enables real-time monitoring of patient–drug interactions throughout their treatment and track disease dynamics (Ray 2015).

The integration of not only genomic but also proteomics and other—omics data allows a more holistic understanding of the diseases (Satagopam et al. 2016), such as cancer, and a better understanding of drug-patient interaction (Zhang et al. 2013; Buescher and Driggers 2016; Chin 2010; Michaut et al. 2016; Wanichthanarak et al. 2015). Companies like Thermo Fisher Scientific, a key player in the NGS space, which provides not only genomics but other—omics technologies, could enable this—omics integration offer.

This genomic and even other—omics data can be integrated with additional patient data from electronic health records like imaging files, and even wearables and sensors that enable a much more holistic vision and understanding of the patient and its disease. This integrated data will be very valuable to the doctor, who can modify the therapy when the first signs of failure of the current treatment appears.

This integrated data will be very valuable also for the pharmaceutical companies (Schumacher et al. 2016; Regan and Payne 2015), which can mine this data and find patterns when comparing different patients' interactions with its drugs along every patient journey. This data can allow pharmaceutical companies to develop algorithms that explore improvements on the drug–patient interaction.

The patient journey can be simulated in a computer (*in silico*). Therefore, while digital therapeutics result of adding digital technologies to traditional therapeutics, *in silico* therapeutics become the result of adding *in silico* technologies, as mentioned in the previous section of this chapter. This approach adds value to therapeutics and translates into better patient treatment and greater profitability for pharmaceutical companies. *In silico* will be the next level of the "digital value added offer" and the driver of personalized medicine that maximizes the way treatment predictions can be made based on each patient's characteristics.

All these developments will benefit the stakeholders of the healthcare ecosystem. Providers will offer better care, patients will receive the appropriate personalized treatment, payers will be able to better allocate funds, and pharmaceutical companies will offer real-time, real-world evidence of their therapeutics' effectiveness.

Deep learning and other computational methods add tremendous value to thera-peutics by providing more precise, timely and personalized modeling of patient state, needs, expectations and experiences, as well as state of health. In a similar way, these methods will also improve the potential of diagnostics.

In Silicon Valley, two diagnostics-based start-ups have recently raised a consid-erable amount of money: Freenome (https://www.freenome.com) $65 M in series A (Ray 2017) and Grail (https://grail.com) $900 M series B (http://ventures.mckes-son.com/grail-closes-900-million-initial-investment-series-b-financing-develop-blood-test-detect-cancer-early/). These companies apply deep learning and other computational methods to their liquid biopsy diagnostic tests (Ray 2017).

Freenome (https://www.freenome.com) is planning to offer a liquid biopsy test that performs lower sequencing coverage of DNA and RNA in plasma, thus requir-ing less quantity of the patient blood sample. They apply deep learning to find pat-terns from the raw patient data and claim that this approach allows the detection of early stage cancer, identification of tissue of origin, and differentiation of respond-ers from non-responders (https://www.freenome.com; Ray 2017).

Grail (https://grail.com), a spin-off of Illumina, a dominant player in Next-generation sequencing (NGS), is also applying deep learning to liquid biopsy data. Their tests will follow a more traditional deep and broad sequencing approach. A considerable amount of Grail's funding has been raised from prominent pharmaceu-tical companies like Merck & Co. Inc., Bristol-Myers Squibb Inc., Celgene Corp., and Johnson & Johnson's venture capital arm (http://ventures.mckesson.com/grail-closes-900-million-initial-investment-series-b-financing-develop-blood-test-detect-cancer-early/). This indicates that pharmaceutical companies realize the importance of drug–patient interaction monitoring through the computational exploration of genomic data.

Another start-up in this space is Deep Genomics (https://www.deepgenomics.com/), based in Canada. It was founded by Prof. Frey, from the University of Toronto, bringing together world-leading expertise in deep learning and genome biology to predict what will happen within a cell when DNA is altered by genetic variation, whether natural or therapeutic.

As Prof. Frey indicated in an enlightening interview (Beyer 2016) with David Beyer, an investor with Amplify Partners: *"we need to bridge the genotype–pheno-type divide." Genomic and phenotypic data abound. Unfortunately, the state-of-the-art in meaningfully connecting these data results in a slow, expensive, and inaccurate process of literature searches and detailed wet-lab experiments. To close the loop, we need systems that can determine intermediate phenotypes, called "molecular pheno-types," which function as stepping stones from genotype to disease phenotype. For this, machine learning is indispensable"* (https://blogs.nvidia.com/blog/2016/07/29/whats-difference-artificial-intelligence-machine-learning-deep-learning-ai/).

As more patients are screened for diseases and monitored through their treat-ment, more genomic data will become available. Companies like Deep Genomics (https://www.deepgenomics.com/) unify meaningfully genomic and phenotypic data. Digital technologies will gather more real-time data from the patient and all these data, properly mined, will allow to model *in silico* the patient journey from beginning to end. Ideally, all this integrated data will allow pharmaceutical companies to develop models that replicate how their drugs interact with patients in very diverse scenarios and consider all different patient characteristics. As these patient journey models evolve and improve, we can only hope for the *in silico* clinical trials concept to become a reality.

The concept of "precision medicine" will also benefit from *in silico* genomic medicine and precision therapeutics: instead of giving drugs in a trial-and-error mode in medical practice, we will be able to gather all the information from the patient first and then very accurately decide which therapy will be most appropriate for its characteristics, anticipating how the patient will respond.

15.6   Conclusion

In conclusion, digital diagnostics and digital therapeutics have a key common objective: Real-time monitoring of the drug–patient interaction along the patient journey. Patient monitoring technology relies on objective continuous data analytics, which provides a foundation for increasing the consistency and efficacy of data use in clinical practice.

Digital therapeutics has successfully proven beneficial to improve those behavioral-based diseases and prevent them in high-risk patients, enhancing traditional therapeutics' effectiveness. Digital tools have also added value to the traditional drug development process by gathering data, for example through wearables, showing real world evidence based data of the interaction drug-patient that can be leveraged by pharma companies.

Digital tools enable the gathering of real-time patient data to better diagnose the patient (digital diagnostics) and better monitor the drug-patient interaction (digital companion diagnostics/therapeutics). They also improve the patient behavior and compliance to the treatment while optimizing the effectiveness of the drugs (digital therapeutics).

While the digital components allow more patient data to be collected, computer tools will let all available patient data and medical knowledge be inclusively accomodated, providing a foundation for increasing consistency and efficacy of data use in clinical practice. Moreover, *in silico* tools allow this data to be mined, and transformed into clinically actionable information that would ultimately enable the modeling of the patient journeys in a way that *in silico* clinical trials and *in silico* companion diagnostics might become a reality. Therefore *in silico* therapeutics and diagnostics will fuel the healthcare revolution from diseases curation to prevention.

Pharmaceutical companies should capitalize on the value of this data and make the investments needed to gather it and develop the algorithms to simulate and predict the impact of their therapeutics in the patients. Integrating all this data and transforming it into actionable information will improve their digital and *in silico* therapeutics offer by showing more real-world evidence of its added value.

Pharmaceutical companies should follow the imperatives of digitalization (De Clerck 2016) and *"in silicatization"* in medicine and partner with diagnostics companies that are taking the initiative in this space, so that both industries complement and enhance each other improving the personalization of medicine. Otherwise, by not doing so, higher costs will be the norm and, even more importantly, the industry will have lost the power to own the data and their critical role in healthcare.

Traditionally, the value of the pharmaceutical companies was in the wet-lab and while this is still important, more and more value will be originated from the *in silico* lab. Therefore, having data ownership will be key. Digital therapeutics will be only the beginning of the *in silico* therapeutics era, where precision medicine will become a reality and prevention enabled by prediction and diagnosis will eliminate unnecessary pain and deaths, improving patient care, health, and well-being.

In silico tools like artificial intelligence and its subset machine learning and deep learning (https://blogs.nvidia.com/blog/2016/07/29/whats-difference-artificial-intelli-gence-machine-learning-deep-learning-ai/; Hof 2017) have proven beneficial for drug discovery (http://berghealth.com/platform/), improving the traditional drug development process, and setting the seeds for future '*in silico* therapeutics'; These *in silico* tools will potentially improve screening and monitoring diagnostics tests to enable early detection of cancer and other diseases, and better control of the drug-patient interaction respectively.

Start-ups might bring the innovation to the traditional pharmaceutical companies enabling their growth into these "digital" and "*in silico*" therapeutics areas. Traditional pharmaceutical companies might help these start-ups with their long history experience and global outreach. However, the key for the success of the "digital" and "*in silico*" therapeutics industry will be real world evidence based value and trustful collaborations, keeping always in mind their ultimate goal that should always be the improvement of the patient care and outcome.

Predicting the future is always challenging. A safe bet is that we will have more data from genomic and from all the -omics technologies, as well as from the digital components added to traditional therapeutics and diagnostics.

In silico tools will help combine this massive data and transform it into medical actionable information that will benefit healthcare stakeholders, especially the patient, by not only improving its diseases, but hopefully preventing them.

The digital and *in silico* therapeutics and diagnostics revolution has only started. It is the duty of all of us, the healthcare stakeholders, to work hard towards a healthier world, keeping always the patient health improvement as our main goal, fueling this revolution from curing diseases to preventing them.

References

Amirah Al Idrus "GSK, Propeller 'smart inhaler' gets FDA green light", Fierce Pharma. 2016. http://www.fiercebiotech.com/medical-devices/gsk-propeller-smart-inhaler-gets-fda-green-light.
David Beyer, "Deep learning meets genome biology". O'Reilly. 2016. https://www.oreilly.com/ideas/deep-learning-meets-genome-biology.

Buescher JM, Driggers EM. Integration of omics: more than the sum of its parts. Cancer & Metabolism. 2016;4(4)   doi:10.1186/s40170-016-0143-y.   https://cancerandmetabolism. biomedcentral.com/articles/10.1186/s40170-016-0143-y. Published: 19 February 2016

Beth Snyder Bulik, "Getting serious about digital: Takeda walks the walk with its digital accelerator model" Fierce Pharma. 2016. http://www.fiercepharma.com/marketing/ getting-serious-about-digital-takeda-walks-walk-its-digital-accelerator-model.

Bruce Carlson, "NGS approvals predict NGS boom" Genet Eng Biotechnol News. 2016. http:// www.genengnews.com/gen-exclusives/ngs-approvals-predict-ngs-boom/77900812.

Lynda Chin, "Integrating genomics with proteomics: towards a comprehensive view of cancer biology" National Cancer Institute. 2010. https://proteomics.cancer.gov/newsevents/eprotein/ november2010/features/chin.

Roberta Codemo, "How digital therapeutics is addressing growing diabetes cases" Fut Business   Tech   (2016)   http://www.futureofbusinessandtech.com/business-solutions/ how-digital-therapeutics-is-addressing-growing-diabetes-cases.

J-P De Clerck. Digitization, digitalization and digital transformation: the differences. Iscoop. 2016. https://goo.gl/oJcwzZ.

Etzioni R, et al. Early detection: the case for early detection. Nat Rev Cancer. 2003;3:243–52. doi:10.1038/nrc1041.

Farr C. Can "digital therapeutics" be as good as drugs? MIT Technol Rev. 2017.; https://www. technologyreview.com/s/604053/can-digital-therapeutics-be-as-good-as-drugs/

Fogel AL, Kvedar JC. Simple digital technologies can reduce health care costs. Harv Bus Rev. 2016.; https://hbr.org/2016/11/simple-digital-technologies-can-reduce-health-care-costs

Fontil V, et al. Adaptation and feasibility study of a digital health program to prevent diabetes among low-income patients: results from a partnership between a digital health company and an academic research team. J Diabetes Res. 2016;2016:8472391. doi:10.1155/2016/8472391. Published online 2016 Oct 27. . https://www.ncbi.nlm.nih.gov/pmc/articles/PMC5102733/

Adriano Garcez. Series: transforming clinical trials with digital solutions–part 1. 2016. https:// www.medullan.com/blog/digital-solutions-improve-clinical-trials-and-reduce-pharmaceutical-costs-so-why-isnt-everyone-on-board.

GenomeWeb. FDA approves roche cobas EGFR mutation test as CDx with AstraZeneca's tagrisso   drug.   2015.   GenomeWeb.   https://www.genomeweb.com/companion-diagnostics/ fda-approves-roche-cobas-egfr-mutation-test-cdx-astrazenecas-tagrisso-drug.

Globenewswire. WellDoc® Raises $22 Million in Series B Funding From Samsung Ventures, Merck Global Health Innovation Fund and Other Leading Venture Groups. Globenewswire. 2015.   https://globenewswire.com/news-release/2015/12/17/796409/0/en/WellDoc-Raises-22-Million-in-Series-B-Funding-From-Samsung-Ventures-Merck-Global-Health-Innovation-Fund-and-Other-Leading-Venture-Groups.html.

Goodwin S. Coming of age: ten years of next-generation sequencing technologies. Nat Rev Genet. 2016;17:333–51.   doi:10.1038/nrg.2016.49.   http://www.nature.com/nrg/journal/v17/n6/full/ nrg.2016.49.html. Published online 17 May 2016

Healthy Ventures. Digital therapeutics vs digiceuticals: defining the software-mediated healthcare landscape. Healthy Ventures. 2016. https://medium.com/@Healthy.vc/digital-therapeutics-vs-digiceuticals-defining-the-software-mediated-healthcare-landscape-fd0eb9dbedec.

Robert D. Hof. Deep learning. MIT Technology Review. 2017. https://www.technologyreview. com/s/513696/deep-learning/.

http://berghealth.com/platform/

http://csdd.tufts.edu/news/complete_story/pr_tufts_csdd_2014_cost_study

http://healthegy.com/digital-healthcare-innovation-summit-2016/presentations/

http://numedii.com

http://ventures.mckesson.com/grail-closes-900-million-initial-investment-series-b-financing-develop-blood-test-detect-cancer-early/

http://www.akiliinteractive.com/

http://www.apa.org/pubs/journals/releases/amp-a0037357.pdf

http://www.atomwise.com

http://www.companiondiagnostics2016.com/wp-content/uploads/2016/04/McKinseyCo_
    Personalized-Medicine_2013_0214-v2.pdf

http://www.decibio.com/market-report/clinical-dianostics/ivd

http://www.healthmine.com

http://www.joslin.org/info/common_questions_about_type_2_diabetes.html

http://www.londonstockexchange.com/exchange/news/market-news/market-news-detail/
    PRTC/12898803.html

http://www.twoxar.com

http://www.who.int/nutrition/topics/2_background/en/

https://a16z.com/2016/10/25/bio-cs-machinelearning-medicine/

https://berghealth.com

https://berghealth.com/berg-initiates-phase-ii-combination-trial-of-bpm-31510-and-gemcitabine-
    in-patients-with-pancreatic-cancer/

https://blogs.nvidia.com/blog/2016/07/29/whats-difference-artificial-intelligence-machine
    learning-deep-learning-ai/

https://chronothera.com/

https://chronothera.com/flagship-product/

https://grail.com

https://molecular.roche.com/news/fda-grants-roche-label-extension-for-the-cobas-egfr-mutation-
    test-v2-for-use-with-plasma-as-a-companion-diagnostic-for-tagrisso/

https://telcare.com

https://www.accessdata.fda.gov/scripts/cdrh/cfdocs/cfpmn/pmn.cfm?ID=K162225

https://www.bighealth.com/

https://www.canaryhealth.com

https://www.cancer.org/research/cancer-facts-statistics/cancer-prevention-early-detection.html

https://www.cancer.org/treatment/survivorship-during-and-after-treatment/when-cancer-doesnt-
    go-away.html

https://www.cdc.gov/healthcommunication/toolstemplates/entertainmented/tips/preventive-
    health.html

https://www.deepgenomics.com/

https://www.fda.gov/MedicalDevices/ProductsandMedicalProcedures/InVitroDiagnostics/
    ucm407297.htm

https://www.fda.gov/NewsEvents/Newsroom/PressAnnouncements/ucm504488.htm

https://www.freenome.com

https://www.genome.gov/10001772/all-about-the--human-genome-project-hgp/

https://www.omadahealth.com/

https://www.propellerhealth.com/2015/12/01/propeller-health-announces-development-agree-
    ment-and-rd-collaboration-with-gsk-to-develop-a-digital-sensor-for-the-ellipta-inhaler/

https://www.science37.com/

https://www.welldoc.com/

https://www.welldoc.com/

Insight Pharma Reports. Global liquid biopsy–market 2017-2021. Insight Pharma Reports. 2017.
    http://www.insightpharmareports.com/Affiliated-Reports/TechNavio/Global-Liquid-Biopsy/

Steve Krupa, David Eichler, Joseph Riley. Digital therapeutics. Psilos Healthcare Outlook 2016.
    http://psilos.com/wp-content/uploads/2016/10/final-psilos_outlook_doc_WEB.pdf.

Heather Mack. FDA clears WellDoc's non-RX version of BlueStar, its mobile diabetes man-
    agement tool. Mob Health News. 2017. http://www.mobihealthnews.com/content/
    fda-clears-welldocs-non-rx-version-bluestar-its-mobile-diabetes-management-tool.

Glen Martin, This company uses AI to accelerate drug discovery. O'Reilly. 2016. https://www.
    oreilly.com/ideas/this-company-uses-ai-to-accelerate-drug-discovery.

Mckinsey & Company. Personalized medicine. Mckinsey & Company. 2016. http://www.companiondiagnostics2016.com/wp-content/uploads/2016/04/McKinseyCo_Personalized-Medicine_2013_0214-v2.pdf.

Michaut M, et al. Integration of genomic, transcriptomic and proteomic data identifies two biologically distinct subtypes of invasive lobular breast cancer. Sci Rep. 2016;6:18517. doi:10.1038/srep18517. https://www.nature.com/articles/srep18517. Published online: 05 January 2016

Ned Pagliarulo. Liquid biopsies: the next frontier in cancer?. BioPharma Dive. 2017. http://www.biopharmadive.com/news/liquid-biopsy-cancer-screening-blood-test/435886/.

Paul S, et al. How to improve R&D productivity: the pharmaceutical industry's grand challenge. Nat Rev Drug Discov. 2010;9:203–14. doi:10.1038/nrd3078. http://www.nature.com/nrd/journal/v9/n3/full/nrd3078.html.

Ray K. Liquid biopsy enables real-time monitoring of molecular alterations in CRC. Nat Rev Gastroenterol Hepatol. 2015;12(372) doi:10.1038/nrgastro.2015.105. http://www.nature.com/nrgastro/journal/v12/n7/full/nrgastro.2015.105.html. Published online 16 June 2015

Turna Ray. Liquid biopsy startup freenome using recently raised funds to show clinical validity, utility. GenomeWeb. 2017. https://www.genomeweb.com/cancer/liquid-biopsy-startup-freenome-using-recently-raised-funds-show-clinical-validity-utility.

Regan K, Payne P. From molecules to patients: the clinical applications of translational bioinformatics. Yearb Med Inform. 2015;10:164–9.

Tom Salemi. Akili brings digital therapeutics to pediatrics. Health News. 2016. http://healthegy.com/akili-brings-digital-therapeutics-to-pediatrics/.

Satagopam V, et al. Integration and visualization of translational medicine data for better understanding of human diseases. Big Data. 2016;4(2):97–108. doi:10.1089/big.2015.0057. PMCID: PMC4932659

Scannell JW, et al. Diagnosing the decline in pharmaceutical R&D efficiency. Nat Rev Drug Discov. 2012;1:191–200.

Schumacher A, Collins M, Fisher-Pollard M Rujan T (2016) Efficient genomic profiling of patients: the benefit of systems interoperability. Featured Article. doi: 10.13140/RG.2.1.3093.4648.

Natalie Sherman. WellDoc announces investment, collaboration with Johnson & Johnson. The Baltimore Sun. 2017. http://www.baltimoresun.com/business/bs-bz-welldoc-johnson-20160301-story.html.

Sliwoski G, et al. Computational methods in drug discovery. Pharmacol Rev. 2014;66(1):334–95. doi:10.1124/pr.112.007336. Published online 2014 Jan. https://www.ncbi.nlm.nih.gov/pmc/articles/PMC3880464/

Bernadette Tansey. Chrono therapeutics scores $47.6M to advance anti-smoking system. Xconomy. 2016. http://www.xconomy.com/san-francisco/2016/09/09/chrono-therapeutics-scores-47-6-m-to-advance-anti-smoking-system/.

The Economist. Will artificial intelligence help to crack biology?. The Economist. 2017. http://www.economist.com/news/science-and-technology/21713828-silicon-valley-has-squidgy-worlds-biology-and-disease-its-sights-will.

Luke Timmerman. Akili interactive seeks to make video games that heal, not harm. Xconomy. 2012. http://www.xconomy.com/san-francisco/2012/03/14/akili-interactive-seeks-to-make-video-games-that-heal-not-harm/via@xconomy.

Tollman P, et al. Identifying R&D outliers. Nat Rev Drug Discov. 2011;10:653–4.

valuatePharma®. World Preview 2015, Outlook to 2020. valuatePharma® (June 2015). http://info.evaluategroup.com/rs/607-YGS-364/images/wp15.pdf.

Vanhaelen Q, et al. Design of efficient computational workflows for in silico drug repurposing. Drug Discov Today. 2017;22(2):211–22.

Viceconti M, Henney A, Morley-Fletcher E. In silico clinical trials: how computer simulation will transform the biomedical industry. Brussels: Avicenna Consortium. 2016. DOI: 10.13140/RG.2.1.2756.6164.

Viceconti M, et al. In silico clinical trials: how computer simulation will transform the biomedical industry international. J Clin Trials. 2016;3(2) doi:10.18203/2349-3259.ijct20161408. http://www.ijclinicaltrials.com/index.php/ijct/article/view/105

Wanichthanarak K, et al. Genomic, proteomic, and metabolomic data integration strategies. Biomark Insights. 2015;10(Suppl 4):1–6. doi:10.4137/BMI.S29511. https://www.ncbi.nlm.nih.gov/pmc/articles/PMC4562606/. Published online 2015 Sep 7

Eric Wicklund. Is digital therapeutics the next big thing in mHealth?. mHealthIntelligence. 2016. http://mhealthintelligence.com/news/mhealth-spotlight-set-to-shine-on-digital-therapeutics.

Woodie A. Accelerating drug discovery with machine learning on big medical data. Datanami. 2015.; http://www.datanami.com/2015/09/24/accelerating-drug-discovery-with-machine-learning-on-big-medical-data.

Zhang G, et al. Integration of metabolomics and transcriptomics revealed a fatty acid network exerting growth inhibitory effects in human pancreatic cancer. Clin Cancer Res. 2013; doi:10.1158/1078-0432.CCR-13-0209. http://clincancerres.aacrjournals.org/content/19/18/4983. Published September 2013

Chapter 16
Biodesign for Digital Health

Bronwyn Harris, Lyn Denend, and Dan E. Azagury

Abstract The biodesign innovation process developed by Stanford Biodesign emphasizes the importance of starting with a well-characterized, compelling clinical need before focusing on the development of any solution. While the initial solutions that emerged from the Stanford Biodesign Innovation Fellowship were traditional medical devices, in the past three to 5 years there has been an increase in solutions related to digital health. This shift from addressing medical needs entirely with traditional medical devices to a mixture of devices and digital solutions reflects the changing healthcare landscape within which care is migrating from the hospital to alternate, more affordable environments. It also shows the timelessness and broad applicability of the biodesign innovation process, which is technology agnostic. By requiring innovators to start with a well-defined clinical need rather than any preconceived invention ideas, the process allows for many different types of solutions to emerge as new care paradigms become possible through the application of emerging technologies. This chapter focuses primarily on the first two stages—*Identify* and *Invent*.

Keywords Biodesign • Innovation • Design process • Needs finding • Medical • Digital health • Brainstorming • Concept generation • Identify • Invent • Implement

B. Harris, M.D.
Stanford University School of Medicine, 300 Pasteur Drive, H3680A, Stanford, CA 94305-5655, USA

L. Denend, M.B.A.
Stanford Byers Center for Biodesign, Stanford, CA 94305-5655, USA

D.E. Azagury, M.D. (✉)
Stanford University School of Medicine, 300 Pasteur Drive, H3680A, Stanford, CA 94305-5655, USA

Stanford Byers Center for Biodesign, Stanford, CA 94305-5655, USA
e-mail: dazagury@stanford.edu

© Springer International Publishing AG 2018
H. Rivas, K. Wac (eds.), *Digital Health*, Health Informatics,
https://doi.org/10.1007/978-3-319-61446-5_16

16.1 History of Biodesign

In 1998 a group of Stanford University faculty, led by Paul Yock, MD, started the Medical Device Network to host seminars and workshops to support faculty and students interested in the development of medical technologies. This network evolved into Stanford Biodesign, whose preliminary mission includes launching a university-based medtech fellowship at Stanford. Josh Makower, MD led development of the Biodesign Innovation Fellowship. The fellowship is a one-year full-time program, which had its first cohort of fellows start in 2001. Fellows with diverse backgrounds are recruited in order to build multidisciplinary teams. A typical team will include physicians and engineers but also fellows with a business or computer science background.

Over time, Stanford Biodesign expanded from just a fellowship to also teaching graduate and undergraduate courses about the biodesign innovation process. The first company initiated based on work from Biodesign students/fellows during their time in the program was founded in 2002. As of June 2016, forty-one companies have been founded out of the program. Collectively, these companies have treated more than 500,000 patients and raised over $370 million in funding. The first digital health company from Stanford Biodesign was incorporated in 2006: iRhythm technologies created the Zio wearable patch to diagnose arrhythmias, which is associated with algorithm-based analytics and a service component to give providers usable information. Since then, four additional projects initiated during the Biodesign Innovation Fellowship are now actively being pursued and are focused on digital health solution. Despite these commercial achievements, the mission of Biodesign is and remains that of a teaching program. This is illustrated by the mission statement, which is grounded squarely in "educating and empowering health technology innovators" (Yock et al. 2015; Biodesign Timeline & History [Internet] 2016).

The biodesign innovation process emphasizes the importance of a well-characterized, compelling clinical need, before focusing on any solution. While the initial solutions identified from the Biodesign Fellowship were typical medical devices, in the past 3 years there has been an increase in the solutions related to digital health. This shift from addressing medical needs with all conventional medical devices to a mixture of devices and digital solutions reflects the changing landscape. It shows the timelessness of the Biodesign process, which starts with a well-defined clinical need, and the solutions will naturally evolve over time as technology changes. This process can be valuable for all innovators in the medical space and anyone can be an innovator.

16.2 Overview

The biodesign innovation process is made of up three phases that are roughly sequential, but often require iteration. The first is the *Identify* phase, which involves identifying many clinical needs and then, through a rigorous screening process,

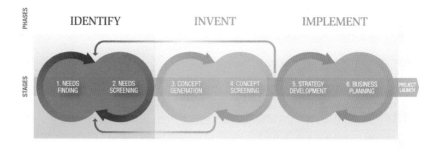

Fig. 16.1 The biodesign innovation process. Reprinted with permission from Cambridge University Press

selecting the top few to advance into invention. The *Invent* phase is when concepts are generated and the top concept is selected based on the most promising overall risk profile. And finally, the *Implement* phase is when strategic and business planning occur in parallel with technical development in preparation for an eventual product launch. These phases are further divided into six stages as shown in Fig. 16.1.

The following sections provide a high-level description of key activities within each of six stages of the biodesign innovation process. Emphasis for the purpose of this chapter is placed on the first four stages, with only a brief summary of the final phase of *Implement*. For more information and specific examples about any of these stages, particularly the last two, please refer to the textbook—Biodesign: The Process of Innovating Medical Technologies (Yock et al. 2015).

16.3   Identify: Needs Finding

The crucial first step in the biodesign innovation process is to identify a compelling clinical need. Identifying an important clinical needs sounds like it should be easy and obvious—why not just ask a physician "what is your biggest problem?" and then move to solve it. However, needs finding is not a simple process and getting it right takes practice and discipline. While it is important to talk to providers, keep in mind that they can be ingrained in the way things currently are done. It is often difficult for them to step back and identify the root of specific problems or even realize that they have some major problems that could potentially be handled differently.

It can be overwhelming to start needs finding, so first identifying a strategic focus can help to initiate this effort. A strategic focus helps the innovator chart a course based on his/her individual mission, goals, and competencies. For example, if an innovator is passionate about children, has a background and/or connections in this field, and/or feels strongly that there should be more solutions designed specifically for this vulnerable patient population, it would be natural to start needs finding in pediatrics. Note that a strategic focus are can also be chosen by a team, with the members jointly evaluating their mission, goals, and competencies to identify common areas of interest, as well as how their strengths and weaknesses may complement one another.

With a specific focus area in mind, an innovator should conduct background research to become knowledgeable in the space. This research is more than just a superficial look. Using the example of pediatrics, it would be important to understand common diseases in the field, the most costly procedures or conditions (some disease, while not common, are extremely expensive), frequent causes of hospitalization, typical pain points for families when seeking care for their child, and other such factors that point to potential innovation opportunities. This research will hopefully lead the innovator to a few particular areas within pediatrics in which to initially focus.

Once this background research is completed the next step is to perform direct observations. If asthma was identified via the background research as a common (and costly) disease within pediatrics, the innovator should seek to visit clinics where asthmatic children are typically diagnosed and treated. S/he should also attempt to observe interactions by the many providers who care for these patients, including general pediatricians, pulmonologists, and allergists to gain a complete picture of the current state of care and the potential problems that these different providers face. Similarly, it is not enough to observe only in the clinic environment. It is important to try to immerse oneself in all care settings, which could include in the pulmonary function lab, emergency room, hospital, and the child's home where routine care is delivered. During these observations the innovator should be looking for specific events that seem problematic. Common "clues" include events where the outcome is not what was expected, the patient or provider experiences uncertainty or fear, or costs are especially high. After each problematic event is observed, the innovator should seek to determine if it was a rare event and/or specific to a particular individual, or if it is a recurring issue that can be seen across different providers, healthcare organizations, and patients, which could mean that it is a true innovation opportunity.

While the innovator is conducting multiple observations and identifying dozens (if not hundreds) of potential problems, s/he can generalize these observations by crafting a need statement from each one. A need statement has three essential components—problem, population, and outcome. For example, the innovator may have observed a patient with congestive heart failure who was admitted to the hospital due to fluid overload. During questioning, it was discovered that the patient had stopped taking his prescribed medications. A need statement crafted from this observation could be, "A way to improve medication compliance (problem) in patients with congestive heart failure (population) that results in decreased hospital admissions (outcome)". Converting an observation into a need statement is an important step, because the need statement makes it clear what issue must be addressed (the problem), the target audience for the intervention (population), and how an improved approach would be measured/assessed (outcome). From a single observation, the innovator may create many different need statements. Taking a preliminary need statement and changing it to evaluate different options for each of the three components is called "needs scoping." For instance, the example need statement given above could be changed to address a more specific patient population if it was clear that part of reason for the medication non-compliance was due to forgetfulness in the elderly. This need statement might read, "A way to improve medication compliance in patients over seventy years of age with congestive heart failure that results in decreased hospital admissions". Alternatively, the outcome could be changed to not just look at hospital admissions, but also to evaluate overall healthcare costs which could also include emergency room visits and clinic visit (Yock et al. 2015).

16.4 Identify: Needs Screening

While it is appealing to find a good clinical need and quickly begin inventing, it is essential for innovators to remain disciplined and carefully evaluate their needs before choosing the most promising one to solve. The needs screening stage of the biodesign innovation process requires innovators to conduct progressively detailed research and compare their needs side-by-side against one another such that the best opportunities rise to the top. There is not one specific formula or method for needs screening, but four key factors should be evaluated as part of this stage—disease state fundamentals, existing solutions, stakeholders, and market analysis.

The first step in needs screening is going back to researching the disease state fundamentals, this time to an even deeper level than was required prior to clinical observations. There are six key areas that should be addressed for each need during this research—epidemiology, anatomy and physiology, pathophysiology, clinical presentation, clinical outcomes and economic impact.

In parallel, it is essential to understand the landscape of existing solutions available to address the problem. The innovator should consider all of the different types of available solutions. For example, with the problem of medication non-compliance, the innovator should explore the strengths and weaknesses of solutions ranging from a piece of paper with instructions and various pill boxes, to combination pills (that allow the patient to take fewer pills), to digital solutions with text reminders. It is also important to also look at emerging solutions so as not to risk being "blindsided" by new approaches that may come to market later in the biodesign innovation process once the innovator begins inventing. Using all of the information gathered, the innovator can create a solution landscape map that combines the disease state and solution research in a pictorial format, making it easy to see competitively crowded areas versus more "open" areas of opportunity.

Stakeholder analysis is another crucial aspect of needs screening that requires the innovator to identify all of the parties involved in addressing each need—this includes both delivering and financing care. Patients and medical providers (ranging from physicians to nurses) are obvious stakeholders and usually the ones that are considered first, but these are rarely the only key players in any given need area. Other examples of stakeholders include family members, patient advocacy groups, professional societies (which can be particularly important when new reimbursement codes may be required), facility administrators, public or private payers, governments, and/or non-governmental organizations. For any specific need area or condition, it is important to think about the entire cycle of care. It is often helpful to map out all of the care facilities, providers, and reasons for medical visits to ensure that all stakeholders have been identified. Another technique is to follow the flow of payments between patients, providers, and facilities to ensure that no stakeholders are overlooked. After identifying the stakeholders, the innovator should assess how a new solution or approach would potentially affect each one: what role each stakeholder might play in delivering a new solution, how each would benefit (or not), which stakeholders would have most to lose if a different approach was adopted, and what the primary "costs" would be (e.g., loss of revenue from fewer procedures or visits, time for providers to learn something new, dynamics associated with changing the venue of care, etc.). This analysis will help the innovator anticipate how receptive or resistant key stakeholders may be to new solutions.

Market analysis helps the innovator estimate the size of the available market associated with each specific need. Importantly, a bigger market does not automatically mean it is better than a smaller one. Other factors, including the costs of bringing a solution to market and how easy/difficult it will be to access the target market, must also be considered above and beyond the size of the market opportunity. The market size estimation is initially very imprecise and will become more and more accurate over the duration of the project with and multiple iterations and increasing data. The innovator can develop a market landscape by looking at the total market and see which segments of the market are available solutions. One approach is to create a map that shows how available and emerging solutions perform on two key criteria: cost and effectiveness. Such a map will help the innovator see potential gaps—opportunities where a new solution with a specific cost/performance profile could address unmet demand. From here, the innovator can make an initial broad assumption about what sort of market penetration may be possible relatively to the rest of the competitive landscape to estimate the market size and growth potential for a new solution to the need. Markets are usually heterogeneous and, as a result, market segmentation—identifying factors that can divide the market into progressively smaller, more homogenous groups that can benefit from a single intervention, will help to identify the most promising initial target market for the innovator to pursue. An example on this type of market segmentation, done by evaluating multiple factors is shown in Fig. 16.2.

Gathering all of the information described above for dozens of needs is no small undertaking. But it is necessary for the innovator to be able to objectively and thoroughly compare his/her needs statements and identify the most promising innovation opportunity. This exercise is accomplished through a comparative filtering approach called "needs selection." As defined in the biodesign innovation process, innovators perform needs selection by choosing various criteria and letting the needs "compete" against them. Common criteria that are considered during need selection include market size, patient impact, provider impact, the competitiveness of the solution landscape, and the presence of stakeholder

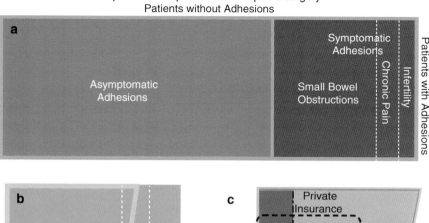

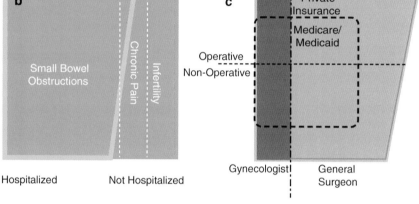

Fig. 16.2 Market segmentation when evaluating a need related to small bowel obstruction and adhesions in the abdomen or pelvis. (**a**) Segmented by symptoms, (**b**) segmented by symptoms and location, (**c**) segmented by provider, operative/non-operative and insurance (courtesy of Andrew Mesher)

support/resistance for new solutions in the need area. Needs selection is an iterative process, with more general criteria used to eliminate the first round of needs and then more detailed, specific criteria used to get to the top few. Importantly, additional research maybe required during the needs selection process to ensure that all needs are being fairly evaluated and ranked. When performing this additional research, innovators should not just rely on literature searches, they should speak directly with stakeholders to validate their research findings. The more someone learns about a clinical need, the deeper he/she can delve into questions when talking to stakeholders. In addition to the criteria discussed above, the team's preferences for what they want to work on and what fits well with their strengths are also important. Figure 16.3 shows one team's example needs screening process, including objective criteria ranked and score generated, but also team specifics, including each team member getting a "kill vote", which removes one need from the list.

Rank	Need statement	Current market size	Competitive /Treatment landscape	Patient impact	Provider impact	Hospital impact	Payer impact	Average Stakeholder	Raw Score	Weighted Score	Kill Vote	Team strengths	Insight
1	A way to diagnose and determine the cause of obstructive sleep apnea in high risk patients to improve specific treatment efficacy.	4	5	4	3	3	3	3.0	22.0	13.0		1	2
2	A way to treat intermittent claudication (Rutherford classification 1–3) in patients with peripheral artery disease to improve pain-free walking distance.	4	5	3	4	3	4	3.7	23.0	12.0		2	1
3	A way to increase adherence to medication use in CHF out-patients to decrease health care cost from non-compliance.	4	4	4	3	4	4	3.7	22.0	11.0		1	1
4	A way to decrease time to complete enrollment in clinical trials to reduce cost of drug/device development.	5	3	3	4	3	4	3.7	22.0	11.0	x	1	0
5	A way to treat gastroesophageal reflux disease refractory to best medical therapy to reduce high grade dysplasia.	4	3	4	4	3	3	3.3	21.0	11.0		1	1
6	A way to prevent deep vein thromboses in patients undergoing abdominal operations to increase therapy adherence(>77%).	4	3	4	3	3	3	3.3	21.0	11.0	x	1	0
7	A way to administer medications to reduce catheter-related blood-stream infections.	4	3	4	3	4	2	3.3	21.0	11.0		0	2
8	A way to treat obstructive sleep apnea in patients 30-60 years old to improve treatment ESS by at least 3.83.	4	3	4	3	2	4	3.0	20.0	11.0		0	2
9	A way to reduce incidence of falls in individuals at home over 65 years to reduce fractures.	4	2	4	4	2	4	3.3	20.0	11.0		1	0
10	A way to treat paroxysmal atrial fibrillation that improves freedom from atrial fibrillation at 1 year (>70-80%).	4	3	4	4	3	2	3.3	20.0	10.0		1	1
11	A way to treat oropharyngeal dysphagia in patients who have suffered a stroke that reduces the incidence of aspiration.	3	3	3	4	3	4	3.3	20.0	10.0		0	0
12	A way to improve the breastfeeding experience that raises the rate of breastfeeding at 6 months to greater than 44%.	3	3	3	4	3	3	3.7	20.0	9.0		1	1
13	A way to coordinate inpatient services to improve resource utilization.	3	2	4	4	4	2	3.7	20.0	9.0	x	1	0
14	A way to improve oxygen supply/demand in post-myocardial infarction patients that improves treatment adherence to at least 45%.	3	3	3	3	4	3	3.3	19.0	9.0		1	0
15	A way to screen pediatric patients and exclude those who do not have an anatomic cardiac abnormality to reduce unnecessary referrals.	3	2	2	3	4	3	3.3	18.0	8.0		0	0
16	A way to detect post-operative wound infections in post-discharge lower extremity vascular procedures to reduce incidence of readmission (<15%).	3	2	3	3	4	3	3.3	18.0	8.0		0	0

Fig. 16.3 Example of needs screening, standard parameters and then the last three individualized to the team. Courtesy of Todd Murphy, William Kethman, Frank Wang and Bronwyn Harris

Once the long list of needs have been screened and the top few have been identified, the innovator's last step before finally beginning to invent is to define need criteria. Need criteria are developed based on what has been learned through all of the research conducted to date. They outline the key requirements that *any* solution to a need must address to have the greatest likelihood of satisfying important stakeholders and convincing them to adopt a new approach. These criteria, which can be organized into "must-have" and "nice-to-have" requirements, are then used to guide the invention process such that the resulting technology has a meaningful chance of improving on the existing standard of care. Accordingly, need criteria should be as specific and measureable as possible to be useful during invention (Yock et al. 2015).

16.5 Needs Selection Case Study: Night Terrors

16.5.1 Identify

While scheduling times to perform observations in specific venues is a great way to identify needs, they also can be identified at any time or place. One of the innovators on a team in the Biodesign Innovation Fellowship witnessed his nephew having night terrors—an event that occurs during sleep where the child appears awake, screaming and crying, but is in fact fast asleep. These events were very disturbing to the entire family, significantly affecting every family member's sleep and their quality of life. As a result of this experience, the fellow came up with the need statement "a way to treat night terrors in children in order to decrease parental concern and nights without night awakening".

During needs selection, the team compared this need to other need statements, including ones addressing adhesive capsulitis, compartment syndrome, and ventilator-associated pneumonia. During disease state research about night terrors the team learned more about what a night terror is, and their incidence. Additionally, despite the common medical teaching that there is nothing that can be done about these events, the team found an article in the medical literature that discussed a small study that showed it is possible to treat night terrors. The team believed that this finding, along with the fact that there were no existing solutions for the condition, to be encouraging and helped to keep this need at the top of their list of potential projects to pursue. The primary stakeholders for a new solution in this space were the parents, since they made treatment decisions and were particularly concerned about the effect of night terrors on their children. The team's market analysis involved looking into parent's awareness of the problem and exploring their willingness to pay for a potential solution to night terrors.

16.5.2 Invent and Implement

The team decided to press forward with this need and founded Lully to develop and commercial their technology to help eliminate night terrors. The technology was validated in a study that demonstrated an 80% reduction in night terrors when used for an 8-week period. The technology was reduced to practice through an under-the-mattress vibrating pod and a smartphone application, and launched as the Sleep Guardian. The Sleep Guardian did not require regulatory clearance allowing Lully to expeditiously bring its product to market. It is positioned a consumer health product and is sold direct-to-consumer through e-commerce channels.

16.6 Invent: Concept Generation

Next comes the fun part—inventing! With a well-defined, well-validated clinical need and well-researched need criteria, the invention portion of the process significantly more likely to be fruitful. Up until this point in the biodesign innovation process, the innovator has been research oriented and logic driven. In contrast, inventing involves letting go of conventional thinking and allowing one's mind to wander. That said, innovators are well served to carefully prepare for each brainstorming session to make the creative process more productive. In addition to referring to the needs statement and need criteria, it is helpful to include a diverse group of participants who can represent multiple perspectives, prepare multiple prompts to stimulate the group's creative thinking, and provide props that can be used to give ideas a physical form. A book written by Tom Kelley, general manager of IDEO, entitled *The Art of Innovation*, gives detailed description of how to conduct effective brainstorming sessions (Kelley et al. 2001). He discusses the importance of the atmosphere and encouraging wild ideas. The number of ideas matter, so Kelley recommends numbering them during the session as motivation, and he suggests encouraging participants to build on each other ideas. He also discusses things that should be avoided in a brainstorming session, such as having a boss speak first, making people wait for their turn, including people all with the same background, or not allowing silly ideas.

Brainstorming may not come naturally to everyone, but people generally get better and more comfortable with it through practice. Tina Seeling, who teaches courses on innovation and entrepreneurship at Stanford University, has written extensively on creativity. She believes that everyone can become more creative and describes various tools and techniques to help people and organizations do so. One approach for unleashing creativity, she says, is to positively affect six key factors: your knowledge, imagination, attitude, resources, culture, and habitat (Seelig 2015).

When brainstorming, it is important to think of all possible solutions for a given clinical need rather than constraining ideation to only the types of solutions the innovator is interested in pursuing (e.g., digital health solutions or a solution that doesn't require regulatory approval). By exploring a full range of ideas, the innovator reduces the risk of overlooking a solution that s/he might not be interested in pursuing but could results in a better overall solution. This leaves the door open to competitors who may ultimately bring forward a superior offering. At this stage, the only constraints that should be considered are the need criteria. Each idea should be evaluated against the need criteria. If it does meet all of the innovator's must-have criteria (and many of the nice-to-have requirements), it should be set aside. Alternatively, the innovator can take the idea back into brainstorming to see how it can be modified to better address the need criteria. Importantly, solution ideas can be modified to address the need criteria, but need criteria should not be adjusted to align with a solution unless the innovator goes back into research mode and identifies that s/he made an error in the initial research.

16.7 Invent: Concept Screening

After multiple brainstorming sessions, hundreds of solution concepts can be identified, ranging from realistic to outlandish. Even after evaluating all of the solution concepts for a need against the need criteria, the innovator is likely to have dozens of possible solutions ideas for any given need. To further screen these ideas and eventually select the most promising solution to take forward to the market, the innovator performance a set of activities referred to as concept screening. There are five major risk factors to evaluate for each solution ideas—intellectual property, regulatory pathway, reimbursement landscape, business model, and technical feasibility.

When evaluating intellectual property, it is important to have a clear understanding of patentability and freedom to operate for a solution idea. Obtaining patent protection in digital health can be more difficult than in traditional medical devices. In particular, recent changes in U.S. Patent and Trademark Office (USPTO) policies have made it more difficult to get protection for certain types of software-related technologies. There are high costs of obtaining patents, but it can be a valuable competitive barrier. Innovators working with digital health concepts should perform an invention audit, where they assess which innovations should be protected by a patent versus a trade secret or no protection. Innovations that should be protected by a patent are ones that provide a competitive advantage, are clearly different from current practice, are easy to reverse engineer, and can be detected if a competitor copies the invention. When pursuing patents, think about design in addition to the technical features of an idea. For example, Apple obtains patents purely on the physical design of their products, as well as their user interfaces. There is a low likelihood of getting a patent granted if it purely focuses on the data used (classified as e-commerce), while the likelihood is much higher if the patent focuses on the underlying technology (Capron and Wells 2016). There was a Supreme Court ruling in *Alice v. CLS Bank* in 2014 about patent eligibility, which ruled that a patent cannot be obtained on an abstract idea that is implemented as software. This ruling has significantly reduced the patents allowed in the e-commerce area. Examples of patents that were successful include Glooko's patent that have inventive concepts and are using specific mathematical data manipulation (Bender 2016).

Understanding the regulatory pathway for a concept idea is important because it reveals a great deal about the timeline and pathway to market—how long it will take and how much funding will be needed. The regulatory authority of the U.S. Food and Drug Administration (FDA) is very broad. In addition to food and drugs, they regulate medical devices ranging from simple items like tongue depressors to complex technologies such as pacemakers. The FDA is different than the Consumer Product Safety Commission (CPSC), which ensures the safety of consumer products (Administration USF and D 2016). As of Fall 2016, the FDA does not regulate low-risk general wellness devices. They define general wellness as "products that meet the following two factors: 1—are intended for only general wellness use, as defined in this guidance, and 2—present a low risk to the safety of users and other persons. General wellness products may include exercise equipment, audio recordings, video games, software programs and other products that are commonly, though not exclusively, available from retail establishments (including online retailers and distributors that offer software to be directly downloaded), when consistent with the two factors above" (U.S. Department of Health and Human Services Food and Drug Administration 2016). Further they stipulate that a general wellness product must have "1—an intended use that relates to maintaining or encouraging a general state of health or a healthy activity, or 2—an intended use that relates the role of healthy lifestyle with helping to reduce the risk or impact of certain chronic diseases or conditions and where it is well understood and accepted that healthy lifestyle choices may play an important role in health outcomes for the disease or condition" (U.S. Department of Health and Human Services Food and Drug Administration 2016). The current guidance from the FDA regarding mobile medical applications is that a majority of them are not medical devices and therefore not regulated by the FDA or another subset that may meet the definition of a medical device, but pose a lower risk, so the FDA intends to not enforce requirements. The intended use is what determines where or not a mobile medical application is classified as a "device". In general if a mobile application is diagnosing a disease, preventing a disease or performing a treatment then it is a medical device. Examples of mobile applications that are medical devices, but the FDA does not plan to regulate at this time—"Help patients self-manage their disease or conditions without providing specific treatment or treatment suggestions, Provide patients with simple tools to organize and track their health, automate simple tasks for health care providers" (U.S. Food and Drug Administration 2015). As these regulations can and likely will change over time, it is essential to review the most current guidelines from the FDA regarding the concept being evaluated to determine what regulatory process, if any, will be needed. For more details on these matters see chapters 16 (Privacy and Security of Patient information in Digital Health) and 17 (Law aspects of Digital Health).

Concept screening also involves looking at the reimbursement landscape to determine where and how a new solution ideas fits in. A great solution cannot become a business without a payment mechanism to support it. The research done in the needs screening process to identify the stakeholders should help identify the relevant payers, which traditionally have been health insurance companies and government insurance programs such as Medicare. When payment will be coming from health insurance programs it is important to understand the process needed to get reimbursed and how this new solution will fit into the existing reimbursement structure in terms of the coding (a specific code is required for any service provided), coverage (insurers decide what codes they will pay for) and payment. If a code does not already exist for the new potential product, it will be a longer (and therefore more expensive) path to reimbursement. Other payment models exist, including self-pay approaches, which are not uncommon in digital health. In this scenario, the burden and risk of obtaining reimbursement is removed, but the innovator faces other obstacles, including the consumer's willingness to pay out of pocket and the added cost of direct marketing expenditures.

Business model analysis for a concept involves defining how a solution will generate revenue and add value for its intended audience. There are many different types of business models, not all of which are applicable to digital health. Common examples include disposable products, services, fee per use offerings, subscriptions, over-the-counter products, prescription products, and physician-sell products. Mobile health applications typically either target consumers directly or physicians/providers. However, with the new healthcare models involving pay-for-performance (instead of fee-for-service) there is a belief that mobile technologies allowing for remote patient monitoring will be more appealing to healthcare organizations as a way to reduce their overall costs. Therefore other larger providers such as healthcare networks or accountable care organizations (ACO's) for example could become significant clients of these technologies. As an innovator evaluates which business model is most appropriate for a concept under consideration, s/he should validate the preferred approach with prospective customers (patients/providers/payers) to ensure there is a willingness to accept the projected business model and make payments at the level necessary to support the model.

In addition to evaluating each concept in terms of key opportunities and risks related to IP, regulatory, reimbursement, and business model, the innovator must assess the technical feasibility of the solution idea through concept exploration and testing. This involves rapid cycles of prototyping and testing to answer key technical questions and retire the most pressing technical risks. In general, innovators are encouraged to build prototypes early and often. Clearly defined questions about a concept can be answered with a well thought-out prototype. Prototypes can also be used to get feedback from stakeholders. This can include building a simple mobile app and putting it in front of the intended user to gather their input. These early prototypes can even be made with paper and other "crude" materials. The key is to get as much user input as possible to identify any major flaws in a concept.

As the innovator gathers all of this information during concept screening, it can be helpful to create a summary that captures the level of risk for each concept under consideration on the aspects of IP, regulatory, reimbursement, business models, and technical feasibility. Many people use a red/yellow/green rating to indicate high/medium/low risk, example shown in Fig. 16.4. They can then evaluate their concepts side-by-side to identify the one with the most promising overall risk profile. While no concept should be expected to have a green rating on every dimension, the innovator will hopefully have at least one idea that has a combination of mostly green and yellow ratings. For example, if one concept has a red for IP, i.e., a very crowded space where there is likely not freedom to operate, that it would potentially

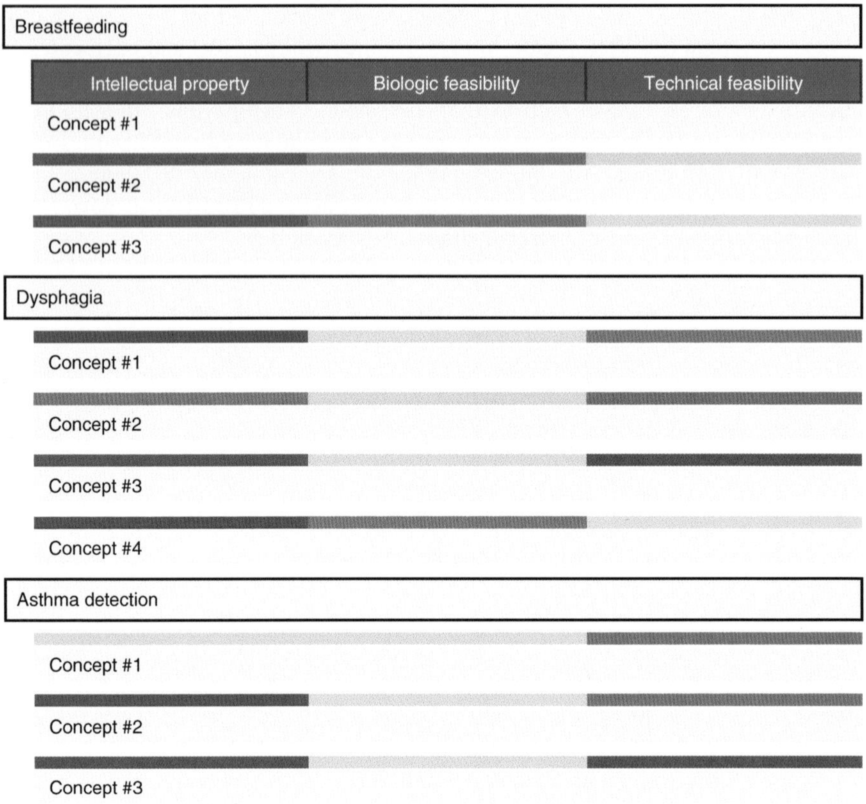

Fig. 16.4 An example where multiple concepts for three different needs are being compared according to intellectual property, biologic and technical feasibility. *Red* high risk, *yellow* medium risk, *green* low risk, *grey* not yet evaluated

be a reason to eliminate that concept. Concepts choosen should be further validated with prospective users and then a final decision made about which one to further develop.

16.8 Concept Generation Case Study: Pediatric Asthma

16.8.1 Identify

During their time as Biodesign Innovation Fellows, a team of innovators was speaking to a pulmonologist about clinical problems and they jointly identified the difficulties providers face in diagnosing asthma and the lack of effective tools for making an accurate diagnosis. The team, which had a specific interest in looking for needs within pediatrics and other underserved populations, went to a pediatric pulmonary clinic to further investigate this need. While in clinic, they spoke to multiple mothers of children with asthma who discussed the challenges of monitoring their children at home, as well as the uncertainty of knowing when their children were getting sick. With additional research into pediatric asthma, the team found that asthma is a chronic and very expensive disease. Multiple medications can be used to control the disease, however, they are often not optimally utilized because the assessment of asthma control is highly subjective. There are few objective indicators of disease status, none of them are reliable in children, and they require active compliance (e.g., the patient must perform a certain activity on a daily basis). Financial analysis indicated that if the disease was better controlled, the total number of exacerbations could be reduced, resulting in a significant cost savings. The need statement they came up with was "A way to monitor and adjust treatment in children with moderate to severe persistent asthma that improves disease control".

16.8.2 Invent

This need statement was taken into a multiple brainstorming sessions. Many ideas came out of the sessions. A few of these general concepts included a passive environmental monitor—a way to identify triggers by tracking data from multiple sources, a sophisticated portable monitor, a wearable monitor, an oral appliance, and a passive bed monitor. These solutions varied greatly, with some more invasive (such as an oral appliance) than others (like a simple tracking application to identify triggers). These concepts were evaluated individually, compared to the needs criteria, and compared to each other. One of the team's must-have need criteria was to create a passive solution, as research clearly showed that adherence to a regimen that requires active daily participation is very low, particularly in children. So this eliminated the portable and wearable monitors. Another must-have was to reduce emergency room utilization by at least 25% relative to other available solutions. It was unclear whether an environmental monitor or trigger identifying application would be able to produce these results. The solutions remaining were an oral appliance and the passive bed monitor. After speaking to children and their families, it was clear that a passive bed monitor would fit much better into their daily lives than an oral appliance. After significantly more detailed research and concept screening, the team decided to move forward with the passive bed monitor idea, *see* Fig. 16.5. They realized that in order to meet the outcome they identified in the need statement—improving disease control, they had to do more than just report values. They decided to

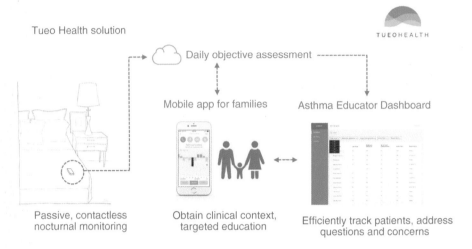

Fig. 16.5 Concept for passive solution to perform monitoring in children with asthma. Courtesy of Tueo Health. *Credits*: The authors would like to acknowledge Todd Murphy for his for his assistance with the case study

provide a service to help families correctly utilize the information and get the outcomes desired. This team has incorporated as Tueo Health and working to implement this solution.

16.9 Implement: Strategy Development and Business Planning

The final phase of the biodesign innovation process is *Implement*. This is the period when the innovator puts concrete plans into place to turn an idea into a business. This phase is very complex and dependent on the specific solution that is being taken forward. As mentioned earlier, a detailed exploration of this last phase is beyond the scope of this chapter and more information is available in the biodesign textbook (Yock et al. 2015). Also, it is rare that the innovators will have expertise in all of the areas necessary, so it is important to rely on outside consultants and/or advisors who can fill in gaps with their prior experiences and knowledge. The work done during the concept screening is a start to now developing more in-depth strategies in the same key areas—intellectual property, regulatory, reimbursement, business planning (marketing, sales and distribution). It will also be important to develop detailed plans for research and development, defining the key technical milestones, and determining how to quickly the address the greatest technical risks. Closely related is clinical strategy, which will help determine what clinical studies are needed to determine a new technology's safety and effectiveness.

16.10 Implement Case Study: Advance Care Planning

16.10.1 Identify and Invent

Vynca is a health information technology company formed by a team out of the Biodesign Innovation Fellowship. During observations in the hospital, the team witnessed multiple individuals with a serious life-limiting illnesses, like advanced, incurable cancer, who were admitted to the intensive care unit and placed on life-sustaining therapies against their wishes. It appeared to be a portability problem of advance care planning documentation that resulted in unwanted and excessive care being delivered. Healthcare providers were not aware of the individual's wishes at the time of the emergency, even if they had completed legal care planning documents. As the team researched the problem further, they recognized many barriers to high quality advanced care planning, including ensuring high quality conversations and accurate documentation. They discovered that up to 87% of paper end-of-life forms were not available in an emergency, (Schmidt et al. 2013) 20% were legally invalid, (Oregon POLST Registry Annual Report [Internet] 2012) and 70% did not accurately reflect all of the patient's wishes (Heyland 2013). From these clinical observations and the team's research they crafted the need statement: "A way to ensure that wishes are honored at the end of life in patients with serious, life-limiting illness, in order to align care preference with care provision". This was an attractive clinical need because there were no other solutions available, no regulatory approval was needed, and all stakeholders—patients, providers and payers—were aligned and would welcome a better solution.

During concept generation for this specific need, the team quickly realized that a digital health solution would be the best way to address this need. The solution the team came up with was a holistic advance care planning solution that is integrated with electronic health records to ensure adoption within the clinical workflow. The team, which founded a company called Vynca, created a technology that helps patients and healthcare providers have meaningful conversations about care preferences, document patient wishes accurately, and most importantly provides real time access to this critical information throughout the care continuum.

16.10.2 Implement

The strategy development for this information technology solution was different than a conventional medical device. While intellectual property is often not emphasized as much in digital health, it is valuable to be able to protect at least some aspects of the solution. The Vynca team was able to develop intellectual property around their system and the method of health information exchange and specific user features. In terms of regulation, their solution did not require (FDA) regulatory clearance, which allowed them to get to market quicker. However, other stringent regulations such as the ones related to the handling of protected health information (HIPAA) were critical and needed to be addressed early on. From a business strategy perspective, the team realized that the primary stakeholders for their solution are the providers who, in turn, would make the technology available to patients, so targeting enterprises would be a more fruitful sales pathway than trying to secure patient-by-patient reimbursement. This strategy also allowed them to tailor their product individually to each health system, ensuring that their specific needs were met. They implemented with one flagship customer, Oregon Health & Science University, a national leader in advanced care planning before expanding to other organizations.

16.11   Conclusion

After reading this chapter, an innovator should have a better understanding of a structured process that can be used to identify important clinical needs, decide which ones to work on and then invent for those clinical needs. This chapter could not comprehensively cover all aspects of this process, so for more detail please refer to the Biodesign textbook (Yock et al. 2015). While the overall biodesign innovation process does not change over time, the digital healthcare landscape and related regulations and patent issues are rapidly changing, so innovators will need to ensure they use the most up-to-date information and counseling on these matters. Now go and invent something great, but first make sure you are working to solve an important clinical need!

Acknowledgements   The authors would like to acknowledge Ryan Van Wert, Rush Bartlett and Frank Wang of Vynca for their assistance with the case study.

References

Administration USF and D. What does the FDA regulate [Internet]. 2016 [cited 2016 Jul 27]. Available from: http://www.fda.gov/AboutFDA/Transparency/Basics/ucm194879.htm.
Bender B. Intangible Assets in Digital Health [Internet]. 2016 [cited 2016 Aug 13]. Available from: https://www.linkedin.com/pulse/intangible-assets-digital-health-brian-bender.
Biodesign Timeline & History [Internet]. 2016 [cited 2016 Jul 8]. Available from: http://biodesign.stanford.edu/about-us/timeline.html.
Capron A, Wells R. How digital health startups can leverage intellectual property. Boston, MA: HIT Consultant; 2016.
Heyland DK. Failure to engage hospitalized elderly patients and their families in advance care planning. JAMA. 2013;173(9):778. Available from: http://www.ncbi.nlm.nih.gov/pubmed/23545563\nhttp://archinte.jamanetwork.com/article.aspx?doi=10.1001/jamainternmed.2013.180.
Kelley T, Littman J, Peters T. The art of innovation: lessons in creativity from IDEO, America's leading design firm. 1st ed. London: Crown Business; 2001.

Oregon POLST Registry Annual Report [Internet]. 2012 [cited 2016 Aug 13]. Available from: http://www.orpolstregistry.org/wp-content/uploads/2013/04/Oregon-POLST-Registry-Annual-Report_2012_FINAL_electronic.pdf.

Schmidt TA, Olszewski EA, Zive D, Fromme EK, Tolle SW. The oregon physician orders for life-sustaining treatment registry: a preliminary study of emergency medical services utilization. J Emerg Med. 2013;44(4):796–805. doi:10.1016/j.jemermed.2012.07.081.

Seelig T. InGenius: a crash course on creativity. New York: HarperOne; 2015.

U.S. Department of Health and Human Services Food and Drug Administration. General wellness: policy for low risk devices [Internet]. 2016 [cited 2016 Jul 29]. Available from: http://www.fda.gov/downloads/medicaldevices/deviceregulationandguidance/guidancedocuments/ucm429674.pdf.

U.S. Food and Drug Administration. Mobile medical applications [Internet]. 2015 [cited 2016 Jul 27]. Available from: http://www.fda.gov/downloads/MedicalDevices/.../UCM263366.pdf.

Yock P, Zenios S, Makower J, Brinton T, Kumar U, Watkins FTJ, et al. Biodesign: the process of innovating medical technologies. 2nd ed. New York: Cambridge University Press; 2015.

Chapter 17
Enhancing Clinical Performance and Improving Patient Safety Using Digital Health

Mitchell G. Goldenberg and Teodor P. Grantcharov

Abstract Patient confidentiality has remained a central issue in the current "big data" era of healthcare. Protections such as the Health Insurance Portability and Accountability Act of 1996 (HIPAA) exist to ensure that digital personal health information (PHI) are legally secure from threats and breaches that would threaten confidentiality. To be compliant with HIPAA regulations, steps must be taken by health care providers and digital health platforms, and these fall under the Privacy Rule, which outlines appropriate uses and disclosures of PHI, and the Security Rule, which lays out with granularity the steps that must be taken to adhere to the HIPAA regulations. Through deliberate design of secure digital health platforms, we can use technological advances in the collection, measurement, and delivery of health care to advance care and improve patient safety. Renewed efforts to optimize and standardize health care delivery has facilitated the implementation of electronic and digital health solutions that benefit medical and surgical training and efficiency while minimizing harm to patients. Cross-industry innovations such as the OR Black Box® will allow us to accomplish these lofty goals. Finally, we must strive to include patients in this digital health movement, as now more than ever we can create knowledge translation solutions that ensure that patients understand their health in a meaningful way.

Keywords Digital health • Patient privacy • Black box • Patient safety • Surgical technology

M.G. Goldenberg, M.B.B.S. • T.P. Grantcharov, M.D., Ph.D., F.A.C.S. (✉)
International Centre for Surgical Safety, Keenan Centre for Biomedical Science,
St. Michael's Hospital, University of Toronto, Toronto, Canada
e-mail: grantcharovt@smh.ca

© Springer International Publishing AG 2018   235
H. Rivas, K. Wac (eds.), *Digital Health*, Health Informatics,
https://doi.org/10.1007/978-3-319-61446-5_17

17.1 What Is the Health Insurance Portability and Accountability Act?

As the world of modern healthcare continues to move toward the use of "Big Data" to guide research and policy-making, it is imperative that systems are developed to not only facilitate analysis of multiplatform data on a large scale, but also ensure that this confidential patient information is kept secure in its transfer and storage. With the introduction of widespread electronic health records (EHR) use in most contemporary health care settings, there has been a subsequent explosion in the availability of raw population-level data (Services DOHAH 2012). The EHR captures demographic, economic, and outcomes-based information, and this heterogeneity has driven stakeholders to create novel and robust methods of analysis that can account for this inherent diversity (Murdoch and Detsky 2013). The concept that Big Data can be used as a measure of healthcare delivery quality is embodied by the National Surgical Quality Improvement Program (NSQIP), (Berwick 2015) which uses a collation of EHR data from 400 United States hospitals in particular to measure hospital outcomes in patient safety. Big Data also has the potential to be used as a means of creating standards in the prevalence of patient morbidity, by accounting for case-mix variation at a hospital-by-hospital level (Bohnen et al. 2016). The use of large-scale, real-world information to drive decision making is important in health care, and this chapter will discuss both the use of clinical data in quality improvement, as well as measures in place to protect its use. We will begin by discussing the Health Insurance Portability and Accountability Act of 1996 (HIPAA) and its implications in the growing field of digital health.

The HIPAA was passed as a two-part Act of The United States Congress, signed by President Bill Clinton in 1996. The second part of the bill, known as the Administrative Simplification (AS) provisions, created a mandate for the Department of Health & Human Services (HHS) to create privacy and security laws regarding the use and transmission of personal health information (PHI) in clinical medicine and research (Nass et al. 2009). The AS provisions contain two primary 'rules' which concern the protection of health data. The first of these, termed *Standards for Privacy of Individually Identifiable Health Information*, or "Privacy Rule" is a set of published standards relating to the disclosure of sensitive patient information (Services UDOHAH 2013). It functions to prevent the disclosure of confidential information by what are called "covered entities," which includes any group that takes part in transactions of PHI (healthcare providers, medical insurers, etc.). It instructs these groups to monitor and ensure that only appropriate employees have access to patient's PHI, and that any disclosures made are as minimal as possible, and only with the patient's consent (Naam and Sanbar 2015; Register 2010). This same rule outlines the exceptions to confidentiality in the United States, for example child abuse and missing person's cases. It further seeks to give the individual control and notice regarding the use and distribution of one's PHI. The second rule outlined by the AS provisions is the *Security Standards for the Protection of Electronic Protected Health Information"*, also called the "Security Rule." This rule relates to the storage and protection of electronic PHI, and serves to standardize security measures around EHR use (Services UDOHAH 2013). Under the security rule, covered entities must maintain the confidentiality, integrity and availability of electronic medical data, and safeguard it against "reasonably anticipated" threats or breaches. It further mandates the need for ongoing risk analysis and management, stating that, "a covered entity regularly reviews its records to track access to e-PHI and detect security incidents, periodically evaluates the effectiveness of security measures put in place, and regularly reevaluates potential risks to electronic PHI (Services UDOHAH 2013)." It also puts forward specific types of protective safeguards that should be employed by a covered entity, including administrative, physical, and technical safeguards. Enforcement of the Security rule is through the Office for Civil Rights (OCR), which is responsible for prosecuting any violations set out in the HIPAA (Stevens 2003). If one's confidentiality is breached by a covered entity, they do not sue the entity based on the HIPAA, rather, they must file a complaint with the OCR in order to trigger an investigation (Nass et al. 2009).

Further action came in 2009, when the Health Information Technology for Economic and Clinical Health Act (HITECH) was passed under the American Recovery and Reinvestment Act. The HITECH contains four "Subtitles," including Subtitle D, a section covering further confidentiality and security regulations around EHR use (Firm 2013). In addition to updating the civil and criminal penalties around breaching PHI, new rules around disclosing a breach in PHI were also implemented, with the HHS issuing guidance around the specifics of keeping information protected to HIPAA levels (Firm 2013). The 2009 update also included rules for "business associates," or those individuals who while not being part of the covered entity, are given access to the data for consultancy purposes. Examples of a business associate as cited by the HHS include a lawyer working for a health plan, or a third party medical transcriptionist (Services UDOHAH 2013). Also included as business associates are those who use eHealth applications or wearable technology (Institute of Medicine (US) Committee 2003). However, not all mobile health applications are covered by HIPAA, including those that collect behavioral and psychometric data from users (Glenn and Monteith 2014). It is important therefore for consumers to understand what the data they provide to third-party software can be used for, including advertising purposes.

17.2 What Makes a Digital Health Platform HIPAA Compliant?

In order for a digital health platform HIPAA compliant, it must satisfy the requirements put forward by the *Security Rule*. Whereas the *Privacy Rule* comprises the principles of use and disclosures of PHI, the Security Rule outlines the measures that must be put in place in order to adequately protect confidential PHI (Bova et al. 2012). However, one important aspect of the Privacy Rule is the Business Associates clause (Institute of Medicine (US) Committee 2003), which as mentioned above, states that a formal contract is needed prior to sharing PHI with a third party that is not part of the covered entity. This is crucial as it is an easily auditable component of your HIPAA compliance and a lack of contractual obligation from a third party to adhere to Privacy Rule guidance is punishable under the HHS.

The Security Rule outlines three main types of "safeguard" that should be implemented in order to ensure the platform is compliant (Services DOHAH 2003). The first are Administrative Safeguards, which according to the HHS are "administrative actions, and policies and procedures, to manage the selection, development, implementation, and maintenance of security measures to protect electronic protected health information and to manage the conduct of the covered entity's workforce in relation to the protection of that information." (Services DOHAH 2003) The Administrative Safeguards are broken down (Table 17.1) into different "Security Standards," which include: Security Management Process, Assigned Security Responsibility, Workforce Security, Information Access Management, Security Awareness and Training, Security Incident Procedures, Contingency Plan, Evaluation, and Business Associate Contracts. These nine Administrative Safeguards contain within them specific implementation requirements, termed "required" and "addressable." The only safeguard which is fully required fall under Security Management Process, which include performing a risk analysis (identifying possible security threats), risk management (reducing vulnerability to a security breach), sanction policy (ensure appropriate sanctions brought on those members of the workforce who fail to follow security procedures) and information system activity review (scheduled review of information systems activity including incident reports). Additionally, three "Contingency Plan" specifications are also deemed mandatory: data backup plan (ensure retrievable electronic copies of medical records), disaster recovery plan (ensure implementable process to restore lost data), and emergency mode operation plan (ability to continue crucial processes in the event of an emergency). All additional specifications listed in Table 17.1 are considered addressable, that is the covered entity must make a determination as to whether this process is *reasonable* and *appropriate* given the operational environment.

The second set of components that ensures a digital health platform is compliant with the Security Rule is the "Physical Safeguards" (Table 17.2). These comprise the "physical measures, policies, and procedures to protect a covered entity's electronic information systems and related buildings and equipment, from natural and environmental hazards, and unauthorized intrusion." (Services DOHAH 2003) The Physical Safeguards are further subcategorized into: Facility Access Controls, Workstation Use, Workstation Security, and Device and Media Controls. The latter contains two "required" specifications. "Disposal" states that all PHI which is to be erased be done in a permanent manner, and "media re-use" ensures that any medium used to store PHI is completely wiped prior to it being re-purposed.

The final set of measures that are put forth in the Security Rule are termed "Technical Safeguards." These comprise five types of technological precautions: Access Controls, Audit Controls, Integrity, Person or Entity Authentication, and Transmission Security (Table 17.3). Adequate technological security is of great importance at a time when cyber-crime continues to evolve in sophistication (Firm 2013). The Security Rule provides a variety safeguards that covered entities can use

Table 17.1 Administrative safeguards in digital health

Administrative safeguard	Description	Implementation specifications
1. Security management process	Internal policies which prevent and protect against security violations	**1. Risk analysis** **2. Risk management** **3. Sanction policy** **4. Information system activity review**
2. Assigned security responsibility	Identification of a individual within the covered entity who will oversee PHI security	None provided
3. Workforce security	Determine which individuals need access to PHI, and ensure they are granted it	1. Authorization and/or supervision 2. Workforce clearance procedure 3. Termination procedures
4. Information access management	The execution of policy for granting access to those individuals needing PHI access	1. Isolating health care clearinghouse functions 2. Access authorization 3. Access establishment and modification
5. Security awareness and training	Ensure all employees and management of covered entity undergoes security training	1. Security reminders 2. Protection from malicious software 3. Log-in monitoring 4. Password management
6. Security incident procedures	Policy and process to address breaches in security practices, covering identification and documentation, and response	None provided
7. Contingency plan	Ensure a policy is in place to respond to system failures, natural disasters, vandalism, etc.	**1. Data backup plan** **2. Disaster recovery plan** **3. Emergency mode operation plan** 4. Testing and revision procedures 5. Applications and data criticality analysis
8. Evaluation	Episodic evaluation of safeguards to ensure policy in place meets the standards set forth by the security rule	None provided
9. Business associate contracts	Ensure written contracts exist between covered entities and third party contractors who will have access to PHI	None provided

bold indicates "required" implementation specifications

for technical protection, but of these only two, "Unique User Identification" and "Emergency Access Procedure," are deemed mandatory. The former instructs covered entities to ensure that each employee and administrator have a unique identification within the electronic information system, both for access security and auditing purposes. The second demands that in an emergency setting (power outage, natural disaster, etc.), access to the electronic PHI is maintained (Services DOHAH 2003).

Table 17.2 Physical safeguards for digital health

Physical safeguards	Description	Implementation specification
Facility access controls	Ensure physical access to HER storage facilities is limited to only those with authorization	1. Contingency operations 2. Facility security plan 3. Access control and validation procedures 4. Maintenance records
Workstation use	Control over the physical properties of a workstation where the EHR is accessed from	None specified
Workstation security	Ensure physical access to workstations is restricted to only those with authorization	None specified
Device and media controls		**1. Disposal** **2. Media Re-use** 3. Accountability 4. Data backup and storage

bold indicates "required" implementation specifications

Table 17.3 Technical safeguards for digital health

Technical safeguard	Description	Implementation specification
Access control	Technical policies that allow PHI access only to those allowed	**1. Unique user identification** **2. Emergency access procedure** 3. Automatic logoff 4. Encryption and decryption
Audit controls	Software that is able to routinely examine activity of an EHR	None specified
Integrity	Prevent unwanted manipulation or destruction of data	1. Mechanism to authenticate electronic protected health information
Person or entity authentication	Verification of employees attempting to access EHR	None specified
Transmission security	Prevent unwanted access to PHI during transmission over an "electronic communications network"	1. Integrity controls 2. Encryption

bold indicates "required" implementation specifications

17.3 How Do We Use Digital Health to Enhance Clinical Performance?

The use of digital health in modern medicine goes beyond the use of technology in medical record keeping. While the EHR has revolutionized modern medicine, there is a multitude of other ways to deploy technology in order to improve our healthcare delivery. According to Eric Topol, author of *The Creative Destruction of Medicine*, digital health is the "…digitization of humans," and through the use of wireless devices, social media, and computer power, we are "...illuminating the human black box" (Topol 2012). In essence, as technology evolves, we are able to capture human metrics in more detail than ever before.

Many examples of how digital healthcare can improve a patient's life are self-evident, from cochlear implants that facilitate hearing, to robots that assist in patient rehabilitation after stroke. We have discussed the EHR and its integral role in modern healthcare, giving stakeholders the ability to rapidly collate large sums of data for quality improvement research. In this chapter however, we will focus on the use of digital data collection in surgery and its use in optimization of healthcare delivery. This is an underexplored field, with recent advances having sent far-reaching ripples through the academic community.

Technology needs to be at the center of quality improvement in surgical care. The most direct way this can be accomplished is through direct improvement of surgeon skill. There are multiple ways in which this can be achieved. As surgery moves from the traditional "open" approach to minimally invasive surgery (MIS), there are more and more procedures being performed with the use of a laparoscope, a small fiber-optic camera that allows the surgeon to see inside a body cavity through an incision only a couple centimeters in width. This use of video-assisted surgery allows for capture of intraoperative, intra-corporeal video. Recording footage from the operating room gives rise to many methods of analysis, from direct assessment and feedback, to tele monitoring and surgical coaching.

Standardized assessment metrics of surgeon technical skill have been used since the mid-1990s. Dr. Richard Reznick's group developed the objective structured assessment of technical skills (OSATS) at the University of Toronto, a simulation-based examination for assessing basic surgical skills (Martin et al. 1997). The introduction of new surgical techniques (laparoscopy, robotics) has demanded the evolution of this type of "global assessment" tool (Vassiliou et al. 2005; Goh et al. 2012). These Likert scale-based assessment instruments allow us to score individual surgeons and trainees in the operating room. Through video analysis, we have moved the arena of surgical assessment from the "bench" to the "bedside." The ability to slow down, stop, or rewind the "game-tape" of a procedure allows for careful analysis of surgeon skill, as well as the use of multiple raters to ensure reliability. The use of video in the operating room also allows for capturing intraoperative errors, defined as ..."any deviation from the normal course of a procedure" (Bonrath et al. 2015a). The development of the Generic Error Rating Tool (GERT) allows for a careful *root-cause analysis* of operative near-misses, errors, and most importantly adverse events, which is imperative for improving surgical care delivery. Additionally, efforts are being made to identify whether a surgeons physiological state in the operating room is of importance to optimizing quality care delivery (Moulton et al. 2007; Ahmidi et al. 2010).

Telemonitoring is another emerging way of using technology to enhance patient care and safety. Multiple companies (News 2013; Storz 2014) are currently working on implementing formal intraoperative telemonitoring, as evidence emerges supporting its use (Shin et al. 2015; Moshtaghi et al. 2015). Google, one of the largest IT companies in the world, developed a program for using Google Glass to capture live surgery (Hashimoto et al. 2015).

Another benefit of retrospective review of surgical performance is that is facilitates peer coaching. Learning surgical technical and non-technical skill, which are determinants of patient outcome (Birkmeyer et al. 2013), in real-time during a procedure is often difficult due to external pressures. According to Bonrath et al. (2015b), a way to enhance trainee and surgeon learning is through "... objective assessment, structured debriefing, feedback, behavior-modeling, and guided self-reflection." This is more feasible in a controlled setting, which the post-operative review session provides. In addition to the aforementioned study, there are other groups showing the benefits of surgical coaching through video analysis (Greenberg et al. 2015).

Another way of improving quality through digital data collection in surgery is the identification of training needs and developing "educational interventions" to address them. This process involves understanding which steps of a procedure are prone to surgeon error and designing a targeted program to address the knowledge or technical deficiencies that led to these errors (Bonrath et al. 2013). One way to approach this is by reviewing error-prone steps of a given surgical procedure with trainees in order to ensure they understand the events that led up to error being committed (Bonrath et al. 2015a). A more technologically advanced means of utilizing error-related data to enhance training is through to creation of simulation models that mimic high-risk steps of a procedure (D'Angelo et al. 2015). This allows for trainees to learn the technical skills needed in order to complete high-risk procedures in a safe, low-risk environment.

Other groups have sought to improve surgeon efficiency in the operating room, through a variety of means. Thalmic Labs (Thalmic Labs, Kitchener, ON, Canada) developed the Myo Armband as a way to control electronic devices wirelessly, through an armband that detects muscle movement in the forearm (Labs 2014). They partnered with TedCas (TedCas Medical Systems, Noáin, Spain), and developed a system for surgeons controlling medical devices such as imaging software, wirelessly and while remaining sterile. A similar endeavor is the GestSure system, which uses a Microsoft Kinect© (Microsoft, Redmond, WA) to interpret surgeon movement in order to control medical software. It was developed to fill a similar niche in surgery, to allow surgeons to remain sterile, while interacting with non-sterile equipment (GestSure 2016). These simple adaptations of existing technology are examples of the 'cross-innovation' that can occur when creative minds draw creative inspiration from other realms of technology.

While these described methods can or may enhance surgeon performance in surgery, one must take a real-world approach that synthesizes these principles, without hindering the day-to-day function of the operative environment. The OR Black Box® has been developed in order to facilitate this, through the input of multiple sources of video, audio, and patient physiological metrics. Complete data capture in the operating room allows for a detailed analysis of the events that lead to an adverse outcome, an process developed and employed by the aviation industry. A holistic approach to intraoperative monitoring allows the OR Black Box® system to conduct complex root-cause analyses, with GERT and other assessment metrics. This multi-modal data can be used for surgeon/trainee/nurse/anesthesiologist assessment, system-wide quality improvement, coaching, and educational interventions, and most importantly ensure patient safety through the study of intraoperative adverse events, including their causes and consequences.

In the United States, efforts have been undertaken to collate high-fidelity intra-operative data capture from multiple sites. Statewide digital health repositories such as the Michigan Bariatric Surgery Collaborative (MBSC) and the Michigan Urological Surgery Improvement Collaborative (MUSIC) have taken advantage of data collected from multiple hospitals in order to analyze and optimize the quality of care being delivered in the state (Birkmeyer et al. 2013; Ghani et al. 2016). Through high-volume analysis, research questions can be approached with high volume data and sufficient power in order to draw meaningful conclusions at a state-wide level. These groups represent a step from *intra-* to *inter-*hospital collaboration and quality improvement initiatives.

Medical education will be revolutionized through the benefits of digital platform development. The shift from the time-base, "Halsteadian" training model (Halsted 1904), to the contemporary Competency-Based Medical Education model (CBME) (Potts 2016) has created a pressing need for robust means of analyzing trainee performance in the clinical environment. Technology such as the OR Black Box® will allow stakeholders to better understand the real-world performance of their trainees, and over time, develop a greater ability to define thresholds for what is deemed "competent" at a given task or procedure (Szasz et al. 2014). We understand that not only is technical skill in surgery is important for high-stakes assessment, but also non-technical skill, and digital platforms that collect both types of data are needed for adequate evaluation of surgical trainees.

17.4   Who Is Ready to Handle Digital Health Information?

As discussed in this chapter, digital health can play a hugely important role in the overall improvement of health care delivery. "Big Data" promises to provide answers for many of the health care challenges we face today. However, it is crucial there is absolute clarity in terms of who has access to this type of data. The legal and ethical implications of allowing open access to patient data are far reaching, and are important to recognize as this field continues to grow. These obstacles may hinder the ability to provide open access to data, and they will be discussed below.

A 2014 systematic review (van Panhuis et al. 2014) describes two types of "legal barriers" that may have implications in data sharing in research. One, "Protection of Privacy," describes the role of the HIPAA and other government organizations around the world that exist to regulate both PHI confidentiality and sharing. In the article, they cite concerns that the borders between fully de-identified data and that which contains some PHI is not always clear, and that this can limit data which can be shared (Wartenberg and Thompson 2010; Lane and Schur 2010). The other barrier described pertains to ownership and copyright concerns. They site a Canadian example of this (Kephart 2002), where in order to amalgamate a nationally collected health survey with provincially collected patient data, individual approval processes were required, province-by-province. This type of legal obstruction leads to increased effort and expense on researchers. As the methods of collecting patient data expands and diversifies, there will be more and more confusion as to who actually is responsible for guardianship of data sets, and this will discourage organizations from sharing data for fear of legal reprimand (Lee and Gostin 2009). As this review points out, this lack of granularity with regard to data ownership leads to inconsistency in guidelines published (Strobl et al. 2000). In the United Kingdom, there was a great amount of uncertainty regarding PHI use in research, following the Data Protection Act of 1998 (Strobl et al. 2000). This lead to the further legislation around the subject of data sharing (Greenough and Graham 2004), and the process there remains disjointed and controversial (Knapton 2016).

The Propublica's "Surgeon Scorecard" is an example of controversial sharing of "Big Data" with the general public. This is a freely accessible database that published surgeon morbidity and mortality statistics, in an effort to increase the transparency of patient outcomes reporting (Allen and Pierce 2015). While a noble pursuit, recent criticism has called the validity of their outcome reporting into question. In a recent article (Ban et al. 2016), Ban et al. conducted an analysis, comparing Scorecard reported "adjusted complication rate" with traditionally studied outcomes from the NSQIP database. They found that ProPublica's exclusion criteria omitted 84% of postoperative complications and correlated poorly with NSQIP outcomes. This critique, in addition to that of the RAND group (Friedberg et al. 2016), have called into question whether this type of data should have been published without first going through a full assessment of validity. While all agree that the public needs to be privy to this type of information, the means by which it is best delivered remains to be answered.

How should patients be integrated in data sharing strategies? A review by de Lusignan et al. in 2014 examined the effect of patient access to the EHR on patient safety, patient experience and satisfaction, adherence, equity and efficiency (de Lusignan et al. 2014). Their group found that patient EHR access fails to impact patient outcomes parameters, except for a possible decrease in prescribing error regarding drug interactions (Staroselsky et al. 2008). Additionally, they found that the literature points to concerns amongst physicians about patient worry or offense taken when accessing their medical file (Haggstrom et al. 2011). Finally, there is general apprehension amongst health care professionals that allowing patient access to EHR data will limit their productivity due to an increase in patient correspondence around test results (de Lusignan et al. 2013). However, other publications have found the inverse to be true (TSO 2012). In an American pilot study in 2013, the Department of Veteran Affairs (VA) offered its patient's full access to their EHR, and assessed overall patient satisfaction. Nearly all patients in the study (90%) felt that this complete transparency improved their overall care (Nazi et al. 2013). A systematic review of the effect of patient access to EHR found that of all endpoints assessed, the strongest evidence showed an improvement in doctor-patient communication when patients were able to see their medical record (Ross and Lin 2003). They found in their review that important factors such as adherence, patient education and empowerment. They also found that in the non-psychiatric patient population, there was not an increase in anxiety or worry around reading medical notes.

The role of robust, highly integrated operative data collection was discussed earlier in this chapter. The OR Black Box® and similar endeavors use real intraoperative footage in its analysis of surgical factors in patient outcomes. This concept of video recording in the operating room comes with some ethical implications that must be addressed. In a recent article from Prigoff et al. (2016), multiple steps are outlined to ensure that video recording is carried out in a way to addresses issues like patient consent and confidentiality. In addition to straightforward concepts, such as ensuring the patient gives *informed* consent and de-identification of video data, the article touches on the important topic of data ownership. If the video is created to be stored in the EHR, then it is considered part of the medical record and is fully accessible to patients. However, if the video is created as part of a quality improvement initiative, then it is considered separate from the medical record (Makary 2013). The legal implication here is that it is considered inadmissible in cases of litigation, unless the court deems its inclusion is necessary for the purposes of discovery. Finally, the article stresses the importance of maintaining security practices that ensure the upholding of patient confidentiality.

17.5   Conclusion

Emerging technologies in data capture and sharing in the medical field open the door for advances in our understanding of healthcare and disease. Big Data has become the mantra of many healthcare researchers who have been tasked with answering the key questions of our day. The use of digital health datasets require highly robust methods of ensuring data security, as well as innovative methods for optimizing patient safety. In this chapter, the concepts of data privacy were covered, focusing on the key aspects of the HIPAA regulations. In addition, novel use of digital health technologies was discussed, highlighting recent innovations in surgery in particular. Finally, the legal and ethical barriers that stakeholders face when interacting with healthcare data was discussed, outlining the roles that both healthcare professionals and patients play as we move further into the era of digital health.

References

Ahmidi N, Hager GD, Ishii L, Fichtinger G, Gallia GL, Ishii M. Surgical task and skill classification from eye tracking and tool motion in minimally invasive surgery. Med Image Comput Comput Assist Interv. 2010;13(Pt 3):295–302.
Allen M, Pierce O. Making the cut. ProPublica Patient Safety. https://www.propublica.org/article/surgery-risks-patient-safety-surgeon-matters. Published July 13, 2015. Accessed July 25, 2106.
Ban KA, Cohen ME, Ko CY, et al. Evaluation of the ProPublica Surgeon scorecard "adjusted complication rate" measure specifications. Ann Surg. 2016;1 doi:10.1097/SLA.0000000000001858.

Berwick DM. Measuring surgical outcomes for improvement: was Codman wrong? JAMA. 2015;313(5):469–70.

Birkmeyer JD, Finks JF, O'Reilly A, et al. Surgical skill and complication rates after bariatric surgery. N Engl J Med. 2013;369(15):1434–42. doi:10.1056/NEJMsa1300625.

Bohnen JD, Chang DC, Lillemoe KD. Reconceiving the morbidity and mortality conference in an era of big data. Ann Surg. 2016;263(5):857–9. doi:10.1097/SLA.0000000000001508.

Bonrath EM, Zevin B, Dedy NJ, Grantcharov TP. Error rating tool to identify and analyse technical errors and events in laparoscopic surgery. Br J Surg. 2013;100(8):1080–8. doi:10.1002/bjs.9168.

Bonrath EM, Gordon LE, Grantcharov TP. Characterising "near miss" events in complex laparoscopic surgery through video analysis. BMJ Qual Saf. May 2015a:1–7. doi:10.1136/bmjqs-2014-003816.

Bonrath EM, Dedy NJ, Gordon LE, Grantcharov TP. Comprehensive surgical coaching enhances surgical skill in the operating room. Ann Surg. 2015b;262(2):205–12. doi:10.1097/SLA.0000000000001214.

Bova C, Drexler D, Sullivan-Bolyai S. Reframing the influence of the health insurance portability and accountability act on research. Chest. 2012;141(3):782–6. doi:10.1378/chest.11-2182.

D'Angelo AL, Law KE, Cohen ER, et al. The use of error analysis to assess resident performance. Surgery. 2015;158(5):1408–14. doi:10.1016/j.surg.2015.04.010.

de Lusignan S, Morris L, Hassey A, Rafi I. Giving patients online access to their records: opportunities, challenges, and scope for service transformation. Br J Gen Pract 2013.

de Lusignan S, Mold F, Sheikh A, et al. Patients' online access to their electronic health records and linked online services: a systematic interpretative review. BMJ Open. 2014;4(9):e006021. doi:10.1136/bmjopen-2014-006021.

Firm WKLB. Modifications to HIPAA privacy, security, and breach notification rules. 2013.

Friedberg MW, Pronovost PJ, Shahian DM. A methodological critique of the ProPublica surgeon scorecard. Santa Monica. Rand Health Q. 2016;5(4, 1)

GestSure. Product information for management. July 2016:1–3. http://www.gestsure.com/product-information-for-management/.

Ghani KR, Miller DC, Linsell S, et al. Measuring to Improve: peer and crowd-sourced assessments of technical skill with robot-assisted radical prostatectomy. Eur Urol. 2016;69(4):547–50. doi:10.1016/j.eururo.2015.11.028.

Glenn T, Monteith S. Privacy in the digital world: medical and health data outside of HIPAA protections. Curr Psychiatry Rep. 2014;16(11):494–11. doi:10.1007/s11920-014-0494-4.

Goh AC, Goldfarb DW, Sander JC, Miles BJ, Dunkin BJ. Global evaluative assessment of robotic skills: validation of a clinical assessment tool to measure robotic surgical skills. J Urol. 2012;187(1):247–52. doi:10.1016/j.juro.2011.09.032.

Greenberg CC, Ghousseini HN, Pavuluri Quamme SR, Beasley HL, Wiegmann DA. Surgical coaching for individual performance improvement. Ann Surg. 2015;261(1):32–4. doi:10.1097/SLA.0000000000000776.

Greenough A, Graham H. Protecting and using patient information: the role of the Caldicott Guardian. Clin Med (Lond). 2004;4(3):246–9.

Haggstrom DA, Saleem JJ, Russ AL. Lessons learned from usability testing of the VA's personal health record. J Am Med Inform Assoc. 2011;18(Suppl 1):i13–7.

Halsted WS. The training of the surgeon. JAMA. 1904;XLIII(21):1553–4.

Hashimoto DA, Phitayakorn R, Fernandez-del Castillo C, Meireles O. A blinded assessment of video quality in wearable technology for telementoring in open surgery: the Google Glass experience. Surg Endosc. 2015:1–7. doi:10.1007/s00464-015-4178-x.

Institute of Medicine (US) Committee on Health Research and the Privacy of Health Information: The HIPAA Privacy Rule. Business Associates. April 2003:1–6.

Kephart G, Canadian institute for health information, initiative CPH. Barriers to accessing and analyzing health information in Canada. Ottawa: Canadian Institute for Health Information; 2002.

Knapton S. Controversial £7.5 million NHS database scrapped quietly on same day as Chilcot Report. *The Daily Telegraph*. http://www.telegraph.co.uk/science/2016/07/06/controversial-50-million-nhs-database-scrapped-quietly-on-same-d/. Published July 6, 2016.

Labs T. See the Myo armband in surgery. November 2014:1–7. http://blog.thalmic.com/myo-armband-surgery/.

Lane J, Schur C. Balancing access to health data and privacy: a review of the issues and approaches for the future. Health Serv Res. 2010;45(5 Pt 2):1456–67. doi:10.1111/j.1475-6773.2010.01141.x.

Lee LM, Gostin LO. Ethical collection, storage, and use of public health data: a proposal for a national privacy protection. JAMA. 2009;302(1):82–4. doi:10.1001/jama.2009.958.

Makary MA. The power of video recording: taking quality to the next level. JAMA. 2013;309(15):1591–2. doi:10.1001/jama.2013.595.

Martin JA, Regehr G, Reznick R, et al. Objective structured assessment of technical skill (OSATS) for surgical residents. Br J Surg. 1997;84(2):273–8.

Moshtaghi O, Kelley KS, Armstrong WB, Ghavami Y, Gu J, Djalilian HR. Using Google glass to solve communication and surgical education challenges in the operating room. *The Laryngoscope*. March 2015: n/a–n/a. doi:10.1002/lary.25249.

Moulton C-AE, Regehr G, Mylopoulos M, MacRae HM. Slowing down when you should: a new model of expert judgment. Acad Med. 2007;82(10 Suppl):S109–16. doi:10.1097/ACM.0b013e3181405a76.

Murdoch TB, Detsky AS. The inevitable application of big data to health care. JAMA. 2013;309(13):1351–2. doi:10.1001/jama.2013.393.

Naam NH, Sanbar S. Advanced technology and confidentiality in hand surgery. J Hand Surg. 2015;40(1):182–7. doi:10.1016/j.jhsa.2014.03.011.

Nass SJ, Levit LA, Gostin LO, Institute of Medicine (US) Committee on Health Research and the Privacy of Health Information: The HIPAA Privacy Rule. Beyond the HIPAA privacy rule: enhancing privacy, improving health through research. 2009. doi:10.17226/12458.

Nazi KM, Hogan TP, McInnes DK, Woods SS, Graham G. Evaluating patient access to electronic health records: results from a survey of veterans. Med Care. 2013;51(3 Suppl 1):S52–6. doi:10.1097/MLR.0b013e31827808db.

News HI. Innovation in telemedicine technology: an entrepreneur's perspective. May 2013:1–19. http://www.healthcareitnews.com/news/innovation-telemedicine-technology-entrepreneurs-perspective.

Potts JR. Assessment of competence: the accreditation council for graduate medical education/residency review committee perspective. Surg Clin North Am. 2016;96(1):15–24. doi:10.1016/j.suc.2015.08.008.

Prigoff JG, Sherwin M, Divino CM. Ethical recommendations for video recording in the operating room. Ann Surg. 2016;264(1):34–5. doi:10.1097/SLA.0000000000001652.

Register OOTF. *Code of Federal Regulations Title 45*. Government Printing Office; 2010.

Ross SE, Lin C-T. The effects of promoting patient access to medical records: a review. J Am Med Inform Assoc. 2003;10(2):129–38. doi:10.1197/jamia.M1147.

Services DOHAH. The security rule. February 2003:1–49.

Services DOHAH. ONC Data Brief Number 1, 2012 Electronic health record systems and intent to attest to meaningful use among acute care hospitals in the U S 2008–2011. February 2012:1–7.

Services UDOHAH. *Summary of the HIPAA Security Rule*. 2013.

Shin DH, Dalag L, Azhar RA, et al. A novel interface for the telementoring of robotic surgery. BJU Int. 2015;116(2):302–8. doi:10.1111/bju.12985.

Staroselsky M, Volk LA, Tsurikova R. An effort to improve electronic health record medication list accuracy between visits: patients" and physicians" response. Int J Med Inform. 2008;77(3):153–60.

Stevens GM. *Compliance with the HIPAA medical privacy rule*. 2003.

Storz K. VISITOR1® from KARL STORZ–TELEMEDICINE EVOLVES into REMOTE PRESENCE. August 2014:1–3. https://www.karlstorz.com/ca/en/visitor1-telemedicine-evolves-into-remote-presence.htm.

Strobl J, Cave E, Walley T. Data protection legislation: interpretation and barriers to research. BMJ. 2000;321(7265):890–2.

Szasz P, Louridas M, Harris KA, Aggarwal R, Grantcharov TP. Assessing technical competence in surgical trainees: a systematic review. Ann Surg. 2014;261(6):1–1055. doi:10.1097/SLA.0000000000000866.

Topol EJ. The creative destruction of medicine. Basic books; 2012.

TSO. The power of information: putting all of us in control of the health. May 2012:1–119.

van Panhuis WG, Paul P, Emerson C, et al. A systematic review of barriers to data sharing in public health. BMC Public Health. 2014;14(1):1144. doi:10.1186/1471-2458-14-1144.

Vassiliou MC, Feldman LS, Andrew CG, et al. A global assessment tool for evaluation of intraoperative laparoscopic skills. Am J Surg. 2005;190(1):107–13. doi:10.1016/j.amjsurg.2005.04.004.

Wartenberg D, Thompson WD. Privacy versus public health: the impact of current confidentiality rules. Am J Public Health. 2010;100(3):407–12. doi:10.2105/AJPH.2009.166249.

Chapter 18
The Evolving Law and Ethics of Digital Health

Nathan Cortez

Abstract Given the novelty of digital health technologies, there remains significant confusion over which laws and regulations might apply to these technologies, and how. This chapter describes the major bodies of state and federal law that can apply, including medical device regulation by the FDA, state and federal consumer protection laws, data privacy and security laws, and potential legal liability for physicians, hospitals, manufacturers, and developers. The chapter examines how awkwardly these laws have adapted to the novel features of digital health, and vice versa. It concludes by detailing how, in the absence of quality screening by the FDA, four alternative methods of quality screening have emerged, including (1) due diligence by venture capital firms, (2) hospital guidelines for users and developers, (3) review by third-parties, such as app review web sites, and (4) coverage policies by health insurers. I call these "surrogate" or "proxy" regulation.

Keywords Law • Ethics • Regulation • Mobile health • Digital health • Predictive analytics • Big data

18.1 Introduction

It is no revelation to say that the laws that apply to the digital health industry were not designed with these technologies in mind. Laws are generally written to address existing technologies, but cannot always foresee future ones. Compounding the lag between law and technology, it can take considerable time to update the law. This dynamic is not at all new. Transportation laws written for railroads could not foresee automobiles or commercial aviation. Communication laws written for the telegraph

N. Cortez
Dedman School of Law, Southern Methodist University,
Dallas, TX, USA
e-mail: ncortez@smu.edu, nathan.cortez@gmail.com

© Springer International Publishing AG 2018   249
H. Rivas, K. Wac (eds.), *Digital Health*, Health Informatics,
https://doi.org/10.1007/978-3-319-61446-5_18

and telephone could not have contemplated the Internet and modern information services (Cortez 2014a). Likewise, the digital health industry—which includes mobile applications, wearables, ingestibles, implantables, and related technologies—is governed by legal frameworks that were largely adopted well before these technologies were even conceived. The recent legal controversies regarding 23 and Me and Theranos demonstrate the unease with which some technology companies have adapted to these legal frameworks, and vice versa.

This Chapter, then, tries to capture a snapshot of the many laws, regulations, and ethical standards that can apply to the digital health industry—both now and as it might exist in the near future. I describe the major bodies of law that can apply, with some ideas on how well these laws accommodate the novel features of digital health.[1] The task is daunting given the scope and complexity of the laws that can apply here, ranging from regulation by the U.S. Food and Drug Administration (FDA) and Federal Trade Commission (FTC), to privacy laws, state licensing laws, medical malpractice, and product liability.[2] To help the reader, and particularly the non-lawyer, understand the laws in this area, I emphasize three themes:

First, categories matter. Categories of products, actors, and activities can have deep legal significance. Hardware or platform companies like Apple and Google can have very different legal obligations from software developers. Physicians, hospitals, and insurers each have very different legal duties, based on historical problems in each industry and on different ideas about they should behave. Likewise, legal expectations for products can diverge greatly depending on whether you wear it, ingest it, implant it, or simply consult it. Lawmaking often relies on using simple, neat categories to determine legal duties, and digital health is no different. So categories matter.

Second, claims matter. What does a digital health product or service claim to do? Why is it useful? How is it valuable? Companies may make claims to a variety of audiences, in a variety of contexts, for a variety of purposes. For example, early-stage companies often face pressure when fundraising to make revolutionary claims about their products. But these claims may be policed by regulators like the FDA, FTC, and SEC (Securities and Exchange Commission), and can create legal problems as the company matures. This Chapter will explain when and how such claims have legal significance.

The third theme of this chapter is that because digital health is relatively new and is developing so rapidly, policymakers have yet to formulate a tailored response. It takes time for the legislative, executive, and judicial branches to fully consider new technologies and business practices. It takes time to update the law—whether it be statutes, regulations, or judicially-created rules. As a result, non-legal mechanisms are filling this void in the digital health industry. For example, venture capitalists, third-party certifiers, product review sites, hospital guidelines, and health insurers

---

[1] I use "digital health" loosely to include mobile health, telemedicine, "big data" analytics, wearables, ingestible sensors, 3D printing, virtual reality, and related health technologies.

[2] Moreover, due to space constraints, I omit discussion of important legal issues like patents, intellectual property, clinical research, discrimination, and cybersecurity that affect the industry.

are serving as quality screening mechanisms in the absence of more tailored regulation. The long-term implications of this are still unclear. But this dynamic is something that everyone in the digital health space should understand.

18.2   Legal Frameworks for Digital Health

Digital health is in many ways the marriage of one sector that traditionally has been subject to very minimal regulation (digital and mobile technology) with another sector that is perhaps the most heavily regulated in our economy (health care). This marriage creates a tension for policymakers on how to calibrate the appropriate amount of "law" that should apply to digital health. Although there are several justifications for adopting a laissez faire approach to foster rapid technological innovation, there are equally persuasive reasons for adopting consumer- and patient-protective regulation given deep uncertainties regarding the safety and efficacy of these technologies. Moreover, there are severe information asymmetries between buyers and sellers that might warrant more government intervention in the digital health market.

But first, the reader should appreciate the volume and variety of legal frameworks that can apply to digital health. These frameworks span both state and federal law, and are created not only by all three branches of government (executive, legislative, and judicial), but also by nongovernmental standard-setting organizations, such as the American Medical Association (AMA):

The next section quickly summarizes each framework and how it applies—or may apply—to the digital health industry.

18.2.1   Medical Device Regulation

Some digital health products will qualify as "devices" subject to regulation by the FDA, the federal agency entrusted with ensuring that medical devices marketed in the United States are safe and effective. FDA regulation relies on an old statute, the 1976 Medical Device Amendments, which itself amended an even older statute, the federal Food, Drug, and Cosmetic Act of 1938, which remains in force today. Although the FDA has been thinking about computer hardware and software in medical devices since the 1970s, the agency has promulgated very few new regulations that are tailored to modern, connected, computerized devices (Cortez 2015). Thus, the FDA applies old statutes to very new technologies.

However, the FDA articulates its approach to digital health products via a series of non-binding guidance documents, which explain the FDA's jurisdiction and its expectations for regulated devices (http://www.fda.gov/downloads/medicaldevices/device-regulationandguidance/guidancedocuments/ucm263366.pdf 2015). Again, both FDA jurisdiction and enforcement depend on categories and claims. Category-wise, the

FDA has clarified that it does not have jurisdiction to regulate many digital health products, particularly those that do not meet the definition of "device" under federal law (21 U.S.C. § 321(h) n.d.). Moreover, the FDA has assured repeatedly that it will not regulate even products that fit the definition of "device" if they pose a low risk to patient safety. Another FDA guidance clarified that the agency would not regulate the vast majority of low-risk "wellness" products, which includes a large proportion of wearables (http://www.fda.gov/downloads/medicaldevices/deviceregulationand-guidance/guidancedocuments/ucm429674.pdf 2016).

Categories also determine how stringently the FDA will regulate devices under its jurisdiction. The 1976 Device Amendments created three "classes" of medical devices depending on their risks: Class I (low risk), Class II (moderate risk), and Class III (high risk) (21 U.S.C. §§ 360c, 360e n.d.). These classes determine not only the product's pathway to market, but also the requirements that apply once a product is lawfully marketed, including registration, adverse event reporting, and quality assurance rules, among many others.[3] The vast majority of digital health products subject to FDA regulation have been classified as Class I or II devices. Still, certain categories of digital health products—ingestibles and implantables, for example—will certainly fall within FDA jurisdiction and receive more careful scrutiny from the agency than other categories of low-risk products.

Likewise, both FDA jurisdiction and enforcement also depend on the claims a product makes and its intended uses (21 C.F.R. § 801.4 2016), and understanding this idea has proven difficult for many companies, notwithstanding the FDA's efforts to clarify. Products that claim to diagnose, cure, mitigate, treat, or prevent specific diseases or otherwise claim to affect a specific structure or function of the body will bring the product within the FDA's technical jurisdiction. But the FDA emphasizes that it will not regulate mobile and digital health products aggressively, and will oversee only those products that are devices *and* also pose a risk to patient safety if they do not function as intended (http://www.fda.gov/downloads/medicaldevices/deviceregulationandguidance/guidancedocuments/ucm263366.pdf 2015). The FDA has assured repeatedly, for example, that it will not regulate mobile device manufacturers like Apple and Samsung if they do not make specific disease claims.

Moreover, the FDA has not been particularly aggressive in enforcing its rules against digital health companies. One example is frequently cited, when the FDA sent a letter to Biosense Technologies after it learned that the company was marketing a urine analyzer app without clearance from the agency (http://www.fda.gov/MedicalDevices/ResourcesforYou/Industry/ucm353513.htm 2013), prompting the company to take the product off the market. However, the FDA only intervened after learning about the product during a congressional hearing, and similar enforcement letters are scarce. Nevertheless, the FDA's high-profile dispute with the consumer genetics company 23andMe, and the ongoing troubles of the blood testing company Theranos, have convinced many in the digital health industry that regulators are

---

[3]Among the requirements include annual registration of manufacturing facilities and listing of device made, labeling rules, quality standards for design and manufacturing, and submission of necessary adverse event reports and corrections.

hyper-skeptical of the industry. However, most data points suggest a much more cooperative posture by regulators like the FDA.

18.2.2 Consumer Protection Laws

A second major legal framework that applies to the digital health industry is consumer protection law, which generally prohibits false advertising and other unfair or deceptive trade practices. Consumer protection laws are enforced federally by the FTC, and at the state level by attorneys general and often by aggrieved consumers who are authorized to sue for state violations of law.

As with medical device regulation, claims matter. Thus, like the FDA, the FTC monitors product claims and will take enforcement action against companies that make unsubstantiated health claims (Cortez 2014b). In fact, the FTC has been more active than the FDA in policing unsubstantiated claims by digital health companies. For example, in 2011, the FTC charged two companies for making unsubstantiated claims that their mobile apps, Acne Pwner and Acne App, could treat acne by displaying flashing colored lights close to the user's skin, with one app claiming support for this technique from a medical journal article (Brown and Pearson 2011; Finkel 2011). The FTC fined both companies for making unsubstantiated claims and subsequently created a Mobile Technology Unit within the agency to develop more expertise on mobile apps and to coordinate enforcement efforts (Carrns 2011). Later, in 2015, the FTC challenged the makers of two melanoma detection apps, MelApp and Mole Detective, for making deceptive claims that the apps could use smartphone images of moles to detect early symptoms of melanoma and calculate a risk score (https://www.ftc.gov/news-events/press-releases/2015/02/ftc-cracks-down-marketers-melanoma-detection-apps 2015). The FTC charged the companies with making claims without adequate scientific evidence, and settlement agreements barred the companies from making further claims not supported by clinical testing (https://www.ftc.gov/news-events/press-releases/2015/02/ftc-cracks-down-marketers-melanoma-detection-apps 2015). The clear message to digital health companies is to have proper substantiation for health claims.

Of course, U.S. consumers are besieged by health claims, and the level of substantiation required by the FTC has been a contentious question. In 2015, the D.C. Circuit Court of Appeals affirmed the FTC's position that products that claim to help treat or prevent diseases or other health conditions must substantiate those claims with competent and reliable scientific evidence, which the FTC interpreted as at least one randomized, controlled clinical trial (POM Wonderful 2015). The case involved POM Wonderful, an aggressive marketer whose advertisements claimed that its pomegranate-based products could help treat, prevent, or reduce the risk of heart disease, prostate cancer, and erectile dysfunction, among several other conditions. Thus, along with the 23andMe and Theranos cases, the POM Wonderful case demonstrates, again, that claims matter.

Yet, as with the FDA, it would be a mistake to view the FTC as "adverse" to the digital health industry. Both agencies have gone out of their way to help well-meaning companies understand their legal obligations. For example, the FTC web site offers a "Mobile Health Apps Interactive Tool," which asks a series of "Yes" or "No" questions and then identifies certain laws that may apply to the mobile app, such as federal privacy law (HIPAA), FDA regulation, and FTC regulation (https://www.ftc.gov/tips-advice/business-center/guidance/mobile-health-apps-interactive-tool 2016). This type of guidance, again, demonstrates how digital health merges a lightly-regulated industry with a heavily-regulated industry, sometimes creating confusion and frustration for those used to minimal regulation.

In addition to federal law, digital health companies should also be aware of state consumer protection laws, which can overlap with federal laws and can vary greatly between states. One particularly important set of state laws is California's, including its Unfair Competition Law (California Business and Professions Code § 17200 n.d.), its False Advertising Act (California Business and Professions Code § 17500 n.d.), and its Consumer Legal Remedies Act (California Civil Code §§ 1750–1784 n.d.), among related statutes. These laws are considered more comprehensive and protective of consumers than in most states. For example, California law prohibits companies from knowingly, or without the exercise of reasonable care, making untrue or misleading claims about their products or services (California Business and Professions Code § 17500 2016). These broad laws are enforced not only by state authorities like the California Attorney General and district attorneys, but also by affected consumers who are authorized to bring suit. For example, consumers in California have sued FitBit under several of these California statutes for making misleading claims about the ability of its devices to accurately track sleep.[4] Although California's Unfair Competition Law is largely modeled on Sect. 18.5 of the Federal Trade Commission Act, it is interpreted and enforced separately, creating multiple layers of legal exposure for companies operating there.

18.2.3 Data Privacy and Security

Many digital health technologies try to make heavy use of consumer health data, promising to collect and deploy such data in novel and useful ways. These data are being used by many non-traditional entities like software companies and data brokers that often operate on the periphery of the traditional health care system, raising corresponding concerns about data privacy and security (Terry 2017). Although both federal and state law govern the collection, use, and disclosure of health data, most non-experts are unaware that the scope of these laws can be exceedingly narrow, and thus that many actors and activities in digital health are not covered by federal or state law.

---

[4] Brickman v. FitBit, Inc., 2016 WL 3844327 (N.D. Cal. 2016).

The federal framework supplied by HIPAA (the Health Insurance Portability and Accountability Act) is relatively well known. HIPAA's privacy and security rules (45 C.F.R. parts 160, 164 2015), enforced by the U.S. Department of Health and Human Services (HHS) Office for Civil Rights (OCR), generally safeguard the collection, use, and disclosure of personal health information, including medical conditions and diagnoses, the care provided, and payment history. However, HIPAA's privacy and security rules apply only to "covered entities" and their "business associates," meaning health care providers, health insurance plans, and persons or organizations that do business with them and receive protected health information electronically. Thus, HIPAA largely focuses on traditional providers and transactions and does not extend to the novel forms of data collection and uses in the digital health sector. For example, wearables and other digital health products that are not operated by hospitals, insurers, or other traditional covered entities are unlikely to be covered by HIPAA's privacy and security rules, perhaps contrary to user expectations (Chen 2016). In short, the primary federal framework for protecting health data does not apply to the vast majority of activities in digital health.

Yet, digital health companies are not entirely unfettered in how they collect and use health data. The FTC can charge companies with violating federal unfair competition statutes (15 U.S.C. § 45 2015) if they fail to secure sensitive consumer information or if they mislead consumers about their privacy practices. For example, the FTC charged a cloud-based health records company, Practice Fusion, with violating the unfair competition statute by soliciting patient reviews of physicians without disclosing that the reviews would be posted online, which resulted in the publication of sensitive patient information (https://www.ftc.gov/news-events/press-releases/2016/06/electronic-health-records-company-settles-ftc-charges-it-deceived 2016). The FTC also brings enforcement actions against more routine failures to protect sensitive personal and medical data, arguing that some data security practices are so inadequate as to be "unreasonable" and thus constitute "unfair" practices in violation of the FTC Act (https://www.ftc.gov/news-events/press-releases/2016/07/commission-finds-labmd-liable-unfair-data-security-practices 2016). Thus, digital health companies that do not adopt reasonable protections for consumer health data, or that do not protect such data in the ways they promise, are subject to FTC enforcement even if they fall outside the scope of HIPAA.

Moreover, as with consumer protection law, there are overlapping state laws that regulate data privacy and security. Again, California law is worth noting because so many digital health companies reside or do business in California, and because California law is more comprehensive and protective of consumers than in most states. California's Confidentiality of Medical Information Act (CMIA) (California Civil Code Part 2.6, §§ 56-59 2016) is broader and in many ways more protective of patient privacy than HIPAA. And, somewhat strikingly, the CMIA specifically addresses the mobile and digital health industry. Section 56.06(b) of the CMIA deems that "[a]ny business that offers hardware or software to consumers, including a mobile application or related device" to make information available to providers or individuals to manage his or her information or to diagnose or treat the individual will be a "provider of health care" subject to the CMIA (California Civil

Code § 56.06 2016). Thus, many digital and mobile health companies will be subject to the CMIA's legal obligations and restrictions, including the restriction against disclosing a patient's medical information without authorization (California Civil Code § 56.10 2016). Again, California law is far ahead of both federal laws like HIPAA and most other state laws in this area.

18.2.4 Licensing and Liability

In addition to device regulation, consumer protection, and privacy, a series of laws govern physicians, nurses, hospitals, and other licensed providers, and thus might create special legal obligations for them when engaging with digital health. In this section, then, I will discuss three distinct but related legal frameworks: state professional licensing; medical malpractice liability; and hospital liability. Again, categories and claims remain important. But there is deep legal uncertainty regarding how digital health products and services might affect existing legal and professional obligations that were developed well before digital health existed.

18.2.4.1 State Professional Licensing

Physicians, nurses, and other licensed professionals[5] are subject to state laws that might create special obligations for them when using digital health products or providing digital health services themselves. The vast majority of digital health technologies do not have corresponding state laws that specifically address their proper use. Again, the law is generally slow to update.

One exception is telemedicine. A growing number of digital health technologies make use of telemedicine—the use of communications technologies by health care professionals to diagnose or treat patients remotely. However, when the remote care is being provided across state lines, or when the patient and provider have not met in person for a physical exam, the provider may run afoul of state licensing rules, including laws prohibiting the unauthorized practice of medicine. Thus, digital health technologies that purport to provide remote diagnoses or treatment may implicate state professional licensing laws.

All but a few states have passed specific laws that address telemedicine directly. These laws may include rules governing licensing, provider conduct, privacy, fraud, referrals, and insurance coverage, among other considerations. Most of these laws try to accommodate the practice of telemedicine, for example by offering an exception for consultations by out-of-state physicians, or by providing a limited telemedicine license for such providers.

---

[5] State licensure is extensive. The state of Texas, for example, applies specific legal requirements on well over two dozen different "health professions," including physicians, nurses, surgical assistants, dentists, and the like. See Texas Occupations Code, Title 3 (Health Professions).

But some states have been more hostile to telemedicine. For example, there are multiple cases in which state medical boards took disciplinary action against physicians for providing telemedicine services without forming a valid doctor-patient relationship (Terry and Wiley 2016). Most cases involved remote prescribing, without an in-person physician office visit. Texas attempted to codify this approach, when the Texas Medical Board revised the Texas Administrative Code in 2015 to prohibit telemedicine providers from prescribing certain drugs and controlled substances without a valid doctor-patient relationship (Texas administrative code § 190.8(1)(L) ("New Rule 190.8") 2015). Later that year, a national telemedicine provider, Teladoc, sued the Texas Medical Board to challenge the rule, arguing that it violated federal antitrust law. A federal court refused to dismiss the case (Teladoc, Inc. v. Texas medical board 2015a), in a victory for telemedicine providers, but the litigation continues on appeal (Teladoc, Inc. v. Texas medical board 2015b).

Thus, although the law of telemedicine is much more well-developed than the law governing other digital health technologies, it continues to change rapidly. Telemedicine and other digital health providers that seek to provide medical care across state lines must continue to monitor state law developments. Although federal law generally favors telemedicine, medical professionals are regulated primarily by states, and thus state laws (particularly state licensing) will continue to predominate in this area.

18.2.4.2 Medical Malpractice Liability

Physicians, nurses, and other health professionals should consider some rather unique medical malpractice risks that may arise from engaging with digital health technologies. The word 'engaging' here is purposefully broad, and is meant to cover the very different roles that health professionals can assume vis-à-vis digital health (Terry and Wiley 2016). For example, some health professionals help design and develop digital health products, serving as consultants, founders, or chief executives for start-up companies. Other health professionals may face liability for using, misusing, or perhaps eventually for declining to use, digital health products for patient care. Still others may face liability risks when recommending or prescribing consumer-facing digital health products to patients. These three types of engagement can raise very different malpractice risks.

To appreciate these risks, one must understand the four elements required for bringing a successful medical malpractice claim. The first element is duty: the plaintiff must establish that there was a valid treatment relationship, such that the health professional owed a duty of care to the patient. The second element is breach: the plaintiff must show that the health professional breached or otherwise fell below the standard of care required in that situation. The standard of care is usually framed as what a competent and reasonable professional with similar skill and training would have done under similar circumstances. The third element is causation: the plaintiff must show that the breach of duty caused the plaintiff's injuries. The fourth is damages: the plaintiff must establish that she suffered some actual damages. Note that damages alone are not sufficient for finding liability, as physicians cannot guarantee results (Terry and Wiley 2016).

These four elements derive largely from state court decisions, some over a century old. Most state legislatures, moreover, have adopted statutes that cap medical malpractice recoveries and otherwise limit when and how plaintiffs can file suit. As a result, medical malpractice law can vary considerably state to state. Another complication is that few if any state medical malpractice cases or statutes contemplate digital health technologies (Terry and Wiley 2016), so there is a great deal of uncertainty regarding what the appropriate legal standards should be, and how old standards apply to very new technologies. The best that lawyers and scholars can do is to extrapolate from analogous cases (Terry and Wiley 2016).

Thus, in the first scenario, when a health professional contributes to the design or development of a digital health product and it injures someone—for example, the product misdiagnoses a medical condition or causes a patient to overconsume a prescription drug—malpractice liability would depend largely on the first element, duty. Did the health professional have a treatment relationship with the user and thus owe a duty of care to that user? For products used by the general public, such as a mobile health app publicly available on the App Store, the likely answer is no. For products used by the physician's own patients, such as when the physician develops a product and then uses it with her own patients, the likely answer is yes. A more difficult question arises when a physician develops a product and then shares it with, or recommends it to, other physicians for patient care (Terry and Wiley 2016). In analogous cases, courts have found a doctor-patient relationship, and thus a duty of care, based on very minimal interaction between the physician and patient. Courts often require the physician to apply her medical judgment to the patient's specific case. For example, in telemedicine cases, courts have found that a single online video consultation or a brief review of radiology images are sufficient to form a doctor-patient relationship (White v. Harris 2011; Bovara v. St. Francis Hospital 1998). But in other cases, courts have found that phone consultations or other remote consultations were not sufficient to form a treatment relationship, particularly when the physician does not apply her medical judgment to the patient's specific case (Terry and Wiley 2016; Jennings v. Badgett 2010; Miller v. Martin 2001). Thus, a physician may be liable if she develops a digital health product that injures one of her own patients, but not for injuries sustained by the general public.[6]

In the second scenario above, when a health professional uses a digital health product to diagnose or treat patients, malpractice liability would depend largely on the second element, breach. A case might arise, for example, when a physician misuses a digital health product or overlooks important data captured by a wearable device and thus fails to provide an accurate, timely diagnosis. In such cases, again, determining breach would require determining the standard of care for using technologies that are not well established (Terry and Wiley 2016). For example, is it

---

[6]Note, however, that the company might still be subject to product liability, as discussed in Sect. 18.2.5 below.

sound medical judgment to rely on a certain mobile health app to diagnose or treat patients? How much time would a reasonable physician spend choosing among different apps, particularly when there may be hundreds or even thousands of options? How much would a reasonable physician educate herself on how to use the product safely and effectively? Would a reasonable physician know, or have reason to know, that a product was defective or unreliable? Courts are unlikely to supply clear and confident answers to these questions.

Finally, in the third scenario, when a health professional recommends or even prescribes a digital health product to her patients, but does not use it herself for patient care, liability will again depend largely on the second element, breach (Terry and Wiley 2016). And again, identifying a baseline standard of care may prove difficult. How much would a reasonable physician investigate a product, including its shortcomings? How many alternatives would a competent physician consider? Is the product reliable? Again, because courts are unlikely to supply clear and confident answers, the outcomes of such cases remain highly uncertain.

18.2.4.3 Hospital and Facility Liability

As with health professionals, hospitals and other licensed health facilities might face unique legal risks from engaging with digital health technologies. And like health professionals, those risks depend on the form of engagement. For example, a growing number of hospitals are developing their own apps to allow medical staff to access electronic medical records (EMRs), medical imaging, and even clinical decision support (CDS) software (Terry and Wiley 2016). Or, in many hospitals, medical staff may rely on apps and other mobile products for patient care without clearance from the hospital and without clear guidelines for their use. Finally, some hospitals offer their own patient-facing apps or recommend certain products to patients (Terry and Wiley 2016). Again, each activity raises discrete legal questions.

Legal liability for hospitals and other health facilities derives largely from state court decisions. Today, the law in most states holds that hospitals are liable for their own negligence and for the negligence of employees (with an important caveat that most physicians are not employees, but independent contractors). Modern liability for hospitals is predicated on the idea that hospitals—and not just health professionals—are responsible for patient care (Darling v. Charleston Community Memorial Hospital 1965). Thus, in most states, courts hold hospitals accountable for maintaining safe and sufficient facilities, enforcing quality and safety rules, selecting and retaining competent medical professionals, and overseeing those professionals (Terry and Wiley 2016). Some jurisdictions deviate downward from these basic expectations, but some deviate upward.

These legal duties for hospitals, logically, would apply when relying on digital health technologies that compromise patient care. For example, hospitals that develop their own apps and other digital health products could be liable—just as any other developer could be—for injuries sustained by users, including physical injuries, data breaches, and the like. Hospitals may also face legal liability for failing to adequately select, screen, or monitor apps and other digital health products used by physicians and other medical staff. Hospitals thus may have to confront questions regarding whether a reasonable hospital would allow the use of certain digital health products, and what due diligence by hospital departments (such as procurement, risk management, and legal) is reasonable before recommending or relying on them. Moreover, several commentators question whether hospitals and health professionals need to obtain informed consent from patients before using novel digital health technologies for patient care (Terry and Wiley 2016). Again, these will remain open questions until courts or legislatures address them.

18.2.5   Product Liability

The parties that manufacture, develop, or market digital health products can face different types of liability than that faced by licensed providers, described above. Products that injure consumers are governed by state product liability law, enunciated primarily through state court decisions, with occasional state statutes that dictate certain requirements. Typically, injured plaintiffs argue that the product was defectively designed or manufactured, or provided insufficient warnings.

Although there is not extensive case law involving injuries from mobile and digital health products, we can forecast how courts might treat these technologies by looking at cases involving more traditional health information technology (HIT) products (Terry and Wiley 2016). Moreover, federal agencies like the FDA and the Office of National Coordinator for Health Information Technology (ONC) (https://www.healthit.gov/sites/default/files/fdasia_healthitreport_final.pdf   2014)   have become more sensitive to safety problems caused by HIT, including errors in data transcription, transmission, and analysis, often exacerbated by software incompatibilities. Others have drawn attention to problems caused by human-computer interaction, including "alarm fatigue," which can also compromise patient safety (Cortez 2014b; Terry 2012). Again, these longstanding safety concerns with HIT Products can apply equally to digital health products.

In what may be a sign of things to come, numerous injuries and deaths are caused each year by exercise equipment (Terry and Wiley 2016), and already, we are seeing product recalls and lawsuits alleging that wearables and digital health products have caused similar injuries. As Nicolas Terry and Lindsey Wiley note, in 2012 the family of an "obsessed" cyclist tried to sue the developer of the cycling app, Strava, after he died trying to break a performance record on the app (Terry and Wiley 2016; Hill 2012). And in 2014, Fitbit recalled one of its activity trackers after thousands complained of blisters and rashes from allergenic materials, mainly nickel (Terry and Wiley 2016; Abrams 2014). As Terry and Wiley observe, courts may look to a wide variety of sources for determining whether such products are "defective," including expectations set by the FDA and the Consumer Product Safety Commission (CPSC), and even by app store developer guidelines (Terry and Wiley 2016).

Finally, state product liability law necessarily intersects with federal product safety regulation, including the frameworks provided by the FDA and CPSC. Although the U.S. Supreme Court has held that the FDA's federal medical device framework preempts state claims (Riegel v. Medtronic 2008), such preemption seems to apply only to devices approved through the FDA's premarket approval (PMA) application process (21 U.S.C. § 360e 2015). Thus, it would not cover the vast majority of digital health products reviewed by the FDA, which are cleared via the much less rigorous 510(k) notification system (21 U.S.C. § 360(k) 2015). Moreover, state claims would not be preempted if the product is not regulated by the FDA at all. Such products would likely be subject to regulation by the CPSC, which, like the FDA, can initiate product recalls. Moreover, consumers can sue manufacturers under the federal Consumer Product Safety Act if it has caused harm (15 U.S.C. § 2072 2015).

In summary, then, although digital health products are novel in many ways, state product liability laws will likely adapt to these technologies more easily than other legal frameworks can. Moreover, manufacturers must keep in mind how federal product safety regulation can overlap with state product liability.

18.3 The Emerging Ethics of Digital Health

Just like the law of digital health seems to be developing slowly, and mostly in reaction to well-known problems rather than as a concerted effort to offer prospective guidance. Another similarity is that ethical standards, like laws, derive from a number of different sources—local, state, and national. However, unlike the law, ethical standards are largely not binding and enforceable in any legal sense, and thus can provide only a "soft" set of standards for using these technologies.

Nevertheless, ethical standards can have a bearing on legal and regulatory actions, when courts and agencies look to professional societies for guidance on the standard of care. And increasingly, federal and state policymakers have incorporated ethical standards and codes of conduct into statutes, or will consider compliance with such standards when contemplating enforcement actions. Thus, although there are very few ethical guidelines for digital health products and services right now, the guidelines that do emerge are likely to reverberate at least somewhat in legal and regulatory matters.

In the meantime, there is considerable lag between the time a digital health technology approaches the mainstream and the time ethical guidelines are finally published. For example, telemedicine has been in use for many years, yet the American Medical Association (AMA) only finalized ethical guidelines for practicing telemedicine in 2016 (http://www.ama-assn.org/ama/pub/news/news/2016/2016-06-13-new-ethical-guidance-telemedicine.page 2016), after three years of consideration. It was not until 2014 that the Federation of State Medical Boards adopted a policy on telemedicine (https://www.fsmb.org/Media/Default/PDF/FSMB/Advocacy/FSMB_Telemedicine_Policy.pdf 2014).

Progress here is thus slow and incremental. Specialty medical societies have adopted their own guidelines, such as the American Psychological Association's *Guidelines for the Practice of Telepsychology* (http://www.apa.org/practice/guidelines/telepsychology.aspx 2013). Moreover, the AMA publishes less authoritative documents online, such as a resource page for "digital health," (http://www.ama-assn.org/ama/pub/advocacy/topics/digital-health.page 2016) which includes resources on electronic health records (EHRs), meaningful use incentives, cybersecurity, and "connected health," which includes statements on telemedicine and mobile health (http://www.ama-assn.org/ama/pub/advocacy/topics/digital-health/connected-health.page 2016).

When viewed from a longer trajectory, one can see an initial reluctance from professional associations like the AMA to embrace telemedicine, which is gradually overcome as the technology matures and as trade associations and industry lobbyists push back. To illustrate, in one of the AMA's earliest pronouncements on telemedicine, in 1994, it prohibited members from providing any clinical services via telecommunications technologies (American Medical Association 1994)—a stark contrast from its current posture. Moreover, industry groups like the American Telemedicine Association (ATA) have worked persistently to ease restrictions on telemedicine imposed by state laws, professional societies, and by others. Thus, our experience with telemedicine may foreshadow how other subsections of the digital health industry will mature.

18.4 Surrogate or Proxy Regulation

The foregoing frameworks may seem to provide sufficient standards for digital health. But recall that medical device regulation is narrow, consumer protection enforcement is sparse, privacy laws cover few digital health technologies, and liability for licensed providers is highly unclear. Thus, the law and ethics of digital health remain unsettled. Compounding matters, no one is anxious to step in and declare what the standards should be.

In the meantime, four mechanisms have emerged to provide surrogate or proxy "regulation" of digital health: (1) venture capital screening; (2) hospital guidelines; (3) app review sites; and (4) health insurance coverage decisions. I use the word 'regulation' here to denote *de facto* mechanisms for reviewing, screening, or otherwise assessing the quality and reliability of digital health technologies, as opposed to more traditional *de jure* regulation, in which a government regulator establishes rules and then enforces those rules legally.

The impetus behind these surrogates or proxies is simple—the sheer volume and variety of digital health products makes it daunting for users to assess each product in a meaningful way and thus choose among what may be hundreds or even thousands of alternatives (Cortez 2014b). For example, a 2015 report estimated that in just one segment of digital health—mobile health apps for smartphones and tablets—there were 165,000 different products available for download (http://www.imshealth.com/en/thought-leadership/ims-institute/reports/patient-adoption-of-mhealth 2015). Even relatively sophisticated users like physicians and hospitals cannot possibly compare all potentially relevant products. Moreover, although academic studies assessing the clinical value of digital health products are being published with more frequency (http://www.commonwealth-fund.org/publications/issue-briefs/2016/feb/evaluating-mobile-health-apps 2016), these too take time and can become outdated as new products are introduced. Thus, the following four mechanisms have emerged as *de facto* screening mechanisms for digital health.

18.4.1 Venture Capital Screens

Shortly after the lab testing start-up Theranos launched in 2014, it faced a series of investigations by newspapers and multiple federal regulators regarding the accuracy of its blood testing technologies. Some of these investigations found that the venture capital firms considered to be most sophisticated and experienced in the biotechnology, life sciences, and health care sectors either did not meet with Theranos or were not persuaded to invest in the company (Farr 2016; Stross 2016). These venture capital firms not only boast numerous staff with an M.D., a relevant Ph.D., or even both (Stross 2016), but they also frequently look for peer-reviewed studies that support a company's claims (Farr 2016; Stross 2016). In fact, many sophisticated investors look for "strong peer-reviewed publications" as "a way of getting expert due diligence at zero cost." (Stross 2016) In fact, some venture firms spend as much as $100,000 in legal and advisory fees and over a year to evaluate start-up companies in the health and biosciences sectors, and expect companies to present peer-reviewed data (Farr 2016). Moreover, a number of start-up "incubators" or "accelerators" serve to connect companies with relevant investors, but also with relevant subject matter experts (http://healthwildcatters.com 2016). Thus, this cadre of investors sophisticated in health and the biosciences provides a screening mechanism for start-up companies seeking to enter the market.

   Of course, the screening provided by venture capital firms is a very imperfect substitute for prospective quality regulation. First, venture capital screening only works for companies that need venture capital. In reality, a large but undetermined portion of digital health technologies are released by individual software developers or by very small firms without being subjected to a multi-tier evaluation by sophisticated investors. Moreover, as in the case of Theranos, there is no guarantee that even high-profile technologies will be kept from the market by failing to attract one of the sought-after venture firms. Thus, although venture capital screening does rely on medical and scientific experts who evaluate peer-reviewed data—something very similar in theory to what the FDA does—not all technologies undergo this type of scrutiny.

18.4.2   Hospital Guidelines

A second surrogate or proxy are hospital guidelines for adopting digital health technologies. In 2016, for example, Boston Children's Hospital published a 14-point
guideline for developing mobile apps intended to be used by staff there (Al Ayubi
et al. 2016). Although designed to address only data privacy and security problems
with the "bring your own device" (BYOD) environment that currently prevails in
hospitals, the guidelines offer a series of measures that hospitals can use to ensure
compliance with HIPAA and other relevant laws, for example by requiring authentication, multiple layers of security, and limits on data storage, caching, printing,
and cloud backup features (Al Ayubi et al. 2016). The guidelines conclude by stating that "Until there are industry-accepted guidelines we will use this … guideline
to inform our enterprise mobile development design approach." (Al Ayubi et al.
2016).

But again, hospital guidelines are an imperfect surrogate or proxy for more comprehensive, prospective oversight. Although early adopters of BYOD policies
showed significant foresight (Sullivan 2014), many hospitals have not begun to contemplate such policies. Second, only a subset of digital health products and services
are designed to be used in hospital settings, and thus will be motivated to consider
hospital guidelines. Finally, although BYOD policies seem relatively well-equipped
to handle data privacy and security, individual hospitals and medical schools do not
have the resources or internal expertise to evaluate the clinical utility of the hundreds of digital health products that might be used in their facilities.

18.4.3   App Review Sites

A third surrogate or proxy for traditional regulation is review by third-party product
review web sites. Perhaps the most prominent and well-established is the site iMedi-
calApps.com, staffed primarily by physician editors with a team of physicians,
health professionals, trainees, and professional writers who collaborate to publish
reviews of mobile health technologies (http://www.imedicalapps.com/about/ 2016).
Although reviews are not as comprehensive and systematic as what a *Consumer
Reports* might provide for everyday consumer products—for example, by surveying
all products in the field—the web site does target more popular apps and offers
curated lists of "top apps" and "top new apps," which are updated periodically.
Moreover, iMedicalApps publishes curated lists of the "top" apps for health professionals in a dozen different specialties, including cardiology, emergency medicine,
and radiology (http://www.imedicalapps.com/about/ 2016). More recently, the site
introduced a new service, called iPrescribeApps, which purports to provide "repu-
table and unbiased" guidance for physicians to "prescribe" apps to patients, including a mechanism for instructing patients on how to use the prescribed app and
reporting their results.

Of course, this was not the first such initiative, and it will not be the last. Happtique initially tried to curate mobile health apps for physicians, before creating a certification program to guide physicians and other prescribers on which apps were "clinically appropriate and technically sound." (Dolan 2016) However, Happtique suspended its certification program after a random review found several security flaws in apps certified by Happtique. Moreover, these kinds of reviews can be very resource-intensive and thus are slow to publish, as experienced by other ambitious app review initiatives like the U.K.'s National Health Service (NHS) Health Apps Library (http://www.nhs.uk/pages/healthappslibrary.aspx 2016).

But these challenges have not deterred others—like Evidation Health (originating at Stanford) and Ranked Health (originating at MIT)—from trying evaluate the efficacy of mobile health apps for physicians, patients, and insurers. Evidation is a partnership between GE Ventures and Stanford Health Care, whose ambition is to provide clinical and economic evidence supporting digital health technologies (http://www.evidation.com/about/ 2016). Ranked Health is operated by the Hacking Medicine Institute, originating out of a program at MIT, and offers to review and rank digital health apps and devices, not only to provide a curated list of clinically effective products, but to highlight "unsafe and ineffective" ones (http://www.rankedhealth.com/about/ 2016). Again, like its predecessors, Evidation and Ranked Health see a clear need, in the absence of more centralized regulation by the FDA, to provide independent, third-party evaluation of digital health products in order to help users navigate the flood of offerings by the industry.

18.4.4 Health Insurers

The fourth and final surrogate that has emerged is review by health insurers, who adopt coverage policies declaring that a health insurance plan will or will not cover a specific digital health technology. Although policies targeting digital health technologies remain somewhat rare, we have examples of both coverage and non-coverage policies—both of which reflect focused scrutiny of a digital health product by a relatively knowledgeable intermediary. For example, in 2014, health insurer Aetna updated its *Clinical Policy Bulletin* on *Cardiac Event Monitors* to cover the ZIO Patch made by iRhythm, which previously had categorized the product as "experimental and investigational." (http://www.aetna.com/cpb/medical/data/1_99/0073.html 2016; Comstock 2014) Conversely, in the same policy, Aetna announces that it still considers a very well-known digital health product, the AliveCor Heart Monitor, to be "experimental and investigational because [its] clinical value has not been established." (http://www.aetna.com/cpb/medical/data/1_99/0073.html 2016) Even more important, perhaps, are the national and local coverage determinations (NCDs and LCDs) issued by Medicare carriers and intermediaries, which are often followed by commercial insurers who do not have the infrastructure to evaluate new technologies on their own.

But again, there are very real limitations in relying on health insurers as a screen for assessing the clinical quality and reliability of digital health products. First, as with third-party product reviewers, health insurers cannot possibly review all products on the market, given their volume and variety. Second, although large insurers like Aetna and Blue Cross Blue Shield have their own internal systems for evaluating new technologies (such as the BCBS Center for Clinical Effectiveness (CCE 2016), formerly known as the Technology Evaluation Center (TEC)) (Comstock 2014), many insurers do not have the infrastructure to independently evaluate new technologies, and often rely on coverage policies published by Medicare, Medicaid, or other public programs. Finally, as with the other three surrogates described above, not all digital health products will rely on insurance reimbursement and thus will be subject to this kind of scrutiny. Each surrogate has major blind spots.

18.5   Conclusion

Digital health technologies are governed by a series of laws, regulations, and ethical standards that were written well before digital health was conceived. Digital health companies have struggled to adapt to these legal frameworks, just as the frameworks have struggled to adapt to these new technologies and business practices. Although over a dozen different legal frameworks can apply to digital health technologies (per Table 18.1 above), it is often unclear exactly how they apply.

Table 18.1 Legal frameworks potentially applicable to digital health

Legal framework	Federal or state law?	Primary regulator(s)
Medical device regulation	Federal	FDA
Consumer protection	Both	FTC, state agencies
Data privacy and security	Both	HHS OCR,[a] FTC, state agencies
Professional licensing	State	State medical and nursing boards
Medical malpractice liability	State	State courts
Hospital, facility liability	State	State courts
Product liability	State	State courts, CPSC[b]
Ethical standards	National, state, local	Professional bodies (*e.g.*, AMA)
Intellectual property[†]	Both	USPTO,[c] state courts
Clinical research[†]	Federal	HHS/CMS[d]
Discrimination[†]	Both	Multiple federal and state agencies
Cybersecurity[†]	Federal	Multiple federal agencies
Securities law[†]	Federal	SEC[e]

[†]Not covered in this chapter
[a]U.S. Department of Health & Human Services, Office of Civil Rights
[b]U.S. Consumer Product Safety Commission, which regulates product safety and provides a private cause of action, as explained in Sect. 18.2.5
[c]U.S. Patent & Trademark Office
[d]Centers for Medicare and Medicaid Services, a sub-agency of HHS
[e]U.S. Securities and Exchange Commission

Thus, there is a great deal of legal, regulatory, and ethical uncertainty regarding how digital health products should be used, and according to what standards. This uncertainty, in turn, has inspired various non-legal mechanisms to offer their own standards, as demonstrated above. Thus, if there is a "law" and "ethics" of digital health, it is emerging slowly, and from a variety of sources. As digital health technologies mature, so, gradually, will the law and ethics that apply to them.

References

15 U.S.C. § 2072. 2015.

15 U.S.C. § 45. 2015.

21 C.F.R. § 801.4. 2016.

21 U.S.C. § 321(h).

21 U.S.C. § 360(k). 2015.

21 U.S.C. § 360e. 2015.

21 U.S.C. §§ 360c, 360e.

45 C.F.R. parts 160, 164. 2015.

Abrams R. After one product recall, fitbit faces a new safety inquiry. New York Times. 2014. http://www.nytimes.com/2014/09/27/business/after-product-recall-fitbit-faces-a-new-safety-inquiry.html.

Al Ayubi SU, et al. A mobile app development guideline for hospital settings: maximizing the use of and minimizing the security risks of "bring your own devices" policies. J Med Internet Res. 2016;4(2):e50. http://mhealth.jmir.org/2016/2/e50/ Accessed 16 Aug 2016

American Medical Association. Opinion E-5.025 (physician advisory or referral services by telecommunications). 1994.

Bovara v. St. Francis Hospital, 700 N.E.2d 143 (Ill. App. Ct. 1998).

Brown K, Pearson GW. dba DERMAPPS, analysis of proposed consent order to aid public comment. 76 Fed. Reg. 57,041. Federal Trade Commission; 2011. https://www.ftc.gov/sites/default/files/documents/cases/2011/09/110915kobebrownfrn.pdf. Accessed 22 July 2016.

California Business and Professions Code § 17200. n.d.

California Business and Professions Code § 17500. 2016.

California Business and Professions Code § 17500. n.d.

California Civil Code § 56.06. 2016.

California Civil Code § 56.10. 2016.

California Civil Code §§ 1750-1784. n.d.

California Civil Code Part 2.6, §§ 56-59. 2016.

Carrns A. F.T.C.: No App to Cure Acne. The New York Times. 2011. http://bucks.blogs.nytimes.com/2011/11/01/f-t-c-no-app-to-cure-acne/. Accessed 22 July 2016.

Chen A. How your health data lead a not-so-secret life online. National Public Radio. 2016. http://www.npr.org/sections/health-shots/2016/07/30/487778779/how-your-health-data-lead-a-not-so-secret-life-online. Accessed 9 Aug 2016.

Comstock J. Aetna now reimburses for iRhythm's ZIO patch. MobiHealthNews. 2014. http://mobihealthnews.com/29484/aetna-now-reimburses-for-irhythms-zio-patch. Accessed 16 Aug 2016.

Cortez N. Regulating disruptive innovation. Berkeley Technol L J. 2014a;29(1):183–6.

Cortez N. The mobile health revolution? UC Davis L Rev. 2014b;47(1173):1201–12.

Cortez N. Analog agency in a digital world. FDA in the 21st Century: the challenges of regulating drugs and new technologies. New York, NY: Columbia University Press; 2015.

Darling v. Charleston Community Memorial Hospital, 33 Ill.2d 326 (1965).

Dolan B. Happtique steps up to certify mobile health apps. MobiHealthNews. 2016. http://mobihealthnews.com/15750/happtique-steps-up-to-certify-mobile-health-apps/. Accessed 16 Aug 2016.

Farr C. The theranos scandal is just the beginning. Fast Company. 2016. http://www.fastcompany.
    com/3059230/the-theranos-scandal-is-just-the-beginning. Accessed 16 Aug 2016.

Federal Food, Drug, and Cosmetic Act of 1938.

Finkel A. Analysis of proposed consent order to aid public comment. 76 Fed. Reg. 57,043. Federal
    Trade Commission; 2011. https://www.ftc.gov/sites/default/files/documents/cases/2011/09/11
    0915kobebrownfrn.pdf. Accessed 22 July 2016.

Hill K. A quantified self fatality? Family says cyclist's death is fault of ride-tracking company
    strava. Forbes. 2012. http://www.forbes.com/sites/kashmirhill/2012/06/20/a-quantified-self-
    fatality-family-says-cyclists-death-is-fault-of-ride-tracking-company-strava/#7ba7e8a42969.

Health Wildcatters. 2016. http://healthwildcatters.com. Accessed 16 Aug 2016.

Aetna. Clinical Policy Bulletin No. 0073: Cardiac Event Monitors. 2016. http://www.aetna.com/
    cpb/medical/data/1_99/0073.html. Accessed 16 Aug 2016.

American Medical Association. Digital health. http://www.ama-assn.org/ama/pub/advocacy/top-
    ics/digital-health.page. Last Accessed 12 Aug 2016.

American Medical Association. Connected health. http://www.ama-assn.org/ama/pub/advocacy/
    topics/digital-health/connected-health.page. Last Accessed 12 Aug 2016.

American Medical Association. AMA adopts new guidance for ethical practice in telemedicine.
    2016. http://www.ama-assn.org/ama/pub/news/news/2016/2016-06-13-new-ethical-guidance-
    telemedicine.page.

American Psychological Association. Guidelines for the practice of telepsychology. 2013. http://
    www.apa.org/practice/guidelines/telepsychology.aspx.

Blue Cross Blue Shield Association. Center for Clinical Effectiveness (CCE). 2016. http://www.
    bcbs.com/cce/. Accessed 16 Aug 2016.

The Commonwealth Fund. Developing a framework for evaluating the patient engagement, qual-
    ity, and safety of mobile health applications. 2016. http://www.commonwealthfund.org/publi-
    cations/issue-briefs/2016/feb/evaluating-mobile-health-apps. Last Accessed 16 Aug 2016.

Evidation Health. About. 2016. http://www.evidation.com/about/. Accessed 16 Aug 2016.

Mobile medical applications: guidance for industry and food and drug administration staff.
    U.S. Food and Drug Administration. 2015 pp 3–36. http://www.fda.gov/downloads/medicalde-
    vices/deviceregulationandguidance/guidancedocuments/ucm263366.pdf. Accessed 22 July
    2016.

General wellness: policy for low risk devices: guidance for industry and food and drug admin-
    istration staff. U.S. Food and Drug Administration. 2016. http://www.fda.gov/downloads/
    medicaldevices/deviceregulationandguidance/guidancedocuments/ucm429674.pdf. Accessed
    5 Aug 2016.

Letter to biosense technologies private limited concerning the uChek urine analyzer. May 21,
    2013. Silver Spring, MD: Food and Drug Administration. http://www.fda.gov/MedicalDevices/
    ResourcesforYou/Industry/ucm353513.htm. Accessed 8 Aug 2016.

iMedicalApps. About iMedical apps. 2016 http://www.imedicalapps.com/about/. Accessed 16
    Aug 2016.

IMS Health. Patient adoption of mHealth. 2015. http://www.imshealth.com/en/thought-leadership/
    ims-institute/reports/patient-adoption-of-mhealth. Last Accessed 16 Aug 2016.

National Health Services. Health apps library. 2016 http://www.nhs.uk/pages/healthappslibrary.
    aspx. Accessed 16 Aug 2016.

Ranked Health. About. 2016. http://www.rankedhealth.com/about/. Accessed 16 Aug 2016.

Federation of State Medical Boards. Model policy for the appropriate use of telemedicine tech-
    nologies in the practice of medicine. 2014. https://www.fsmb.org/Media/Default/PDF/FSMB/
    Advocacy/FSMB_Telemedicine_Policy.pdf.

Federal Trade Commission. FTC cracks down on marketers of "Melanoma Detection" Apps.
    2015. https://www.ftc.gov/news-events/press-releases/2015/02/ftc-cracks-down-marketers-
    melanoma-detection-apps. Accessed 22 July 2016.

Federal Trade Commission. Electronic health records company settles FTC charges it deceived
    consumers about privacy of doctor reviews. 2016. https://www.ftc.gov/news-events/press-
    releases/2016/06/electronic-health-records-company-settles-ftc-charges-it-deceived. Accessed
    22 July 2016.

Federal Trade Commission. Commission finds LabMD liable for unfair data security practices. 2016. https://www.ftc.gov/news-events/press-releases/2016/07/commission-finds-labmd-liable-unfair-data-security-practices. Accessed 9 Aug 2016.

Federal Trade Commission. Mobile health apps interactive tool. 2016. https://www.ftc.gov/tips-advice/business-center/guidance/mobile-health-apps-interactive-tool. Accessed 22 July 2016.

Food and Drug Administration, Federal trade commission, and office of national coordinator for health information technology. FDASIA Health IT Report. 2014. https://www.healthit.gov/sites/default/files/fdasia_healthitreport_final.pdf.

Jennings v. Badgett, 230 P.3d 861 (Okla. 2010).

Medical Device Amendments of 1976.

Miller v. Martin, 754 N.E.2d 41 (Ind. Ct. App. 2001).

POM Wonderful, LLC v. F.T.C., F.3d 483–84 (D.C. Cir. 2015).

Riegel v. Medtronic, 552 U.S. 312 (2008).

Stross R. Don't blame silicon valley for theranos. N Y Times. 2016. http://www.nytimes.com/2016/04/27/opinion/dont-blame-silicon-valley-for-theranos.html. Last Accessed 16 Aug 2016.

Sullivan T. The fine art and hardest part of crafting BYOD policy. MobiHealthNews. 2014. http://mobihealthnews.com/news/fine-art-and-hardest-part-crafting-byod-policy. Accessed 16 Aug 2016.

Teladoc, Inc. v. Texas medical board, 112 F.Supp.3d 529 (W.D. Tex. 2015a).

Teladoc, Inc. v. Texas medical board, 2015b WL 8773509 (W.D. Tex. 2015) (pending before the Fifth Circuit Court of Appeals as of August 2016).

Terry N. Regulatory disruption and arbitrage in healthcare data protection. Yale J Health Policy L Ethics. 2017 (forthcoming).

Terry N. Foreward: drug-drug interaction warnings as technological iatrogenesis. St Louis J Health L Policy. 2012;5:251–5.

Terry N., Wiley L. Liability for mobile health and wearable technologies. Ann Health Law. 2016 (forthcoming).

Texas administrative code § 190.8(1)(L) ("New Rule 190.8"). 2015.

White v. Harris, 36 A.3d 303 (Vt. 2011).

Chapter 19
Digital Health Entrepreneurship

Hubert Zajicek and Arlen Meyers

Abstract Digital health is the application of information and communications technologies (ICT) to exchange biomedical and clinical information with the goal of improving population health, the doctor–patient experience, and lowering aggregate costs. Digital health entrepreneurship is the pursuit of opportunity within healthcare characterized by scarce and uncontrolled resources, with the goal of creating user-defined value through the design, development, roll out or launch, and harvesting of digital health innovative products, services, platforms, and models. Digital health technologies, and the digital health entrepreneurs who create them, are rapidly changing the practice of medicine and the doctor–patient relationship. This chapter presents a Digital Health Innovation Roadmap and the opportunities and challenges confronting digital health entrepreneurs.

Keywords Digital • Health information systems • Health • Innovation • Entrepreneurship • Telemedicine • Data • Analytics • Remote sensors • Electronic medical records • Social media • Mobile medical applications

19.1 Introduction, Issues, and Opportunities

Not since the invention of books has medicine and the dissemination of information been as profoundly changed as in our lifetimes. With vast opportunities to innovate available to virtually everyone, change is the only constant.

Digital health, which can be defined as the application of information and communications technologies to exchange biomedical and clinical information, is no exception. While the barriers to innovation via digital health are extremely low, the

H. Zajicek, M.D., M.B.A. (✉)
Health Wildcatters, Dallas, TX, USA
e-mail: hubert@healthwildcatters.com

A. Meyers, M.D., M.B.A.
Society of Physician Entrepreneurs, South Norwalk, CT, USA

© Springer International Publishing AG 2018   271
H. Rivas, K. Wac (eds.), *Digital Health*, Health Informatics,
https://doi.org/10.1007/978-3-319-61446-5_19

barriers to success are much higher than in the non-health related world. A high school student can innovate and create a digital health solution that solves his or her observed problems, usually from a healthcare consumer point of view (Palfrey and Gasser 2008). It doesn't get any more democratic than that. To succeed in the healthcare industry properly, however, the regulations that have to be understood and comprehended include: complying with the Healthcare Insurance Portability and Accountability Act of 1996 (HIPAA), the Federal Drug Administration's (FDA) rules, Stark laws (Physician self-referral laws), etc. Moreover, the complex healthcare delivery systems and intricate reimbursement models paired with disparate groups of stakeholders create a maze that makes entrepreneurship anything but democratic. In a nutshell, it isn't hard to spot a problem in healthcare that needs a solution, but it is immensely difficult to create a compliant, functional solution that becomes a commercial success and that has a viable business model.

For example, two emergency doctors observed that patients were going to inappropriate places for care. The result was an application, iTriage, that informs patients about where they should go for care.

The US healthcare system is, in reality a sick care system, since most of the over 3T is spent taking care of sick patients, not on wellness, prevention and health maintenance. The challenge for digital health entrepreneurs, like other stakeholders, is to change a provider centric, fee for service, low quality, high cost, specialty driven, outcomes disparate system to a patient centric, value based, healthcare system that eliminated health outcome disparities based on geography, race, gender, insurance coverage and other socio-economic drivers (e.g. nutrition, housing and education), of outcomes disparities.

19.2   Digital Health

This topic touches anything that puts 1s and 0s between healthcare and humans. Today, digital health touches almost every aspect of the physician–patient interaction, as patients have evolved into healthcare consumers.

There are several categories of digital health technologies, applications and intended uses. They include:

1. Remote sensing and wearables.
2. Telemedicine.
3. Data analytics and intelligence, predictive modeling.
4. Health and wellness behavior modification tools.
5. Bioinformatics tools (-omics).
6. Medical social media.
7. Digitized health record platforms.
8. Patient -physician patient portals and consumer experience.
9. DIY diagnostics, compliance and treatments.
10. Decision support systems.
11. Population health.
12. Workflow improvement.

With these consumers in charge, digital health requires the patients' interactions and consent, not just when in the hospital or at the doctor's office. The very basic question has to be: "Who, if not the individual, can best carry the burden and responsibility of taking charge of the healthcare of that individual?" Accountable Care Organizations (ACO's) are taking a stab at it, but there is a fine balance between best care and best affordable care when institutions are in charge. To a certain degree, the ACO model (or Euro-model light), can work for a group. These models are ultimately subject to a host of ethical questions as profits and individual interests collide. Digital health empowers individuals; however, it also enables a host of controls whereby health systems can discern the "compliance" of individuals with their own healthcare. Conflicts here are inevitable. With the increased use of digital health monitors, we can not only monitor our health, but we may also gain an ability to intervene early and innovate totally new models to treat certain diseases. Big data plays an important role in discerning population trends, and genomics data can assist with patient-level decisions.

19.3   The Entrepreneur

Here is the dilemma: many innovations in digital health are best approached from a consumer perspective, because that is where the pain often lies.

Now, one other way to approach this subject is to simply assume that consumers should go ahead and just innovate. One argument holds that consumers will become so powerful or so influential that they will change "the rules." One would think that in a patient-centered environment, consumers could apply enough pressure to "change the rules" and make information sharing simpler. Recent examples like the shutdown/warning letter (U.S. Food and Drug Administration 2013) of 23andme, for instance, have demonstrated that the entrenched rules continue to apply no matter how much consumers would like more information sharing.

When deciding to start a digital health startup, it would be advisable to stay within the bounds of the various healthcare laws (U.S. Food and Drug Administration 2017). This is important for many reasons, one of which is to garner significant financial backing to grow the startup.

Digital Healthcare entrepreneurs often have a healthcare background. In part this is necessary to identify the problems, in part it is necessary to execute in the much more complex world of laws, rules and regulations. So who is a typical successful healthcare entrepreneur? Does he or she come from a professional healthcare background, a healthcare system, or is he or she more likely to be an empowered healthcare consumer? The reality of many successful startups is that at least one of a basic team of two entrepreneurs has a healthcare background and can reasonably navigate the maze of existing rules and regulations. There are notable exceptions, but it is hard to bet on a team that has no background in healthcare. That said, I see fewer physician inventors and more allied health and other healthcare professionals who play at the intersection of health, technology and entrepreneurship (Table 19.1).

Table 19.1 Digital health gaps: needs finding and how to identify voids

The most invested YTD markets according to Startup Health's Mid-year 2016 report are
1. Patient/consumer experience
2. Wellness
3. Personalized health/quantified self
4. Big Data/analytics
5. Workflow
6. Clinical decision support
7. Medical device
8. E-commerce
9. Research
10. Population health

These trends are reflected in the Health Wildcatters application pool this year as well, in addition to the medical device candidates and other applicants. We have also seen a number of blockchain and artificial intelligence startups, undoubtedly a trend that will continue. We definitely see distinct trends over the last few years from a surge in health and wellness apps to more of a big-data/machine-learning focus in digital health. In the last year, we have seen a multitude of tech-enabled services exploit the fact that in so many verticals, nothing has changed in decades. For instance, app-based house calls, home health services, long-term care solutions, etc. are all at one's fingertips, allowing innovative companies to capture market share just as Uber did in the limo/taxi world.

For the individual entrepreneur, finding problems in healthcare takes little more than going to a doctor's office and observing the archaic processes deployed there. We often meet entrepreneurs who have done just that and have come up with a new form of EHR or digitized patient intake form. What most innovators fail to understand, however, is that the challenge is not simply to solve technical shortcomings and create a better EHR. Instead, the challenge is to fulfill the needs of both the hospital/physician's office/insurer as well as those of the patient/consumer with a fully integrated solution. In the end, only the large hospital systems or insurers themselves are able to devise and adopt new EHR solutions, as they must consider compatibility with the multi-million dollar systems already in place. This makes it nearly impossible for the entrepreneur to come in with a solution derived solely from the healthcare consumer's point of view, despite the many frustrations that come from the lack of a simple, functional and readily accessible repository of Electronic Health Records.

At Johns Hopkins, the Biodesign course in the field of Bioengineering, Innovation, and Design teaches students a sophisticated method of identifying and tackling problems. One of our startups at Health Wildcatters came from this program and ultimately commercialized their solution to an inefficient process they had observed at Johns Hopkins. It is often best to assemble a startup team from members of diverse, yet relevant backgrounds. At Stanford University, for instance, the Byers Center for Biodesign, students in the Biodesign course may come from the bio-engineering program, but also from the medical school. Residents, fellows and/ or fully-trained physicians also participate. "Needs finding" is taught systematically through observation of clinical settings and interviews over a 4-week period. Paul Yock, Director at Stanford Biodesign, puts it this way: "A well characterized need is the DNA of a good invention." After the need is discovered, execution follows and much iteration takes place before an invention hits the first beta testers. I won't go into the process in detail here; however, I recommend a perusal of *Biodesign: The Process of Innovating Medical Technologies* 2nd edition by Yock et al. (2015). What's important to understand is that the process by which one would assess "need" is the same as with any other biomedical invention. When a need is translated into a business opportunity, designing the right business model and surveying the market for demand are completely separate tasks which should be pursued with equal persistence and open mindedness. The key difference is that when pursuing the business model, you have to spend a lot more time with outside parties that would be your end-user purchasers. These users can have vastly different ideas about what it means to deliver value to them. Here, the bottom line, not just the challenge of building a better mousetrap, matters greatly. This means spending time with and gaining an understanding of the different ideas of outside parties. It is these outside parties who will become end-user purchasers, so delivering a product of value to them is critical.

We have been hearing a lot about digital health and electronic medical records over the past few years and, given the rapidly evolving state of technologies and rules, we are likely to continue to do so in the future. The bugaboos are well known, but it seems there is more momentum to plug the gaps, particularly since taxpayers have spent billions to subsidize digitizing healthcare information.

As a result, patients, doctors, and now the US government are putting more and more pressure on the health information technology industry to get it right. They want these gaps closed.

1. The technology development gap, where designers don't communicate or collaborate with end users.
2. The access gap, where both providers and patients get access to the internet and to enough bandwidth to manage the increasing amount of data. This is but one of many digital divides. The issues become even more pressing when we note that there are four billion people on the planet who are not connected. Getting to them and to those in underserved areas of more developed countries will have to address three main problems: affordability, relevance, and unfamiliarity.
3. The manpower gap, where we don't train enough clinical informaticians or data scientists in a reasonable amount of time instead of requiring an MD, MBA, or Masters in Information Systems or Computer Science.
4. The interoperability gap, where information can be globally exchanged from one patient or provider to another. Protect but share has not worked.
5. The data security gap, where almost every day we read about another hack of patient data.
6. The censorship gap, where some think EHRs are a threat to academic freedom and free speech.

7. The EHR data ownership gap, where patients want to "own" their data and not relinquish it to vendors, doctors, or hospitals.
8. The usefulness gap, where electronic records are bill-collecting and profit-generating instruments not designed to maximize patient care and reduce costs.
9. The aim gap, where the triple aim omits the experience of the healthcare users. There should be a quadruple aim.
10. The cost gap where, particularly for small, independently owned practices, the costs of electronic medical data systems has become prohibitively expensive and another federal unfunded mandate further threatening private practice.
11. The health IT gender pay gap. There is also a significant policy research gap confounded by poor research design or conflicts of interest.

So what is the treatment for digital health 'gaposis'?

1. Focus on making digital health a sub-segmented academic domain.
2. Write an online textbook and case book.
3. Craft a specific value proposition for the scientists, engineers, lawyers, businesspeople, and health professionals.
4. Create free, faster, smarter, more secure WiFi networks.
5. Create better knowledge exchange programs.
6. Offer better experiential learning opportunities.
7. Focus on creating user-defined value, not investor-defined companies.
8. Prototype and simulate to verify and validate.
9. Expand bioentrepreneurship education and training programs.
10. Reward faculty digital health innovation scholarship.
11. Here are some other solutions suggested by the Commonwealth Fund:

    "To move forward with consumer-mediated health information exchange, several steps will be required. First, the federal government needs to more aggressively enforce HIPAA's information-sharing provisions. Second, we need a new cohort of health-data stewards who can help patients manage their own data. Some process of private certification or public regulation will likely be necessary to assure that these new entities can be trusted to discharge this sensitive and complex responsibility. Third, we will need to perfect the technical ability of these new data stewards to access the electronic-data repositories of health-care providers."

Doctors are spending too much time as data managers overseeing patients as data points using dysfunctional systems. As a result, we are getting the garbage out we would expect.

19.4   The Digital Health Innovation Roadmap

Bioscientists, engineers, non-healthcare entrepreneurs, and health professionals have many ways to practice biomedical and clinical entrepreneurship, e.g., in biopharma, medical device and diagnostics, small business medical practice, educational technologies, and social entrepreneurship and intrapreneurship. Digital health entrepreneurship is another pathway.

As noted, digital health is the application of information and communications technologies (ICT) to exchange medical information. Like all other areas of biomedical entrepreneurship, digital health entrepreneurs pursue opportunities with scarce resources with the goal of creating user/patient/customer/stakeholder-defined value through the design, development, testing, validation, and deployment of digital health products and services.

In some instances, digital health products and services can be stand-alone offerings, usually providing the intended user with information, a communications interface, and education that are not defined as drugs or devices and, therefore, not subject to regulatory requirements. Some, on the other hand, become a new part of a drug or device, e.g., a remote sensor in an orthopedic implant or a "smart" pill or other innovative drug delivery device.

Much like the medtech innovation roadmap, the digital health innovation roadmap has several stops along the way that can take several months, if not years, to arrive. They include:

1. Early stage or prototype product development, customer discovery and development, and validating the parts of the business model canvas. If you don't do this right, then there is not much point in moving to the next steps. In fact, not having a viable business model is the main reason companies, including digital health companies, fail.
2. Design and reduction to practice using established quality system controls, including technical validation and verification.

    The terms "verification" and "validation" are commonly used in software engineering to mean two different types of analysis. The usual definitions are:

    - Validation: Are we building the right system?
    - Verification: Are we building the system right?
    In other words, validation is concerned with checking that the system will meet the customer's actual needs, whereas verification is concerned with whether the system is well-engineered, error-free, and so on. Verification will help determine whether the software is of high quality, but it will not ensure that the system is useful.

    The distinction between the two terms is largely due to the role of specifications. Validation is the process of checking whether a specification captures the customer's needs, whereas verification is the process of checking that the software meets the specification.

3. Following the appropriate regulatory approval pathway, when appropriate.
4. Securing intellectual property protection, when appropriate (Capron and Wells 2016).
5. Translational and human subjects research, when appropriate.
6. Launch, marketing, and sales.
7. Post-marketing surveillance.

While the path may be clear, the journey is difficult and filled with hazards.

19.5 Digital Health Entrepreneurship Trends

There have been several recent trends in physician entrepreneurship. Most of the activity has been around medical practice and process entrepreneurship and digital health entrepreneurship. More specifically, here are some highlights:

1. As biomedical entrepreneurship education programs evolve, more are offering specific interdisciplinary courses and degrees in data science and digital health entrepreneurship.
2. Physician digital health entrepreneurs and trainees are getting more and more involved in the early stages of new product design and development as founders, advisors, or consultants.
3. Some medical students are electing to not do a residency after medical school to pursue startup opportunities.
4. Digital health entrepreneurs are starting to understand the importance of demonstrating clinical validity of products and services by testing them in human subjects. Like many other therapeutic interventions, dose matters.
5. Investors are increasing their bets on digital health entrepreneurs.
6. The barriers to digital health entrepreneurship are falling due to increasing collaboration of members of emerging national digital health ecosystems.
7. Academic medical centers are changing to move from predominantly drug discovery and development interest to include digital health ideas and inventions. Several have rebranded their technology transfer offices into innovation centers with a focus on inside–outside collaboration.
8. The IP and regulatory landscape of digital health is coming more and more into focus and importance.
9. Bottom up, patient- and physician-centered digital health collaborations are becoming a major component of product development and deployment.
10. Generational digital native knowledge, skills, and attitudes are driving the adoption and penetration of digital health.
11. Remote sensing, pattern recognition, and machine learning will change telediagnostics to a consumer electronics platform, further disintermediating doctors.
12. The driverless electric car and sharing economy model has come to medicine. Machine learning and deep intelligence is forcing us to deal with the medical machine problem.

19.5.1 Digital Health Innovation Is Different from Biomedical Innovation

There are two basic categories of medical entrepreneurship-biomedical and clinical. There are significant differences in the innovation pathways for the two:

1. Intellectual property protection usually is of more importance in biomedical entrepreneurship.
2. Regulatory approval can be a long, expensive and risky process for drugs and devices.

3. Reimbursement and payment for biomedical innovations are often dependent on getting the appropriate codes and third party payments at high enough amounts to generate a profit.
4. Business models differ and are constantly changing.
5. The amount of capital necessary to get a drug or device to market is frequently higher than health innovation by several orders of magnitude.
6. The FDA may not have jurisdiction over many health innovations, for example a digital health app that is not deemed to be a medical device but rather something that provides information and education to users.
7. The customers vary depending on whether you are deploying a biomedical or health product.
8. Validating your business model using lean startup methodologies will vary and can be more challenging for biomedical innovators.
9. Biomedical entrepreneurship often requires a different skill set than health entrepreneurship.
10. Biomedical entrepreneurship is riskier.

Health or clinical entrepreneurs focus their activities on digital health, care delivery models, business or clinical processes, or policy. Furthermore, digital health can be further subdivided into segments:

1. Remote sensing and wearables.
2. Telemedicine.
3. Data analytics and intelligence, predictive modeling.
4. Health and wellness behavior modification tools.
5. Bioinformatics tools (-omics).
6. Medical social media.
7. Digitized health record platforms.
8. Patient -physician patient portals.
9. DIY diagnostics, compliance and treatments.
10. Decision support systems.

Unlike bioimedical entrepreneurs who are trying to get drugs, devices, diagnostics,vaccines and biologics to patients, digipreneurs have to face the facts that:

1. There is a difference between an industry and a market. Those companies that provide products and services comprise the industry. The customers who use those products and are looking for ways to get a particular job done are the market. However, both the digital health industry and digital health users are a complex combination of providers, payers, industry partners in interface technology industries and patients, some of whom are customers or consumers while others are influencers.
2. Like all investors, digital health investors are looking for the highest rate of return with the least amount of risk. Given the foggy legal, regulatory and reimbursement atmosphere, it's too early to tell which dogs will eat the food. There has already been high profile digital health failures, roll ups, IPOs and consolidation as the industry and markets continue to mature.

3. Most digital health technologies have not been clinically validated nor are they required to do so. However, other regulatory agencies, like the FTC or the Consumer Products Safety Commission, are wary about digital health product claims that are not supported by research.

4. The FDA continues to offer periodic guidance documents and regulations that contribute to a level of uncertainty when it comes to defining what is a medical device and what is not. That makes the hair stand up on the back of investor's necks.

5. Given the multiple stakeholders in healthcare—payers, providers, patients, partners and others—it's hard to target any one customer. Several need to see the value for any given product or service.

6. The industry is too new and there is too little research to know which customers/ patients/stakeholders will adopt a product and why.

7. Scale trumps innovation. The single most important characteristic of those companies that have received substantial follow-on investments are those that have scaled their customer rate rapidly by at least 70% a year.

8. Doctors don't have the information they need to know whether to prescribe or use a given digital health technology.

9. Most doctors don't get paid to use digital health technologies, they disrupt workflow, and there are nagging behavioral and emotional barriers to adoption by both patients and their families and their doctors.

10. There are significant confidentiality, security and data privacy issues still lurking.

11. Patent protection is not as important in digital health as it is in biopharma or medtech. Things move much more quickly, the product life cycles are much shorter and time is of the essence when it comes to getting adaption and penetration in the patient/consumer or medical community.

12. Business models are evolving and change on a regular basis, sensitive to the protean tastes of Internet junkies.

For these and other reasons, non-sickcare entrepreneurs fail despite their previous track records of success in other consumer markets.

Here is the story about how many came together to create the Colorado digital health cluster.

Digital health is the new New Thing. Like all new things, it is surrounded by hype and hope. Whether digital health can bend the cost curve and help patients or is just another tech bubble remains to be seen. Digital health entrepreneurs need to do their due diligence with both eyes open and their wallets protected until they are convinced they can overcome the risks.

Digital health entrepreneurs have a big challenge. Digitizing sick care, while inevitable, has already seen its share of failed products, bad rules, and dysfunctional ecosystems (Biselli 2016). Most have failed because they did not achieve the 4Vs of sick care innovation.

For sick care innovation to be truly transformative, innovators need to demonstrate four main things:

Their solution need to be validated and verified Many innovators confuse the two. Here's one explanation of the difference.

The terms Verification and Validation are commonly used in software engineering to mean two different types of analysis. The usual definitions are:

- Validation: Are we building the right system?
- Verification: Are we building the system right?

In other words, validation is concerned with checking that the system will meet the customer's actual needs, while verification is concerned with whether the system is well-engineered, error-free, and so on. Verification will help to determine whether the software is of high quality, but it will not ensure that the system is useful.

The distinction between the two terms is largely to do with the role of specifications. Validation is the process of checking whether the specification captures the customer's needs, while verification is the process of checking that the software meets the specification.

In sickcare, since we are creating products and services that impact patients directly, you need to validate and verify your solution not just at the technical and commerical level, but at the clinical level as well. Sick care entrepreneurs, particularly non-sick care entrepreneurs, don't do the latter due to cost, regulatory risk, delays in time to market or simple ignorance about how to design, execute, analyze and report human subject trials.

Something that creates a significant multiple of user defined value in relation to a competitive offering, the status quo or non-users. Here are ten things physician entreprneurs need to know about value. Defining and comparing end user value is tricky and filled with wrong turns that make innovators believe they have reached their destination, when, in fact, they are lost. Innovation has both a qualitative and quantitative part. End users won't switch to your product unless they perceive at least a 5× greater multiple of value. You should shoot for much higher multiples.

It needs to go viral. In other words, it needs to get traction, overcome the barriers to widespread adoption and penetration, be applicable to populations for the intended use and, ultimately, become the standard of care.

There are other reasons why digital health entrepreneurs fail:

1. They fail to understand what it takes to cross the chasm generally and, specifically, digital health adoption and penetration. They think that because they were successful in other industries and that sick care is a million years behind the times and ripe for change that they can make it happen and move on.
2. They erroneously think that consumer product strategies can easily be transposed to sick care products and services.
3. They don't understand human subject clinical trials or how to demonstrate clinical effectiveness.
4. They are confused by FDA mandates and guidance documents regulating mobile medical apps.

5. They consider reimbursement or revenue generation as an after-thought instead of as part of their initial commercial feasibility assessment and business model canvas assumptions.
6. They ignore the intellectual property protection issues.
7. They stumble over how to deal with doctors as part of their business to business model and think that doctors are lousy business people, know-it-alls and too smart for their own good.
8. They don't satisfy all the sick care stakeholders (patients, payers, providers, and partners) and instead focus on just one.
9. They are investor and technopreneur driven, instead of end-user driven. They don't understand what makes patients and doctors tick or how to navigate the last mile.
10. They have a hard time penetrating a clinical culture that is resistant to change and has a not-invented-here mindset.We are in the early stages of digital health entrepreneurship and trying to figure out what works and what doesn't, what rules and regulations we need and which we should revise, and the impact on society and the medical profession.

19.6   Business Models

The business model can be described as: create, deliver, and capture value (Myler 2014). Things are NOT different as far as the basics go in healthcare. Just like in all other industries, a business model has to deliver value that ultimately can be captured. In healthcare, the capture piece can be extremely tricky. Think of long sales cycles, slow paying, difficult pricing models, insurance reimbursement percentages, and so forth. Think of a diverse set of customers with various incentives to buy or not. To call this a maze is an understatement. That is why it is so critical for digital health startups to do a thorough analysis and assessment of the business model, including an extensive dive into who the customers are, who captures the value on the customer side, and who ends up paying for the services. Being off just a tad bit can result in a failed startup.

Some digital health solutions are stand-alone while others need to be integrated into healthcare systems, medical devices, pharma, or other regulated products. When we are dealing with stand-alone systems, it usually has to do with a single information exchange connection that needs to be made. This often occurs between new players, as in the case of data retrieved from consumer-worn health trackers or other health related gadgets. The beauty with these digital health startups is that they generally don't fall under FDA guidelines or are treated like any other consumer good (U.S. Food and Drug Administration 2017).

The situation looks decidedly different when we involve regulated devices or other products. Not just are we dealing with the associated regulatory burdens, but if we're talking about communicating with health information systems, then we are also dealing with transmitting sensitive information into possibly rather complicated networks. The whole solution becomes decidedly more difficult to plan, execute, or sell.

As you create value with a digital health solution, you are likely to encounter significant differences to the classic medical device or pharma startup. The good news is that you are less likely dealing with intellectual property, an arduous, costly and long regulatory pathway and clinical validation as you would with a device, for instance. All this translates into lower costs, less time, and likely fewer barriers to entry for others to do exactly what you are doing. On the other hand, besides lower barriers to entry, you will likely be dealing with having to figure out your business model, which is much less straightforward, and integration issues with hospital or other systems. The person tackling a digital health solution has to have a quite different skill set, but it is hard to say what the ideal background for that entrepreneur or team may be. A good understanding of health systems, data, and workflow are a good start. As always, the core entrepreneurial team should have access to the right people they need to be selling and providing value to as well as be able to speak their "language." Very likely, one on this entrepreneurial team will have a professional healthcare background.

A business model is the plan implemented by a company to generate revenue and make a profit from operations. The model includes the components and functions of the business as well as the revenues it generates and the expenses it incurs. A key step for startups and scaleups is to create a business model and validate the underlying assumptions as quickly and as cheaply as possible.

However, there are many options when it comes to creating a model and a startup entrepreneur has to decide which to deploy and test. By applying certain screens or criteria to your model, you can make it VAST:

1. Validity—Regardless of which elements of your model you choose, they have to be valid. In other words, the dogs have to eat the food. When the dog won't eat the food, you'll have to change your approach and try again.
2. Automaticity—At the very start of planning your venture, you should think about how you are going to work on your business, not in it. Reducing hands-on time to manage operations will give you more time to lead the company and create strategies for growth and give you more personal time to enjoy the fruits of your success. Outsourcing, automating or using technologies to ramp up operations, sourcing, and distribution are key parts of scaling and something that investors want to see...which brings us to the next piece.
3. Scalability—Your business model is primarily a way to create a business machine that can produce an infinite number of products. Think of it as a device that takes in customers and generates profits out the other end, and can do so at an increasing rate.
4. Time and Traction—Finally, your model needs to create as much profit as quickly as possible with a growing customer base that is loyal to your brand.

The building blocks of any business have to do with problem seeking, problem solving, a team that can create and deploy a VAST business model, and an exit strategy.

If you want to accelerate, then build a machine that will respond to the accelerator.

19.7 Financing Digital Health Ventures

According to Rock Health (Tecco 2017), digital health funding has increased from $1B in 2011 to $4.2B in 2016 Data from Startup Health (Mack 2016) for 2016 showed a record setting pace of funding at over $8.1B.

The overall most active markets for funding are patient experience, wellness, personalized health/quantified self, big data and analytics, workflow, clinical decision support, medical device, e-commerce, research, and population health. Dealwise, the coasts continue to dominate the larger deals, with six of the largest hubs located on the East or West coasts (Wang et al. 2015).

Digital health technologies, which apply information and communications technologies to improve care outcomes, reduce per capita costs, and improve the doctor–patient experience, continue to hit the market at breakneck speed.

While the venture investments are well documented, what is happening at the seed stage and pre-angel investment level is a lot less well documented. By definition, these fundings are too small to be captured, but some trends emerge nevertheless. The funders of early stage digital health ventures tend to be healthcare angel investors, and some of the venture arms of the larger hospital groups. Needless to say, digital health startups, that can provide value to hospitals and insurers garner their attention and have a ready made- built in customer in their strategic investor.

Major categories include wearables and biosensing, analytics and big data, patient engagement, telemedicine, employee wellness, EHR, and workflow.

Here's how I segment the industry:

1. Remote sensing and wearables.
2. Telemedicine.
3. Data analytics and intelligence, predictive modeling.
4. Health and wellness behavior modification tools.
5. Bioinformatics tools (-omics).
6. Medical social media.
7. Digitized health record platforms.
8. Patient–physician patient portals and consumer experience.
9. DIY diagnostics, compliance, and treatments.
10. Decision support systems.
11. Population health.
12. Workflow improvement.

If you are thinking about investing in the digital health industry, then keep a few things in mind:

1. There is a difference between an industry and a market. Those companies that provide products and services comprise the industry. The customers who use those products and are looking for ways to get a particular job done are the market.

2. Like all investors, digital health investors are looking for the highest rate of return with the least amount of risk. Given the foggy legal, regulatory, and reimbursement atmosphere, it's too early to tell which dogs will eat the food.

3. Most digital health technologies have not been clinically validated.

4. The FDA continues to offer periodic guidance documents and regulations that contribute to a level of uncertainty that makes the hair on the backs of investors' necks stand up. In addition, other regulatory agencies, like the FTC and Consumer Product Safety Commission, have started poking their noses under the tent.

5. Given the multiple stakeholders in healthcare, like payers, providers, patients, partners, and others, it's hard to target any one customer. Several need to see the value for any given product or service.

6. The industry is too new and there is too little research to know which customers/patients/stakeholders will adopt a product and why.

7. Scale trumps innovation. The single most important characteristic of those companies that have received substantial follow on investments are those that have scaled their customer rate rapidly by at least 70% per year.

8. Doctors don't have the information they need to know whether to prescribe or use a given digital health technology. In many instances, they have too much data and not enough actionable information.

9. Most doctors don't get paid to use digital health technologies, they disrupt workflow, and there are nagging behavioral and emotional barriers to adoption by patients, their families, and their doctors.

10. Significant confidentiality, security, and data privacy issues are still lurking.

Fitbit went public and was valued at $4.1B. However, they face competition from Apple and other mobile platforms.

Here is a due diligence checklist for digital health products and services investors

1. Payment opportunities.
2. Impact of product design and functionality on regulatory requirements.
3. Design for safety.
4. Interoperability with other data.
5. Design for privacy and security.
6. Security and breach mitigation.
7. FCC equipment authorization.
8. Accurate and truthful advertisements.
9. Intellectual property rights.
10. Consider license and service agreements.

We are moving down the digital health hype cycle curve (Fig. 19.1).

Digital health is the newest new thing and, like all new things, it is surrounding by hype and hope (Panetta 2017). Whether digital health can achieve its goals or is just another tech bubble remains to be seen. Digital health investors need to do their due diligence with both eyes open and their wallets closed until their risk hurdles are met. *Caveat Digemptor*.

19.8 Summary

Digital health is the application of information and communications technologies to exchange biomedical data and information. Digital health entrepreneurship is the pursuit of opportunity using scarce resources with the goal of creating user-defined value through the deployment of digital health innovation.

Closing digital health gaps and creating products and services that are technically, commercially, and clinically valid will be a challenge and an opportunity for the foreseeable future.

Core strategies should include:

1. Reinventing the core, including a digital strategy and eCare.
2. Pursuing adjacencies.
3. Building talent and capabilities.
4. Revamping IT and building a whole product solution.
5. Starting with the patient/customer and working back.

References

Biselli M. How to build a thriving startup ecosystem anywhere. 2016. https://www.entrepreneur.com/article/282859. Accessed 28 Sept 2017.

Capron A, Wells R. How digital health startups can leverage intellectual property. 2016. http://hitconsultant.net/2016/01/18/digital-health-startups-intellectual-property/. Accessed 28 Sept 2017.

Mack H. Startup Health: $3.9B in digital health funding for 2016's first half. 2016. http://www.mobihealthnews.com/content/startup-health-39b-digital-health-funding-2016s-first-half. Accessed 28 Sept 2017.

Myler L. 3 Steps to an irresistible business model. 2014. https://www.forbes.com/sites/larrymyler/2013/08/01/3-steps-to-an-irresistible-business-model-multiple-authentication-methods/#5626b5473c6c. Accessed 28 Sept 2017.

Palfrey JG, Gasser U. Born digital: understanding the first generation of digital natives. New York, NY: Basic Books; 2008.

Panetta CK. Top trends in the Gartner Hype Cycle for emerging technologies. 2017. http://www.gartner.com/smarterwithgartner/top-trends-in-the-gartner-hype-cycle-for-emerging-technologies-2017/. Accessed 29 Sept 2017.

Tecco H. 2016 Year end funding report: a reality check for digital health. 2017. https://rockhealth.com/reports/2016-year-end-funding-report-a-reality-check-for-digital-health/. Accessed 29 Sept 2017.

U.S. Food and Drug Administration. Digital health. 2017. https://www.fda.gov/medicaldevices/digitalhealth/. Accessed 28 Sept 2017.

U.S. Food and Drug Administration, Center for Drug Evaluation and Research. 23 and Me DN: GEN1300666 warning letter, November 22, 2013. www.fda.gov/ICECI/EnforcementActions/ WarningLetters/2013/ucm376296.htm (2013).

Wang T, King E, Perman M, Tecco H. Digital health funding: 2015 year in review. 2015. https://rockhealth.com/reports/digital-health-funding-2015-year-in-review/. Accessed 28 Sept 2017.

Yock PG, Zenios S, Makower J, Brinton TJ, et.al. Biodesign: the process of innovating medical technologies. 2nd ed. Cambridge, UK: Cambridge University Press; 2015.

Chapter 20
Who Will Pay for Digital Health?
The Investor Point of View

Mussaad Al-Razouki

Abstract The beauty of investing in digital health is that it combines the high-risk/high-reward paradigm, synonymous with the tech industry, and the stability/defensiveness paradigm of the healthcare industry, thereby hedging or mitigating the investor's risk and providing an ideal counterbalance to future rewards. While many investors from Wall Street to Wuxi are singularly driven by maximizing profit, a great number of healthcare and digital health investors are driven by the tandem outlook of both financial profitability and improved societal benefits.

In this chapter, we will view the digital health industry through the lens of an investor, starting with the investor's contribution throughout the entrepreneurial life cycle and ending with the main drivers behind digital health investing. The investor perspective will often provide key insights for budding digital health entrepreneurs and will share with them some tricks-of-the-trade. This chapter will also provide them with insights into the inner workings and motivations of the different types of investors. The chapter will also cover the current state of digital health investors and discuss some of their investments. We will also cover some of the current and future models of digital health finance.

Perhaps the best way to summarize this chapter is that the greatest investors, like the best spouses, always see the potential of the person in front of them rather than their current status. Technical terms, such as top line revenue, net present value, P/E (price:earnings) ratio, and buzz words such as traction, big data, and brighter days ahead, play second-fiddle to the all-important truth in investing: you invest in the potential of the team.

Keywords Digital health investment • Total addressable market • Entrepreneurial life cycle • Seed stage • Angel investing • Crowdfunding • Venture capital • Private equity • IPO • Fundamental law of growth

M. Al-Razouki
Kuwait Life Sciences Company, Sharq, Kuwait
e-mail: Mussaad@klsc.com.kw

© Springer International Publishing AG 2018
H. Rivas, K. Wac (eds.), *Digital Health*, Health Informatics,
https://doi.org/10.1007/978-3-319-61446-5_20

20.1   The Economic Impact of Digital Health

Healthcare is one of the world's largest industries. Globally, the size of the health-care market is estimated to be between five trillion and six trillion dollars. Three trillion (Centers for Medicare & Medicaid services n.d.), or over half this amount is spent in the United States; that is, just 5% of the world's population, accounts for over 50% of the world's total health bill. To further compound the impact of health-care on the US economy, it is well known that the US spends anywhere between 16 and 18% of its GDP on healthcare (Centers for Medicare & Medicaid services n.d.), which is over twice what most developed countries spend (Organization for Co-operation and Development n.d.). Just as one example of how large the health-care industry actually is globally, one should consider this: all spending on products and services concerning the heart (pharmaceuticals such as beta-blockers, cardio-vascular surgery procedures, etc.) is actually larger than the entire automotive industry. Therefore, it is no wonder that investors have traditionally looked at healthcare as a lucrative industry in which to invest.

Investors typically start most business assessments by calculating the Total Addressable Market (TAM), which is simply the total size of the market (in terms of revenue potential) that a new product or service or, in our case, the digital health industry, can potentially achieve. So what is the TAM for digital health and how does this potential impact the healthcare economy?

Many would argue that the TAM for digital health is actually the entire health-care industry itself. That we will one day wake up to robo-diagnosticians that will prescribe 3D-printed pills delivered by automated drones and robo-surgeons that splice our DNA while uploading nanoparticles through the complex Internet of Things (IoT). Those who are slightly more conservative might limit digital health to disrupting the 30% administrative cost that currently plagues the healthcare industry (Woolhandler et al. 2003), making the global TAM for digital health to be roughly around two trillion USD. So, regardless of the side of the spectrum, it is clear that the potential for digital health is substantial and that the economic implications of disruptive digital health technologies are vast.

More importantly, is the rate of innovation and digitization in healthcare trails in comparison with other industries that have adopted these disruptive digital technologies at a much more rapid pace. Consider all the banking transactions available in the palm of your hand, or the thousands of hours of digital simulation training pilots must master prior to their first test flight. Many digital pundits believe that if healthcare had embraced the adoption of all things digital at the same rate of, say, the banking industry, then patients today should be able to perform heart surgery... on themselves.

The state of the digital health industry today in terms of size and funding is as follows. Globally, the digital health industry is calculated to be between 55 and 67 billion USD (Global digital health market size, share, development, growth and demand forecast to 2022 – industry insights by technology (Digitized Health System, Telemedicine, mHealth, Health Analytics and Others) n.d.), with roughly 1–1.5% of the global

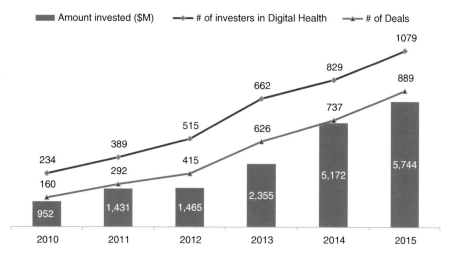

Fig. 20.1 Digital health funding trends: deals, digital health investors and dollars invested (Source: CB Insights)

healthcare industry and is estimated to be growing at a rate of 20–25% annually (Global digital health market size, share, development, growth and demand forecast to 2022 – industry insights by technology (Digitized Health System, Telemedicine, mHealth, Health Analytics and Others) n.d.) and growth rate that is likely to be just as aggressive in the next 5 years. To capture the growth of this industry, investors poured in over 5.7 billion USD into 889 digital health companies in 2015 and over 17 billion USD since 2010 into over 3000 companies (Digital health funding hits new highs in 2015, reaching nearly $6B n.d.). In 2015, there were over 1000 companies and investors that made an equity investment in at least one digital health company, up more than 361% from the 234 that invested in digital health in 2010 (Fig. 20.1) (Digital health funding hits new highs in 2015, reaching nearly $6B n.d.)

Digital health is certainly a hot subsector of the healthcare economy. Over 7600 digital health start-ups were in operation around the world in 2015 and the market for investing in them is quite bullish and optimistic (Start-up Health, LLC 2015). Moreover, the United States' dubious designation as the larger contributor to global healthcare costs reflects its leadership in digital health investing, responsible for nearly 80% of all global digital health funding through 2015 (GP Bullhound 2015; Hathaway and Rockwell 2015).

20.2 Making Money in Digital Health Investing

As mentioned earlier, digital health investors typically do have a tandem outlook of both profitability and social impact, but investors still need to make money. Broadly speaking, investors typically look for two types of returns when investing in a company: dividends or exit multiples. Similar to buying a house, it can either be rented to generate steady profits (dividends) or re-sold (exit) and the profits generated by the sale to buy another house.

Generally, investors typically use the word "play" to describe the type of investment or even the industry of the investment. An investment in company A could be both a digital health play and a dividend play.

Typically, the earlier in the *entrepreneurial life cycle* an investor invests, the more likely he or she or it ("it" being an institutional investor, i.e., investment company) is looking for an exit play as opposed to a steady dividend play later on in the entrepreneurial life cycle. The entrepreneurial life cycle is summarized in Fig. 20.2.

Companies, like living organisms, move through different stages in their development. The merits of this particular framework differ from the typical "Start-up Financing Life cycle," which plots a snaky S curve that starts in the dreaded "valley of death" and climbs upward as higher revenue targets dictate funding rounds across an axis of time. Today, investors encourage entrepreneurs to be more milestone-driven, not time-driven, and digital ventures are becoming increasingly less dependent on revenue when raising multiple rounds of financing.

20.2.1 Pre-seed Stage

All companies start out as ideas and, from an investor's point of view, the ability to invest in hard-working teams with bright ideas is known as the "Seed Round," where investors and entrepreneurs plant the seeds to sow future success. Prior to the seed round, there typically exists a *Pre-Seed Round,* where entrepreneurs may or may not have an idea or corporate license, but exhibit the entrepreneurial spirit and are ready to venture off on their own into the world of business. This round is also comically known as the FFF round, which endearingly refers to the Friends, Families, and Fools that typically invest in the earliest primordial days of the company. Also common in the pre-seed round (and of particular relevance to digital health) are the many grants (typically government) and competitions that entrepreneurs sign up for that offer "free" money, i.e., money that is typically gifted to a promising idea or prototype without any (or very limited) reciprocation required from the entrepreneur.

Crowdfunding is an emerging mechanism that is becoming increasingly the *maluit iter*, or preferred path in pre-seed/seed rounds, especially for digital health entrepreneurs building hardware-focused platforms. Entrepreneurs can now leverage a slew of websites and marketplaces that connect would-be sellers with would-be buyers. Sellers can essentially pre-order a given product (and sometimes even a service) ahead of its final production. Entrepreneurs can then use the collective proceeds from pre-sales to scale their operations and start manufacturing *en masse*. This method, however, does not always work as efficiently as envisioned. There are examples of companies, even well-funded companies that take an exorbitant amount of time to deliver their products. A well-known example is that of **Oculus VR** who,

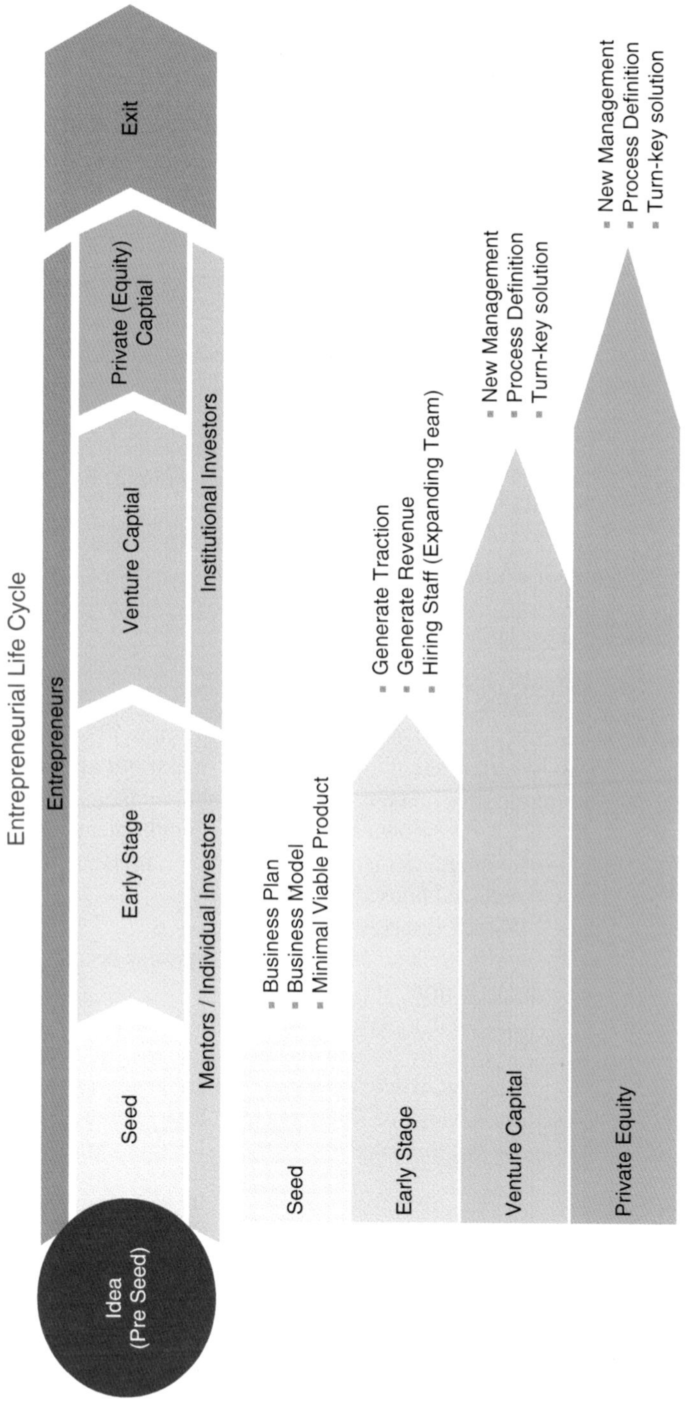

Entrepreneurial Life Cycle

Fig. 20.2 Entrepreneurial life cycle

despite a very popular **Kickstarter** campaign in August 2012 and a massive two billion dollar buy-out from **Facebook Inc.** in early 2014, kept consumers waiting **3 years, 7 months, and 27 days** to receive the first consumer-ready Oculus Rift VR headsets.

Crowdfunding can also be used to collect many smaller tickets (dollar size of an investment) from a multitude of individual investors and there are many websites and businesses focused on this community form of investing.

Digital health pioneered a new process of crowdfunding known as "regulation crowdfunding," when **Beta Bionics**, a company creating an "artificial pancreas" aimed at diabetes type 1 patients, became the first startup to raise $1 million using a new type of online stock sale open to the public at large. Using the crowdfunding portal **Wefunder**, 775 members of the public put up an average of $1300 each on Beta Bionics stock (Artificial pancreas is first to raise $1 million under new crowdfunding rules n.d.).

Beta Bionics opted for the crowdfunding route as it considers itself a "public benefit corporation," meaning the company's charter is to act in the best interests of people with type 1 diabetes at the expense of short-term profits. This means it was seeking investors motivated by idealism or who have been affected by type 1 diabetes. Indeed, many investors turned out to be scientists or people involved with diabetes research, or even family members of those affected (Artificial pancreas is first to raise $1 million under new crowdfunding rules n.d.).

A few *key terms* that entrepreneurs should familiarize themselves with at the pre-seed stage are described below.

Burn rate is the monthly cost of maintenance (cash outflow) of the company. This gives investors an idea of when the enterprise is running out of cash. A common mistake many entrepreneurs make is that they do not pay themselves a salary at the start, or even account for their own monthly living requirements. After all, as Napoleon once said, an army marches on its stomach, so entrepreneurs must ensure that they are well fed, clothed, and housed as well.

Option pool is shares of stock reserved for employees of the company and used to attract talent. The amount of stock an employee gets typically decreases polynomially throughout the entrepreneurial life cycle.

Boot-strapping is a term used to symbolize self-reliance. The analogy is to extract one's boot from the mud by pulling on the bootstraps. Boot-strapping is analogous also to self-sufficiency, where entrepreneurs are encouraged to venture on their own using whatever savings or resources they have accumulated prior to their entrepreneurial exercise without accepting any outside financial investment.

20.2.2 Seed Stage

There are no set amounts for each of the investment rounds that delineate the different stages of the life cycle as it is really more of an art than a science—a balance between the vision of the founders and the investors, market conditions (what other founders/investors have raised) combined with the requirements of the business from a financial perspective; i.e., how much money the entrepreneur needs to execute his or her vision and business plan. Having said that, seed rounds in the digital health space typically range from 50,000 to 150,000 USD for a 5–10% equity stake (shares) of the company. It is at this stage where both the founders and the potential investors must concern themselves with the two M's—Market and Money—so far as to outline if there is a given market opportunity for this venture and if this venture can (eventually) turn a profit or be profitably sold to another investor or company.

Seed rounds are also the stage at which entrepreneurs may elect to join an incubator, accelerator, startup foundry, or co-working space. While small distinctions exist between these platforms, the common denominator entrepreneurs can basically expect to part with a small minority of their equity (usually 3–7%) in exchange for mentorship, cross-pollination of ideas, experiences with other entrepreneurs (usually in the same industry; however, the argument could be made that inter-industry cross-pollination might be more fruitful than intra-industry pollination), and some cash, typically in the range of 50,000–150,000 USD. Perhaps the most important benefit of joining these collective entrepreneurial groupings is the promise of leveraging the contacts and experiences of the principals of these platforms who then can provide valuable introductions and act as much-needed sounding boards to continuously vet different ideas suggested by the founders.

Accelerators and incubators are often assumed to represent the same concept. However, there are a few key distinctions that first-time founders should be aware of if they are planning on signing up (Accelerators vs. incubators: what start-ups need to know n.d.). Breaking it down into simple terms, accelerators "accelerate" the growth of an existing company, whereas incubators "incubate" disruptive ideas with the hope of building a business model and, eventually, a company. So, accelerators typically focus on scaling a business while incubators are often more focused on innovation. Another big difference is in how the individual programs are structured. Accelerators usually have a set timeframe in which individual companies spend from a few weeks to a few months working with a group of mentors to build their business and navigate the different challenges of launching a product/service. Indeed, the goal of an accelerator is to help a startup achieve roughly 2 years of business building in just a few months (Accelerators vs. incubators: what start-ups need to know n.d.).

Accelerators can either be generalist in nature (but usually focused on tech), such as **Y Combinator** and **Techstars,** or focused on a particularly industry or industry subset. **Rock Health** and **Blueprint Health** are examples of digital health-focused accelerators.

Accelerators start with an application process, but the top programs are typically very selective. Y Combinator accepts only about 2% of the applications it receives and Techstars has to fill its ten spots from around 1000 applications (Accelerators vs. incubators: what start-ups need to know n.d.) for each rotation.

The end of an accelerator program is typically concluded by entrepreneurs presenting (pitching) their ventures at some sort of demonstration (demo) day attended by select investors and, more often than not, the media as well.

Table 20.1 List of selected digital health accelerators, incubators, startup foundries, and co-working spaces (mostly within the US)

	Name of the accelerators/ incubators	Location	Notable digital health investments
1	Rock Health	San Francisco, CA	Aptible, Studio Dental
2	Health Wildcatters	Dallas, TX	Orb Health, Obaa, Get Fitter
3	Startup Health	New York, NY	Valera Health, Aver, Mouth Watch
4	Blueprint Health	New York, NY	Medicure, OhMD, Medpilot
5	HealthBox	Chicago, IL	Tute Genomics, HomeTouch
6	New York Digital Health	New York, NY	iQuartic, Wellth
7	Y Combinator	Mountain view, CA	Drchrono, Spire
8	WestHealth	La Jolla, CA	Svelte Medical Systems, SoteraWireless
9	Illumina Accelerator Program	San Francisco, CA	Vitagen, Nextgen
10	DigitalHealth, London	London, UK	Revere Care, SBRI Health
11	Dubai 100	Dubai, UAE	Sihatech.com, OTTA

Incubators, on the other hand, typically begin with companies that may be earlier in the process and they usually do not operate on a set schedule. If an accelerator is a greenhouse for young plants to get the optimal conditions to grow, then an incubator matches quality seeds with the best soil for sprouting and growth (Accelerators vs. incubators: what start-ups need to know n.d.).

While most incubators operate independently, there are some that can also be sponsored or run by venture capital (VC) firms, government entities, and major corporations. In the case of digital health, these corporations typically include hospital groups or large pharmaceutical companies (also known as "Big Pharma"). Some incubators have an application process, but others only work with companies and ideas that they come in contact with through trusted partners (Accelerators vs. incubators: what start-ups need to know n.d.).

Similar to accelerators, incubators can too be either generalist in nature (again, usually focused on tech), such as **IdeaLab,** or focused on a particularly industry or industry subset. **Start-up Health**, **HealthBox,** and **InnovateNYP** are examples of digital health-focused accelerators (Table 20.1).

20.2.3 *Early Stage*

Once digital health companies are seeded, accelerated, or incubated, they enter the *Early Stage* part of the life cycle where the entrepreneurial team begins to develop customer validation of their product/service and demonstrate some traction and, ideally, some revenue, thus proving their business model.

Traction can be a tricky thing to measure, especially when it comes to digital health. Traction can simply mean acquiring customers; however, in an increasingly complimentary digital world, customers do not necessarily need to purchase products or services right away. Instead of money, metrics to measure traction include acronyms such as MAUs, MPVs, MUVs, and MRGs, which, respectively, represent Monthly Active Users (MAU), Monthly Page Views (MPV), Monthly Unique Visitors (MUV), and Monthly Registered Users (MRU). These acronyms, or their daily counterparts (e.g., Daily Active Users—DAUs), are particularly important for digital health businesses with a B2C (business-to-consumer) business model. Ventures focused on the enterprise (or selling to other businesses or B2B) or governments (B2G) typically tend to focus on signed contracts based on both volume and, more importantly, value. In many cases, the size of the client counterpart is also of particular importance as investors place a higher intrinsic value on large corporate customers. The larger the customer, either in terms of employee number, revenue, or market share, the more valuable the contract. A broad traction truism is that a steady stream of revenue from a contract is usually preferred to a one-shot signing of epic proportions—as the aphorism states: slow and steady beats large and in charge.

For many digital health companies, a few key terms are important to consider when defining the business model for either consumer or corporate clients.

Per Member Per Month (**PMPM**) finds its origins in the health insurance industry where it can refer to capitation payments as in a Health Maintenance Organization (HMO), where an insurance company pays a PMPM amount to a primary care physician based on the number of members on the physician's panel, regardless of whether the physician has an encounter with the patient that month or not. It also can refer to a measure of cost where total yearly healthcare costs for a group are divided by the number of members, then divided by 12 to calculate healthcare costs for a group PMPM.

Many digital health entrepreneurs have adopted this terminology when providing their products and services to various hospital systems or healthcare insurance payers.

Software as a Service (SaaS) is simply when companies license their software to end users on a subscription basis. The software can either be hosted on the client's servers or, more commonly, on the cloud. Usually, a maintenance fee is also priced into the SaaS contract.

Freemium is a model pioneered by internet firms in general, whereby basic services are provided free-of-charge and more advanced features are usually then offered at a price.

The early stage round is typically dominated by **Angel Investors**—wealthy people that like to invest early in startups. Just like accelerators and incubators, angel investors can either be generalists or focused on a particular industry. They may also be principals of either an accelerator or incubator (or both) or even executives in a venture capital firm or large corporation. In the United States, angel investors are defined by the Securities and Exchange Commission (SEC) as individuals with over one million dollars in liquid assets or an annual income of over $200,000 a year if single or $300,000 if married. However, the SEC is required to re-examine the definition of "accredited investor" every 4 years. The intent of the review is to determine whether the definition should be modified "for the protection of investors, in the

public interest, and in light of the economy (Crowd Funding Legal Hub n.d.)."
Indeed, in lieu of new disruptive technologies that we have already covered in this
chapter, such as crowdfunding, the SEC planned to revise the financial thresholds
for individuals to qualify as accredited investors and the list-based approach for
entities to qualify as accredited investors. Indeed, a major shake-up in the crowdfunding industry did occur when the SEC approved Title III of the 2012 Jumpstart
Our Business Startup Act ("JOBS Act") in October 2015. Passage of the JOBS Act
dramatically changed the way startups could raise capital for new ventures, making
it possible for any company to raise up to $1 million annually through equity crowd-
funding without having to endure the red tape of registering those securities with the
SEC (The rising billions and healthcare's expanding global market n.d.). For over
80 years, investors have been limited by provisions in the Securities Act of 1933,
which enforce strict regulations on the advertisement and sale of securities to the
public. Title II of the JOBS Act eased these restrictions, but only for accredited
investors. In October 2013, the SEC proposed rule changes for Title III of the JOBS
Act that would open up the crowdfunding arena to non-accredited investors. Now,
anyone can invest in startups, small businesses, or even real estate through crowdfunding, with some protective limitations based on an investor's income and net
worth (The rising billions and healthcare's expanding global market n.d.). **AngelList**,
an online platform that connects startups with angel capital, is one example of the
enormous growth in angel financing. Since it launched in 2010, thousands of companies have raised capital using the platform and startups now raise more than $10
million a month (Six myths about venture capitalists n.d.).

20.2.4 Venture Capital (VC) Stage

The Venture Capital (VC) stage is when the real money starts coming in for many
entrepreneurs. It is, however, also the stage at which entrepreneurs are expected to,
at the bare minimum, demonstrate considerable growth of their company and ideally start to turn a profit and become cash flow positive.

The top venture capital firms are often structured as partnerships and are formed
by a group of seasoned investors, many of whom are either former entrepreneurs or
influential corporate executives themselves. These partners are known as the General
Partners or GPs. VC firms then go and raise massive amounts of money from other
investors, known as Limited Partners or LPs, who typically include sovereign wealth
funds (government-owned investment vehicles), pension funds, mutual funds and
ultra-high-net worth individuals (UHNWI). These investments are usually grouped
into funds with a certain investment horizon and investment strategy that typically
ranges from 5 to 7 years. Most VC firms follow the "2 + 20 rule," which corresponds
to the GP's taking 2% of all committed capital over the life of a fund to cover the
firm's operating expenses and then 20% of the profits generated by investing the
capital as what is known in the industry as "carried interest" or "carry." This means
that a VC firm that has raised a one billion dollar fund and charges a 2% fee would

receive a fixed fee stream of $20 million per year to cover expenses and compensation. VC firms raise new funds about every 3 or 4 years, so let us assume that 3 years into the first fund the firm raises a second one billion dollar fund. That would generate an additional $20 million in fees, for a total of $40 million annually and two billion dollars to spend.

In return, the GPs promise the LPs significant returns that beat the market and must consistently strive to make investments in ventures that can generate significant multiples of return—the much sought-after tenfold return or a unicorn (any private company who achieves a valuation above one billion USD). You will see that VC's are very fond of the letter X, considered by many to be a symbol of the multiplier for wealth. *Forbes* identifies the top individual VCs on its Midas List, implicitly crediting them with a mythical magic touch for investing. The story of venture capital appears to be a compelling narrative of bold investments and excess returns (Six myths about venture capitalists n.d.). The VCs' use of the alphabet also extends to symbolizing their different rounds of investment. The Series A round signifies the first funding round led by venture capitalists and other institutional investors, and may be either followed by a Series B round or the cheekier Series A1. Similar to the stages of the entrepreneurial life cycle, there is no strict science or agreed upon industry standards that delineate the size or timing of the round. However, these alphabet rounds generally tend to be 1–2 years apart, whereas an A1 or B1 round might be only 6–12 months after the formal A or B round. More importantly, both the size of the round and the frequency with which a company raises the said round are a combination between investor interest in the company and the industry and the founding team's own rush to achieve their corporate vision. An important quote on these constant and multiple VC rounds was made by the former Chief Executive Officer of Allscripts and current digital health maven, Glenn Tullman, who tongue-in-cheek mentioned that he had never heard of a "Series J1 Preferred" round until he was brought on to lead Allscripts as CEO.

Another very important quote that both entrepreneurs and investors must keep in mind is from legendary tech entrepreneur, venture capitalist, and Y Combinator founder, Paul Graham, who likens the various rounds of VC to the gears of a car, where *"a typical startup goes through several rounds of funding. Each round you take just enough money to reach the speed where you can shift into the next gear."*

Indeed, there are certain truisms when it comes to the frequency of raising outside capital for large swaths of equity. These include:

Raise Money Before You Need It—opportunities either come too early or too late, which means that an entrepreneur must have enough capital in reserve to act on these opportunities.

A Piece of a Cake is Better than a Cookie—cakes are always larger than cookies (sorry cupcakes and pizzookies); thus, entrepreneurs must make peace with the fact that owning a piece of a growing company (ideally with support from multiple stakeholders) is empirically much better (and safer) than owning majority equity in a small, stagnant, venture.

Smart Money Above All Else—smart entrepreneurs seek smart money, which basically means investors that can add some strategic value other than just contributing capital. In digital health, smart money can mean former hospital or health insurance executives that can help entrepreneurs navigate complicated reimbursement cycles or simply former digital health entrepreneurs who have "been there and done that" and might help the founders save valuable time and avoid costly pitfalls common to the industry.

Equity for Passion and Ideas—in today's increasingly materialistic world of mercenaries, one could argue that essentially everything could be bought in exchange for a fee, so why give away valuable equity. Ideally, there are many entrepreneurs that ascribe to the philosophy that equity should only be awarded to like-minded individuals that passionately share the vision of the enterprise.

Time Value of Money—similar to the first truism, but more concerned with the financial fact that a dollar today is worth more than a dollar tomorrow. This is also of particular importance in highly competitive industries, where raising money from investors becomes increasingly expensive given unfavorable and highly competitive macroeconomic conditions.

20.2.4.1 Fundamental Law of Growth

Similar to accelerators, venture capitalists rely on their vast industry experience and networks to source the best investment opportunities. However, it is not all gut feeling and logo buying. Venture capitalists employ detailed calculations and assumptions, an example of which is known as the Fundamental Law of Growth (Fig. 20.3) (Medium Corporation n.d.).

Like Newton's laws of gravity and momentum, most tech startups that sell directly to customers—both enterprises and consumers—must eventually obey the Fundamental Law of Growth: LTV/CAC > 3. There's a lot of nuance as to why (The rising billions and healthcare's expanding global market n.d.), but suffice to say that the LTV/CAC ratio speaks to a startup's revenue trajectory, capital needs, and, in turn, how much irrational exuberance is demanded of its investors (Medium Corporation n.d.). The lower the LTV/CAC ratio, the less efficient a company is at

The Fundamental Law of Growth

$$\frac{LTV}{CAC} > 3$$

$$\frac{LTV}{CAC} = \frac{\text{Customer Lifetime x ARPU X Margin \%}}{\text{Marketing Expense / New Customers}}$$

Life Time value of Customer

Customer Acquisition Cost

*Companies whose value is not predicated on revenue (e.g., disruptive technologies, monopolies, social networks, intellecutal property) as well as companies where revenue is achieved indireclty (e.g., ad-tech networks, certain marketplaces, certain viral growth startups) or discontinuously (e.g., government contractors) typically do not follow this rule

Fig. 20.3 Fundamental law of growth

deploying capital and the more money it needs to fuel growth; conversely, the higher the LTV/CAC ratio, the more efficient the company is and, thus, the more value it creates for the same amount of capital. Though this can be derived, it has been observed empirically that 3× is roughly the threshold needed to build big, sustainable businesses (Medium Corporation n.d.).

Exceptions to the Fundamental Law of Growth include companies whose value is not predicated on revenue (e.g., disruptive technologies, monopolies, social networks, intellectual property) as well as companies where revenue is achieved indirectly (e.g., ad-tech networks, certain marketplaces, certain viral growth startups) (Medium Corporation n.d.).

As we will later cover, assessing a company's valuation is a discipline on its own and growth is only one factor in that calculation. However, for simplicity's sake, one can assume that tech companies who don't obey the Fundamental Law of Growth will eventually lose access to capital, drastically slow their growth, and watch their valuations plummet (Medium Corporation n.d.).

Below are presented two case studies of digital health companies and how they fared against the Fundamental Law of Growth.

Case 1: Clover Health (Health Insurance Payer)

Clover Health is a "new-age" health insurance company currently valued at just less than one billion USD and with a focus on utilizing technology, services, and data to humanize healthcare. Applying the Fundamental Law of Growth to Clover Health, one may get:

- Customer Lifetime—Clover is a Medicare Advantage plan, so when seniors switch to a plan, they tend to stay there. Three years is used even though the true lifetime may be longer.
- Average Revenue Per User—Medicare Advantage average payments are publicly available and average around 10,000 USD per user.
- Margin %—incumbent healthcare insurance payers have gross margins in the 5–10% range with a maximum of 15% as mandated by the US Affordable Care Act (known loosely as "Obamacare"); thus, 15% is assumed.
- Customer Acquisition Cost (CAC)—Medicare Advantage fixes brokers' commissions on a state-by-state basis (<$550); additional channels, such as direct-to-consumer, are likely more expensive, so $800 is assumed for the blended CAC.

LTV/CAC = 3 years × \$10,000/year × 15%/\$800 = 5.6×

Further potential upside can be expected as Clover Health's expansion in the US reduces costs and as it works directly with healthcare service (provider) networks.

Case 2: ZocDoc (Online Doctor Appointments)

ZocDoc is an online platform where patients can find in-network neighborhood doctors, instantly book appointments online, see reviews by other patients, get reminders for upcoming appointments and preventive checkups, and fill out part of their paperwork. ZocDoc is also based in New York City and is currently valued at 1.8 billion USD. Applying the Fundamental Law of Growth to ZocDoc, one gets:

- Customer Lifetime—ZocDoc has traditionally targeted standalone physician practices (they are now trying to target more established healthcare provider networks). These doctors typically opt out of the 300 USD per month subscription per physician once they have established a sizable patient base within a year. Again, to be conservative, a lifetime of 2 years is assumed.
- Average Revenue Per User (ARPU)—$3000 as reported publicly by ZocDoc.
- Margin (%)—since ZocDoc is an SaaS company at its core, with light-touch customer service, it should probably achieve a margin of 60–80%; thus, a very high margin of 80% is assumed.
- Customer Acquisition Cost (CAC)—Selling to physician practices is challenging and the founders of ZocDoc have many incredible stories of being literally escorted out of physicians' offices by security; therefore, like any high-touch inside sales operation, ZocDoc's CAC probably ranges from the $1 to 10K range. Here, we will assume $3K as it is closer to the bottom of the range (SaaS Metrics 2.0 – a guide to measuring and improving what matters n.d.).

LTV/CAC = 2 years × $3000/year × 80%/$3000 = 1.60×

Even with a very conservative CAC, the results show a very optimistic profit margin. We must also keep in mind that as competition increases, customer lifetimes and pricing erode as well, further driving down the LTV/CAC ratio. We can now clearly see why ZocDoc is shifting sales to hospital system customers, which would probably result in a 1000× higher LTV and only 20× higher CAC (SaaS Metrics 2.0 – a guide to measuring and improving what matters, n.d.).

It is important to note, however, that there are also some VCs that believe that a lack of understanding customer acquisition costs and life time value is driving companies to premature failure and that focusing on a large LTV/CAC ratio can be a trap, especially when the payback period may be long even if LTV/CAC is large.

Fundamental Law of Growth

So why do investors sometimes grant multibillion dollar valuations if the Fundamental Law of Growth displays an LTV/CAC below three? The answer is most likely a combination of optimistic upside predictions of Brighter Days Ahead (BDA), downside protections, and what can only be described as Fear of Missing Out (FOMO) (Medium Corporation n.d.) on a "hot" company that is set to disrupt a market with a multibillion or even trillion dollar Total Addressable Market (TAM).

Downside protections are when early stage investors insulate themselves from potential future losses using some techniques we will cover shortly. This allows VCs to hedge their large investments and, at the same time, fully benefit from the positive press their investment will generate for the entrepreneurs and their ventures.

With regard to optimistic upside predictions, both investors and entrepreneurs especially must always remain eternally optimistic—expecting CLVs to extend, ARPUs to increase, margins to expand, and CACs to decline (The rising billions and healthcare's expanding global market n.d.).

Perhaps the most important tool in the VC's arsenal, especially when it comes to downside protection, is the **term sheet**, which is a legally binding document that

Table 20.2 Difference between pre- and post-money valuations

Pre-money valuation			Post-money valuation		
	Value	Percent		Value	Percent
Entrepreneur	$1000,000	80	Entrepreneur	$750,000	75
Investor	$250,000	20	Investor	$250,000	25
Total	$1,250,000	100	Total	$1000,000	100

outlines the terms by which an investor will invest cash into a company in exchange for equity. Investors use the term sheet to protect their investment in a venture. Term sheets usually comprise three major sections: funding, corporate governance, and liquidation.

When it comes to funding, an important distinction that entrepreneurs need to familiarize themselves, at this stage of the entrepreneurial life cycle, is the difference between a pre-money and a post-money valuation. Let us say that a venture achieves an important milestone and now needs to raise 250,000 USD to achieve the next set of milestones. It is agreed between the entrepreneur and potential investor(s) to value a startup at one million USD—but is this a pre-money or a post-money valuation? The difference could mean an extra 5% worth of equity to the entrepreneur, who can use the pre-money valuation as shown in the Table 20.2. All things considered, if the investment amount is the same, a pre-money valuation usually favors the entrepreneur, whereas a post-money valuation usually favors the investor.

VC investors are also typically issued shares of preferred stock, not common stock. Preferred stock, as the name suggests, is preferable because it grants certain key rights to the holders, which makes it far more valuable than common stock. One of those rights is a liquidation preference.

Liquidation Preferences are one of the essential components of preferred stock and are generally considered to be the second most important deal term in a VC investment term sheet (the first being the company's valuation prior to the investment, which we now know is commonly referred to as the "pre-money valuation" or "pre").

An example would be a simple 1× liquidation preference. This means that if the company is sold, then the investors get the higher of either the amount of their investment or their ownership percentage of the sale value. In the worst case, if the company is wound down (or bankrupt) with very little left, then anything left (after the creditors clear liabilities) would be distributed to the investors in proportion to their ownership.

To further complicate matters, there are three main types of liquidation preferences:

- **Straight (or non-participating) preferred** is the most favorable to the **entrepreneur**. Upon the sale of the company (or any other liquidation), the preferred stockholders would be entitled to the return of their entire investment (plus any accrued dividends) prior to the distribution of any proceeds to the common stockholders. Alternatively, the preferred stockholders could choose to convert their preferred stock to common stock and simply be treated the same as the common stockholders (letting them share ratably in the proceeds).

- **Participating preferred** is the most favorable to the **investor** (and is sometimes referred to as "double-dip preferred"). Similar to straight preferred, the preferred stockholders would be entitled to the return of their entire investment (plus any accrued dividends) prior to the distribution of any proceeds to the common stockholders. However, preferred stockholders would then also be treated like common stockholders and would share ratably in the remaining proceeds—in effect, being paid twice (or "double"). Issuing participating preferred has the same economic effect as issuing a promissory note and shares of common stock (or a warrant) to the investor.
- **Capped (or partially) participating preferred** is the "Goldilocks" option and is often viewed as an **intermediate approach**. The preferred stockholders have the same rights as participating preferred (i.e., return of investment, plus share ratably in the remainder), but their aggregate return is capped. Once they have received the capped amount, they no longer have the right to share in the remaining proceeds with the other common stockholders.

The next major block of the term sheet concerns governance, or how the entrepreneur and the investors will interact together to govern the growth of the company through various mechanisms, relations, and processes. Usually this is personified by the Board of Directors (BoD), which acts as a legislative oversight body when compared with the more execution-focused management team. In digital health startups, the BoD usually includes members from the founding team as well as VC general partners, or maybe even an early angel investor or independent industry expert. The idea is to provide a fair platform of accountable dialogue where all opinions can be shared. This platform must also carefully balance and protect the many interests of all the stakeholders of the corporation. Usually, these boards are odd in number to ensure major decisions are met democratically. In the case where the number of board members is even, a single person, usually the Chairman of the Board, is often given veto-like powers through a casting vote (simply a vote that is worth two votes), or the group can agree that any major decisions require an outright or total majority.

Below are a few other important terms that any entrepreneur should familiarize themselves with prior to meeting with VCs.

Signed vs. Closed vs. Funded—Signing is for the term sheet, closing is when the money is in the bank and funded is when the round has closed.

Reps—Representations are assurances that the entrepreneur gives to the investors that what they are saying is true. Normally, investors have the right to financial claims against the founders if they have misrepresented the business; however, the right to claim is only against the company, not the founders, and the amount *should* not be more than the amount invested.

Warrants are effectively a form of bonus for the VC investor in the event that the enterprise performs well. Warrant holders will exercise their warrants and buy shares when the value of the company has increased beyond the exercise price (per share) specified in the warrant. This gives them a larger share in the company at what is effectively a discounted price.

Pre-emption Rights—Ideally, all shareholders, including the founders, should have the right to invest in future financing rounds to avoid being diluted. This doesn't mean shareholders have to put more money in, but if they want to and are able to, they have the right to maintain their ownership in any future funding round.

RoFR—The Right of First Refusal or Co-Sale is when any shareholder wants to sell their shares to someone else. Under RoFR, any other investors have the option to buy those shares on the same terms or to sell those shares again on the same terms.

Drag/Tag Along—If shareholders owning more than 50% (or another predetermined equity stake) of the shares in the company want to sell their shares (typically to accept an acquisition offer), then, if approved by the board and investors, all other shareholders must also sell their shares. This protects all shareholders from, say, one small, stubborn shareholder refusing to sell their shares in an acquisition offer and blocking a deal.

Rights and Covenants—These are used by investors as restrictive levers to protect their investment, e.g., not allowing the entrepreneur to found a competing company. These restrictions usually apply as long as the entrepreneur is employed by the company or holds at specific pre-determined equity stake or right as an investor to monthly updates.

Vesting—This is another way investors protect their investment by encouraging Founders Shares to vest, whereby they earn their shares monthly across multiple years (usually 2–3 years). If the founder quits, then the company can buy back the outstanding shares.

20.2.4.2 Simple Agreement for Future Equity (SAFE) Thinking

An increasingly popular way to avoid negotiating complicated term sheets involves using a Simple Agreement for Future Equity (SAFE). Coined by Y Combinator, a SAFE is usually employed early in the entrepreneurial life cycle, during the early or even seed stage, whereby an investor makes a cash investment in a company, but gets company stock at a later date in connection with a specific event, usually the Series A round or the first Institutional or VC round.

A SAFE is **not a debt instrument**, but is intended to be an alternative to a convertible note. It is usually beneficial for both founders and investors, with the usual path to agreement requiring the negotiation of only one item: the "valuation cap," which is the maximum valuation an early investor will use to convert their investment into shares. The valuation cap is usually significantly lower than the Series A valuation and, for respectable digital health startups, is usually in the range of 5–10 million USD.

20.2.5 Later Stage or Private Equity Round

The penultimate stage of the entrepreneurial life cycle can be described as the **Later Stage** or **Private Equity** round, where both entrepreneurs and their early investor counterparts typically look to either achieve financial stability to maintain their accelerating growth. This growth can either continue organically, e.g., by adding more employees or more revenue, or inorganically, e.g., by acquiring other companies. The motivation for acquisition, especially in the world of tech, can be viewed from three different perspectives, aptly named the "Three T's":

1. *Technology*—is the Intellectual Property, whether software source code or a physical product that a company has innovated.
2. *Talent*—is the most talented founders, who will only join a new company if they are offered a significant equity stake. Buying their company and then "acqui-hiring" the founders and their team is looked upon as a worthy signing bonus to bring in much needed talent.
3. *Trouble*—is caused by competitors. Some companies, especially large incumbents in a given industry, make it common practice to buy and essentially quietly kill competing smaller companies, flushing out their disruptive technology to maintain their own hold on the market. This so-called "acqui-dire" strategy can be counterintuitive and antithetic to the innovative spirit; however, in the ruthless corporate world, it is a sure-fire way to ensure market hegemony.

The following chart (Fig. 20.4) provides an overview of the different funding stages of the previously mentioned 3000 digital health companies from 2010 to 2015, keeping in mind that many digital health companies have gone through multiple rounds of investment.

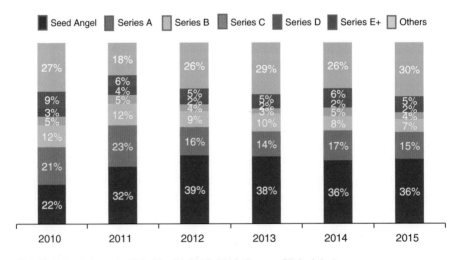

Fig. 20.4 Deal shares in digital health 2010–2015 (Source: CB Insights)

20.2.6   Exit Stage

The final and most important event of the entrepreneurial life cycle is the stage that truly captures the imagination and motivates many "serial entrepreneurs" to start the life cycle all over again: the **Exit Stage**. Just as the "E" in exit is closely juxtaposed to the X multiplier of wealth, entrepreneurs and their investors must keep their exit strategies in mind throughout each stage of the entrepreneurial life cycle.

Exits can be broadly classified into two distinct opportunities:

1. Strategic or secondary sale
2. Public markets

A strategic sale is simply when a company is bought by another company from the same or similar industry. Public markets, also known as capital, equity, or stock markets, are where the company's shares are listed and certain company information becomes available to the general public through an Initial Public Offering (IPO). Founders will typically work with their investors and an investment bank to decide upon the new valuation of both the company and the price and number of shares to be sold. These shares are then issued and traded either through exchanges or over-the-counter markets. Private equity or venture capital companies can still play a role in these listed companies post-IPO through Private Investments in Public Equity (PIPE).

It is interesting to note that many companies see the progression into the realm of public markets as a natural flow that will ensure the future sustainability of the company. It does, in fact, go back to that promise of partnership, whereby now, as a listed company, the founders must continue their pact with both their customers and investors in a transparent manner that is focused on value creation.

Indeed, the digital health industry has attracted increasing interest from both strategic and financial investors. In 2014, digital health was the fastest growing subsector in terms of mergers and acquisitions (M&As) in the United States (Irving Levin Associates n.d.), where the number of digital health deals increased from 68 to 112 in the previous year, representing a 65% increase and second only in number after the number of biotechnology deals (126). The total number of M&A exits in the US in 2014 was 1208. Overall, health care M&A activity grew by 14% in 2015, to 1498 transactions, setting a new record for healthcare M&A deal volume. In 2014, which held the previous record, 1318 deals were announced across 13 health-care subsectors. Spending in 2015 reached $563.1 billion, which was another new record (Table 20.3). That total represents a 45% increase over the $387.7 billion spent in all of 2014 (Irving Levin Associates n.d.).

When it comes to the digital health industry, nearly half (47%) of venture-backed healthcare exits in 2014 were IPOs, which is an increase of 30% from the previous 2 years (Start-up Health Insights 2015). In 2015 alone, five venture-backed healthcare startups went public (CB Insights n.d.) (see end of chapter for select list of publically listed digital health companies) (Fig. 20.5).

Table 20.3 Healthcare M&A Market with deal volume by deal sector

	Q3:14	Q2:15	Q3:15	Change	Change	2014	2015	Change
				Q2–Q3	Q3–Q3			
	Deals	Deals	Deals	(15)	(14–15)	Deals	Deals	(14–15)
Services								
Behavioral healthcare	4	6	10	67%	150%	24	38	58%
Home health and hospice	15	6	9	50%	−40%	70	47	−33%
Hospitals	19	24	33	38%	74%	99	102	3%
Labs, MRI, and dialysis	8	15	16	7%	100%	33	52	58%
Long-term care	85	65	90	38%	6%	302	356	18%
Managed care	5	8	12	50%	140%	22	45	105%
Physician medical groups	14	22	15	−32%	7%	60	88	47%
Rehabilitation	5	6	7	17%	40%	19	30	58%
Other	36	40	46	15%	28%	136	177	30%
Services subtotal	**191**	**192**	**238**	**24%**	**25%**	**765**	**935**	**22%**
Technology								
Biotechnology	27	34	41	21%	52%	136	158	16%
Digital health	**34**	**34**	**33**	**−3%**	**−3%**	**118**	**123**	**4%**
Medical devices	26	29	31	7%	19%	111	113	2%
Pharmaceuticals	67	38	42	11%	−37%	188	169	−10%
Technology subtotal	**154**	**135**	**147**	**9%**	**−5%**	**553**	**563**	**2%**
Grand total	**345**	**327**	**385**	**18%**	**12%**	**1318**	**1498**	**14%**

Source: Health Care M&A News 2015, Health care M&A News 2016

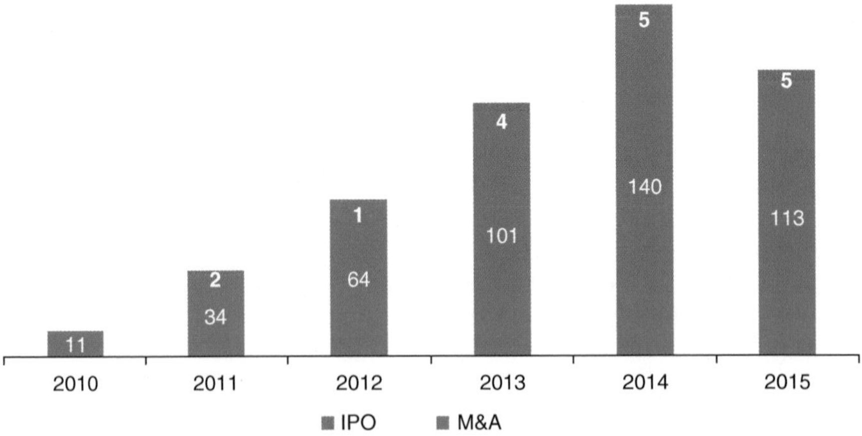

Fig. 20.5 Number of digital health exits 2010–2015 (Source: CB Insights)

20.3   Trends Sought by Digital Health Investors and Entrepreneurs

As a forward-looking conclusion to the Chapter, we would like to mention a few of the current trends shaping the digital health industry. These are described below.

20.3.1   Accountability

Accountability is perhaps one of the most interesting recent global trends in healthcare and forms the crux of Obamacare in the US. The main idea is that healthcare practitioners will no longer profit from the sickness of patients, but, instead, be incentivized to keep patients healthy and encourage preventative and evidence-based medicine. This is nothing new: in the days of the Fertile Crescent in the seventeenth century BC, the Code of Hammurabi called for physicians to be paid only if their patients remained healthy.

Recent political policies related to health, including evidence-based medicine (EBM) and precision medicine, are pseudo-prescient buzzwords and battle-call banners for rallying armies of entrepreneurs and their capital-providing commanders.

20.3.2   Consumerism

Consumerism is another interesting global trend in healthcare that has affected other industries, such as travel and tourism. Consumerism represents a paradigm shift whereby patients take increasing ownership of their own healthcare needs. Whether it is shopping via the phone or online for the best-priced healthcare service, or even self-diagnosing themselves prior to a doctor's visit by browsing the multitude of online healthcare resources, the traditional paternal model of medicine, where the physician's word is unequivocal, is eroding. In particular, price transparency is an increasingly important global sub-trend since consumers have greater access to pricing information prior to obtaining medical services.

This healthcare consumerism is accentuated in developing markets, where many medical portals do not have the proper oversight or peer-reviewed integrity of Western websites. This is also enhanced by the high mobility of patients who are not limited by the primary care gate-keeper model of medicine and, instead, prefer to be seen directly by a specialist or plunge themselves directly into an emergency room when a routine primary care visit would suffice.

Another issue is the lack of coordination of care when it comes to the medical consumer. The average person in the US will see about 18 different doctors in their lifetime (Practice Fusion surveys patients, highlights the inefficiency of paper records and the need for electronic medical records in the US n.d.).

20.3.3 Medical Inflation

The healthcare sector has outpaced the Consumer Price Index (CPI) by almost 700% over the past 40 years (Bureau of Labor Statistics n.d.). Within health-care, the largest cost bucket is typically the remuneration of healthcare workers. Whether it is the salaries of healthcare executives, clinicians, or administrative staff, it is costing more and more to staff healthcare facilities; moreover, tech-nology still has not been as disruptive in healthcare as in other industries, with only around 50% of doctors in the US using some form of electronic health record (EHR) according to US-based Practice Fusion (Why 'one patient, one chart' is still far off n.d.), and this number is substantially lower across the GCC. Another cost barrier is the high administrative cost associated with health-care. This is estimated to be between 24 and 31% in the US (Woolhandler et al. 2003), which many experts agree is the world's most bloated healthcare system with spending between 16 and 18% of GDP (Organization for Co-operation and Development n.d.).

20.3.4 Predictive Analytics

Predictive Analytics is the analysis of large quantities of data, otherwise known as "Big Data," for the purpose of providing a data-driven prediction/solution or to assess the likelihood of occurrence of a future event. In digital health, predictive analytics is applicable across the entire spectrum of the health economy, for example:

- Model drug development collaborations that maximize IP and drug discovery
- Simulate PRO (Patient Reported Outcomes) for care quality improvement and outcomes
- Accelerate time-to-market (TTM) for new therapies with strategic portfolio modelling.
- Predict market access and optimize resource allocation for new therapies
- Predict high-risk patients for ACO (accountable care organization) and hospitals
- Leverage advanced analytics to reduce hospital readmissions. This is perhaps one of the most important benefits of predictive analytics in healthcare as hospi-tal readmissions are a costly and usually avoidable healthcare expense that both regulators and payer strive to avoid.
- Simulate connected health consumers and recommend technology interventions that drive healthy behavior change, i.e., preventative healthcare measures. This is also becoming increasingly popular as insurers are pressured by the increased competition in the payer space to find more creative ways to limit their MLR (medical loss ratio) by encouraging prevention and, thus, keeping their plan members outside of the healthcare service providers.

- Simulate the financial risks and incentives of emerging reimbursement models for ACO. Again, the trends of accountability and pay for performance are becoming increasingly favored by both regulators and payers as a means to reduce the cost burden of the healthcare system.
- Quantify health costs and productivity of simulated workforce while recommending the most appropriate wellness intervention or disease management. This is particularly important in an industry where a lack of data and industry information is commonplace. In addition, most private insurance companies across the globe have yet to fully utilize the potential of disease management, whereby the patient's treatment plan is thoroughly assessed according to international best practices and clinical guidelines before approval by the case manager of the insurance company.

20.3.5   Passion

While passion is the more abstract concept of the drivers, it is perhaps the most important. The term "passion" in this context means the entrepreneur's zeal for change and the investor's eye for deal-making in an industry that literally tugs at the heart strings of almost every individual.

Appendix

Profiles of Select Digital Health Accelerators

Y Combinator

Overview
Investments: 961 Investments in 885 Companies
Exits: 1 IPO & 117 Acquisitions
Founders: Naveen Jain, Paul Graham, Jessica Livingston, Robert Morris, Trevor Blackwell
Headquarters: Mountain View, CA
Funds raised: $700M
Categories: Finance, Venture Capital, Consulting
Description: Y Combinator is a startup accelerator based in Mountain View, CA
Employees: 1193
Company valuation: $20M
Website: http://www.ycombinator.com
Investor Details
Founded: March 1, 2005
Aliases: ycombinator, YC

Contact: info@ycombinator.com

Y Combinator is a startup accelerator based in Mountain View, CA. In 2005, Y Combinator developed a new model of startup funding. Twice a year they invest a small amount of money ($120K) in a large number of startups (most recently 68). The startups move to Silicon Valley for 3 months. The YC partners work closely with each company to get them into the best possible shape and refine their pitch to investors.

Successful exits by Y Combinator-funded companies include Reddit, Heroku, and OMGPOP. Other successful companies that went through Y Combinator include Dropbox, Airbnb, Stripe, Loopt, Justin.tv, Weebly, and Scribd.

Blueprint Health

Overview

Investments: 51 Investments in 50 Companies
Exits: 2 Acquisitions
Founders: Brad Weinberg, Mathew Farkash
Category: Healthcare
Description: Blueprint Health is a mentorship-driven startup accelerator program supporting companies at the intersection of health and technology.
Website: http://www.blueprinthealth.org
Employees: 5
Valuation: $3.2M
Investor Details
Founded: 2011
Contact: info@blueprinthealth.org

Blueprint Health is geared toward healthcare companies seeking to benefit from our intensive 3-month program focused on acquiring clients and capital. Blueprint is a Charter Member of the Global Accelerator Network and started by TechStars. Selected companies range from one founder with an idea to businesses that have customers, investors, and significant revenue. Blueprint's seventh class began on February 2, 2015.

Rock Health

Overview

Investments: 93 Investments in 80 Companies
Exits: 9 Acquisitions
Founders: Halle Tecco, Nate Gross
Headquarters: San Francisco, CA
Funds raised: Undisclosed
Categories: Mobile, Apps, Venture Capital, Healthcare

Description: Rock Health is an accelerator and seed fund investing in digital health startups
Website: http://rockhealth.com
Employees: 50
Valuation: $81.56M
Investor Details
Founded: 2010
Contact: hello@rockhealth.org
Founded in 2010, Rock Health is the first seed fund focused exclusively on healthcare technology. Rock Health provides entrepreneurs with funding ($250K), strategic and operational support, co-working space, and access to a top-tier network of partners, academic medical centers, and clinicians.

Profiles of Select Digital Health Venture Capital Firms

Sequoia

Overview
Investments: 1149 Investments in 661 Companies
Exits: 54 IPOs & 146 Acquisitions
Founder: Don Valentine
Headquarters: Menlo Park, CA
Funds raised: $4.12B
Category: Venture capital
Description: Sequoia helps founders turn imaginative ideas into enduring companies.
Website: http://www.sequoiacap.comInvestor
Employees: 134
Valuation: $78.9M
Investor Details
Founded: November 1, 1972
Contact: (650) 854-3927
Type: Venture Capital that does seed, early stage venture, and later stage venture investments
Investment size: $1–100M
Sectors: Energy, Enterprise, Financial, Healthcare, Internet, Mobile
Regions: China, India, Israel, United States
The Sequoia team helps a small number of daring founders build legendary companies. We spur them to push the boundaries of what's possible. In partnering with Sequoia, companies benefit from an unmatched community and the lessons learned over 40 years working with Steve Jobs, Larry Ellison, John Morgridge, Jerry Yang, Elon Musk, Larry Page, Jan Koum, Brian Chesky, Drew Houston, Adi Tatarko, and Jack Dorsey among many others.

New Leaf Venture Partners

Overview
Investments: 109 Investments in 59 Companies
Exits: 12 IPOs & 9 Acquisitions
Founder: Philippe Chambon
Headquarters: New York, NY
Funds raised: $1.03B
Description: Healthcare-focused VC firm
Website: http://www.nlvpartners.com
Employees: 16
Valuation: $75M
Investor Details
Founded: 2005
Aliases: Sprout Group
Contact: info@nlvpartners.com
Type: Private equity firm that does early stage venture, later stage venture, private equity, and debt financing investments
Sectors: Biotechnology, Healthcare, Pharmaceuticals
Region: United States

New Leaf Venture Partners is a venture capital firm that invests primarily in healthcare technology. The company typically focuses on later stage biopharmaceutical products, early stage medical devices, and laboratory infrastructure technologies.

The New Leaf Ventures (NLV) team has been built over a decade, originating within Sprout Group, the venture capital affiliate of Credit Suisse First Boston. Sprout Group was formed in 1969 and has historically been one of the leading venture capital firms in the country.

Trident Capital

Overview
Investments: 185 Investments in 107 Companies
Exits: 6 IPOs & 42 Acquisitions
Founders: Donald Dixon, John Moragne, Don Dixon
Headquarters: Palo Alto, CA
Funds raised: $750M
Description: Trident Capital is a venture capital and growth equity firm investing in software, business services, and internet-focused companies.
Website: http://www.tridentcap.com
Employees: 15

Valuation: $51.4M
Investor Details
Founded: 1993
Contact: info@tridentcap.com
Type: Venture capital that does early stage venture, later stage venture, and debt financing investments
Region: United States
Trident Capital is a venture and growth equity firm investing in Software, Services and Internet. Trident focuses on companies addressing the major technology challenges facing today's enterprise, including cloud computing, IT security, digital monetization, and healthcare IT. We target growth equity investments up to $30 million in rapidly growing companies, often as the first institutional investor. Founded in 1993, Trident has raised $1.9 billion of capital and is currently investing its $362 million Fund VII. Investing region—North America and are headquartered in Palo Alto, CA.

OrbiMed

Overview
Investments: 166 Investments in 112 Companies
Exits: 36 IPOs & 22 Acquisitions
Headquarters: New York, NY
Funds raised: $4.27B
Description: OrbiMed is a healthcare-dedicated investment firm, with approximately $5 billion in assets under management.
Website: http://www.orbimed.com
Employees: 80
Valuation: $97.3M
Investor Details
Founded: 1989
Contact: info@orbimed.com
Type: Private equity firm that does early stage venture, later stage venture, private equity, debt financing, and post-IPO debt investments
Sectors: Biotechnology, Healthcare, Health and Wellness
Region: United States
OrbiMed is a healthcare-dedicated investment firm, with approximately $5 billion in assets under management. OrbiMed's investment advisory business was founded in 1989 with a vision to invest across the spectrum of healthcare companies: from private start-ups to large multinational companies. OrbiMed manages the Caduceus Private Investments series of venture capital funds and a family of public equity investment funds.

Profiles of Select Digital Health Publically Listed Companies

Athenahealth

Overview
Acquisitions: 5 Acquisitions
IPO/Stock: Went public on Sept. 20, 2007 (ATHN)
Headquarters: Watertown, MA
Description: Athenahealth provides cloud-based services for physician practices, such as electronic health records and practice management.
Founder: Todd Park
Category: Enterprise software
Website: http://www.athenahealth.com
Employees: 3676
Private company valuation: $241M
Public company valuation: $5.28B
Company Details
Founded: 1997
Contact: (800) 981-5084

Athenahealth is a leading provider of internet-based business services for physician practices. The Company's service offerings are based on proprietary web-native practice management and electronic health record (EHR) software, a continuously updated payer knowledge-base, integrated back-office service operations, and live patient communications services.

Castlight Health

Overview
Investments: 2 Investments in 1 Company
IPO/Stock: Went public on March 17, 2014 (NYSE:CSLT)
Headquarters: San Francisco, CA
Description: Castlight Health develops a web application that provides information to its users about healthcare costs, usage, coverage, and choices.
Founders: Todd Park, Bryan Roberts, Giovanni Colella
Category: Healthcare
Website: http://www.castlighthealth.com
Employees: 466
Private company valuation: $44.3M
Public company valuation: $9.6B
Company Details
Founded: 2008
Aliases: Castlight Health, Inc., Ventana Health Services, Inc.
Contact: info@castlighthealth.com|(415) 829-1400

Castlight Health, Inc. develops a Web application that provides consumers with clarity around their healthcare costs, usage, coverage, and choices. It enables employers and employees to make choices and lower costs. The company's products are used in various visionary companies in the United States. The company was founded in 2008 and is based in San Francisco, California.

Cerner

Overview

Acquisitions: 1 Acquisition
IPO/Stock: Went public on Dec. 12, 1986 (CERN)
Headquarters: Kansas City, MO
Description: Cerner Corporation is a supplier of healthcare information technology solutions, services, devices, and hardware.
Category: Software
Website: http://www.cerner.com
Company Details
Founded: 1979
Contact: 1(816) 221-1024
Employees: 22,220
Private company valuation: $25M
Public company valuation: $837M

Cerner Corporation is a supplier of healthcare information technology solutions, services, devices, and hardware. Cerner solutions optimize processes for healthcare organizations. These solutions are licensed by 9300 facilities globally, including more than 2650 hospitals; 3750 physician practices 40,000 physicians; 500 ambulatory facilities, such as laboratories, ambulatory centers, cardiac facilities, radiology clinics, and surgery centers; 800 home health facilities; 40 employer sites and 1600 retail pharmacies. It operates in globally, which includes revenue contributions and expenditures linked to business activity in the US, Argentina, Aruba, Canada, Cayman Islands, Chile, Puerto Rico, Saudi Arabia, Singapore, Spain, and the United Arab Emirates. On May 23, 2011, it acquired Resource Systems, Inc. On October 17, 2011, it acquired Clairvia, Inc.

Editas

Overview

IPO/Stock: Went public on Feb. 3, 2016 (NASDAQ:EDIT)
Total equity funding: $210M in 3 Rounds from 17 Investors
Headquarters: Cambridge, MA
Description: Editas Medicine is engaged in discovering and developing a novel class of genome-editing therapeutics.
Founders: Feng Zhang, Jennifer A. Doudna, George Church, J. Keith Joung

Categories: Healthcare, Biotechnology
Website: http://www.editasmedicine.com
Company Details
Founded: 2013
Contact: info@editasmed.com|(617) 401-9000
Employees: 66
Private company valuation: $50M
Public company valuation: $16M

The company's mission is to translate its genome-editing technology into a novel class of human therapeutics that enable precise and corrective molecular modification to treat the underlying cause of a broad range of diseases at the genetic level. The company has generated substantial patent filings and has access to intellectual property covering foundational genome-editing technologies, as well as essential advancements and enablements that will uniquely allow the company to translate early findings into viable human therapeutic products.

Fitbit

Overview
Acquisitions: 1 Acquisition
IPO/Stock: Went public on June 19, 2015 (NYSE:FIT)
Headquarters: San Francisco, CA
Description: Fitbit offers compact, wireless, wearable sensors that track a person's daily activities in order to promote a healthy lifestyle.
Founders: James Park, Eric Friedman
Categories: Healthcare, Hardware, Fitness, Personal Health, Wearables
Website: http://www.fitbit.com
Company Details
Founded: May 1, 2007
Contact: info@fitbit.com
Employees: 980
Private company valuation: $26.6M
Public company valuation: $969.7M

Fitbit inspires people to exercise more, eat better, and live healthier lifestyles. The company is developing an ultra-compact wireless wearable sensor, called the Fitbit Tracker, which automatically tracks data about a person's activities, such as calories burned, sleep quality, steps, and distance.

The Fitbit Tracker collects activity data automatically while it is worn all day by the user. The collected data is wirelessly uploaded to a website where the wearer can see their data and track their progress toward personal goals.

Health stream

Overview

IPO/Stock: Went public on Apr. 20, 2000 (HSTM)

Total equity funding: $2.4M in 1 Round

Headquarters: Nashville, TN

Description: HealthStream, Inc. (HealthStream) provides internet-based learning and research solutions to meet training, information, and education needs.

Category: Enterprise software

Website: http://www.healthstream.com

Company Details

Founded: 1990

Contact: info@healthstream.com

Employees: 972

Private company valuation: $15.8M

Public company valuation: $463.5M

HealthStream (NASDAQ:HSTM) is dedicated to improving patient outcomes through the development of healthcare organizations' greatest asset: their people. Healthstream's unified suite of solutions is contracted by healthcare organizations in the U.S. for workforce development, training and learning management, talent management, credentialing, provider enrollment, performance assessment, and managing simulation-based education programs. Healthstream's patient experience/research solutions provide valuable insight to healthcare providers to meet CAHPS requirements, improve the patient experience, engage their workforce, and enhance physician alignment.

Illumina

Overview

Investments: 9 Investments in 8 Companies

Exits: 1 Acquisition

Founders: David R. Walt, Larry Bock, John Stuelpnagel

Headquarters: San Diego, CA

Description: At Illumina, the goal is to apply innovative technologies and revolutionary assays to the analysis of genetic variation and function.

Website: http://www.illumina.com

Employees: 4600

Private company valuation: $37.6M

Public company valuation: $241.9M

Investor Details

Founded:

Accelerator that does early stage venture and later stage venture investments. At Illumina, the goal is to apply innovative technologies and revolutionary assays to the analysis of genetic variation and function, making studies possible that were not even imaginable just a few years ago. These studies will help make the realization of personalized medicine possible. With such rapid advances in technology taking place, it is mission critical to have solutions that are not only innovative, but flexible, scalable, and complete with industry-leading support and service. As a global company that places high value on collaborative interactions, rapid delivery of solutions, and prioritizing the needs of its customers, they strive to meet this challenge.

Teladoc

Overview
Acquisitions: 3 Acquisitions
IPO/Stock: Went public on July 1, 2015 (NYSE:TDOC)
Headquarters: Purchase, NY
Description: Teladoc is a telehealth services company providing medical care for adults and children via video conferencing and telephone consultations.
Founder: George Byron Brooks
Categories: Healthcare, mHealth
Website: http://www.teladoc.com
Company Details
Founded: 2002
Aliases: 835-2362835-2362
Contact: marketing@teladoc.com | (800) 835-2362
Employees: 219
Private company valuation: $36.4M
Public company valuation: $194.9M

Teladoc, Inc. (NYSE:TDOC) delivers on-demand healthcare anytime, from almost anywhere via mobile devices, the Internet, secure video, or phone. Teladoc provides consumers with access to its network of more than 2650 board-certified, state-licensed physicians and behavioral health professionals who provide care for a wide range of non-emergency conditions. Teladoc is certified by the National Committee for Quality Assurance (NCQA) for its physician credentialing process.

WebMD

Overview
Acquisitions: 6 Acquisitions
IPO/Stock: Went public on Sep. 29, 2005 (WBMD)
Headquarters: New York, NY
Description: WebMD provides timely and credible health information and services to consumers and healthcare professionals.

Founder: Ann Mond Johnson
Category: Curated web
Website: http://www.webmd.com
Company Details
Founded: 1996
Employees: 1638
Private company valuation: $53.2M
Public company valuation: $3.47B
WebMD is the leading provider of health information and services to consumers and healthcare professionals. WebMD works closely with CBS News and provides health news and features for CBS News programs. WebMD helps consumers take an active role in managing their health by providing objective healthcare information and lifestyle information.

Profiles of Select Digital Health Private Companies

DrOnDemand

Overview
Headquarters: Skokie, IL
Description: DocOnDemand delivers enterprise-wide telemedicine services for health systems.
Category: Healthcare
Website: http://www.docondemand.com/
Company Details
Founded: Dec. 1, 2010
DrOnDemand delivers enterprise-wide telemedicine services for health systems. It helps health systems create, expand, complement, and replace services with online delivery alternatives and achieve significant outreach, cost, and customer service gains.

eClinicalWorks

Overview
Headquarters: Westborough, MA
Description: eClinicalWorks provides ambulatory clinical information systems such as electronic medical records systems and community applications.
Category: Software
Website: http://www.eclinicalworks.com
Company Details
Founded: 1999
Contact: sales@eclinicalworks.com

Employees: 2237
Private company valuation: $39.7M
Public company valuation: $27.1M
eClinicalWorks is a privately held, leader in ambulatory clinical solutions. Its solutions extend the use of electronic health records beyond practice walls with the latest technologies and create community-wide records. The company has an established customer base of more than 50,000 providers and 225,000 plus medical professionals across all 50 states. Revenues for 2009 exceeded $100 million.

MEDtrip

Overview
Total equity funding: $500K in 1 Round
Most recent funding: $500K Seed on Nov. 4, 2012
Headquarters: Lakewood, CO
Description: MEDtrip is the world's premium medical tourism portal.
Founders: Jason Coppage, Greg Mogab
Category: Healthcare
Website: http://www.MEDtrip.com
Company Details
Founded: Nov. 1, 2012
Aliases: HealthcareAbroad.com
Contact: info@medtrip.com | (720) 257-5277
Employees: 11
Private company valuation: $5M
MEDtrip is a comprehensive and unbiased directory connecting patients directly to clinics and hospitals worldwide. MEDtrip was created to help patients receive the best care possible, anywhere in the world. It is run by an amazing team made up of talented health and technology professionals.

Practice Fusion

Overview
Acquisitions: 2 Acquisitions
Total equity funding: $155.02M in 10 Rounds from 29 Investors
Headquarters: San Francisco, CA
Description: Practice Fusion provides a free, web-based electronic health record (EHR) system and medical practice management technology to physicians.
Founders: Ryan Howard, Matthew Douglass
Categories: Medical, Healthcare
Website: http://www.practicefusion.com
Company Details
Founded: July 10, 2005
Contact: (415) 346-7700

Employees: 358
Private company valuation: $13.6M
Public company valuation: $24.3B
Practice Fusion provides a free, web-based EMR system to physicians. With medical charting, scheduling, e-prescribing (eRx), lab integrations, referral letters, Meaningful Use certification, unlimited support, and a Personal Health Record for patients, Practice Fusion's EMR software addresses the complex needs of today's healthcare providers and disrupts the health IT status quo. Practice Fusion is the fastest growing electronic medical record community in the country with more than 150,000 users serving 50 million patients. Practice Fusion's mission is to connect doctors, patients, and data to drive better health and save lives. The mission drives company culture and passion is the biggest requirement.

Theranos

Overview
Total equity funding: $88.4M in 6 Rounds from 5 Investors
Most recent funding: Private equity on June 12, 2014 (undisclosed amount)
Description: Theranos' mission is to make actionable health information accessible to everyone at the time it matters.
Founder: Elizabeth Holmes
Categories: Biotechnology, Healthcare, Health Diagnostics
Website: http://www.theranos.com
Company Details
Founded: 2003
Aliases: RealTime Cures
Contact: info@theranos.com
Employees: 141
Private company valuation: $27.5M
Public company valuation: $22.1M
Headquartered in Palo Alto, Theranos, Inc. is a consumer healthcare technology company. Theranos' clinical laboratory offers comprehensive laboratory tests from samples as small as a few drops of blood at unprecedented low prices. Founded in 2003 by Elizabeth Holmes, Theranos' mission is to make actionable health information accessible to people everywhere in the world at the time it matters, enabling early detection and intervention of disease, and empowering individuals with information to live the lives they want to live.

WellDoc

Overview
Total equity funding: $54.93M in 6 Rounds from 9 Investors
Most recent funding: $7.5M Series B on March 1, 2016
Headquarters: Baltimore, MD

Description: WellDoc is a health care technology company that develops solutions to transform the management of chronic disease.

Founders: Ryan Sysko, Suzanne Sysko Clough, Yves Nordmann

Categories: Medical, Healthcare, Real-Time

Website: http://www.welldoc.com

Company Details

Founded: March 1, 2005

Aliases: Welldoc Communications, Inc., WellDoc, Inc.

Contact: (443) 692-3100

Employees: 72

Private company valuation: $8.8M

Public company valuation: $45.6B

WellDoc is developing the next generation of technology solutions to support chronic disease management. They do integrating clinical, behavioral, and motivational applications with everyday technologies, like the internet and cell phone, to engage patients and healthcare providers in ways that dramatically improve outcomes and significantly reduce healthcare costs.

ZocDoc

Overview

Total equity funding: $223M in 4 Rounds from 11 Investors

Most recent funding: $130M Series D on August 20, 2015

Headquarters: New York, NY

Description: ZocDoc is the beginning of a better healthcare experience for millions of patients every month.

Founders: Cyrus Massoumi, Oliver Kharraz, Nick Ganju

Categories: Medical, Dental, Healthcare

Website: http://www.zocdoc.com

Company Details

Founded: September 18, 2007

Contact: service@zocdoc.com | (855) 962-3621

Employees: 773

Private company valuation: $27.5M

Public company valuation: $101.8M

ZocDoc is the tech company at the beginning of a better healthcare experience. Each month, millions of patients use ZocDoc to find in-network neighborhood doctors, instantly book appointments online, see what other real patients have to say, get reminders for upcoming appointments and preventive checkups, fill out their paperwork, and more. With a mission to give power to the patient, ZocDoc's online marketplace delivers the accessible and simple experience patients expect and deserve. ZocDoc is free for patients and available across the United States via ZocDoc.com or the ZocDoc app for iPhone and Android.

References

Bureau of Labor Statistics. Measuring price change for medical care in the CPI. http://www.bls.gov

CB Insights. Healthcare start-up boom: 2015 could see more than $12B invested into VC-backed companies. https://www.cbinsights.com

Centers for Medicare & Medicaid services. https://www.cms.gov

Crowd Funding Legal Hub. Changes to "accredited investor" definition recommended by SEC staff; the good, the bad and the ugly. https://crowdfundinglegalhub.com

GP Bullhound. Digital healthcare-local challenges, global opportunities. 2015. http://www.gpbullhound.com

Hathaway, Ian and Jonathan Rockwell. A cure for health care inefficiency? The value and geography of venture capital in the digital health sector. Brookings. 2015. http://www.brookings.edu

Why 'one patient, one chart' is still far off. VB. http://venturebeat.com

The rising billions and healthcare's expanding global market. Forbes. http://www.forbes.com

SaaS Metrics 2.0 – a guide to measuring and improving what matters. for Entrepreneurs. http://www.forentrepreneurs.com

Practice Fusion surveys patients, highlights the inefficiency of paper records and the need for electronic medical records in the US. PR Newswire. http://www.prnewswire.com

Accelerators vs. incubators: what start-ups need to know. Techrepublic. http://www.techrepublic.com/

Six myths about venture capitalists. Harvard Business Review. https://hbr.org

Digital health funding hits new highs in 2015, reaching nearly $6B. https://www.cbinsights.com

Global digital health market size, share, development, growth and demand forecast to 2022 – industry insights by technology (Digitized Health System, Telemedicine, mHealth, Health Analytics and Others). https://www.psmarketresearch.com

Artificial pancreas is first to raise $1 million under new crowdfunding rules. https://www.technologyreview.com/

Irving Levin Associates. Health care M&A deal volume and value exploded in 2015. http://www.levinassociates.com

Medium Corporation. Unicorns vs. Donkeys: your handy guide to distinguishing who's who. https://medium.com.

Organization for Co-operation and Development. http://stats.oecd.org/

Start-up Health Insights. 2015. Digital health funding rankings - 2015 mid year report. https://www.start-uphealth.com

Start-up Health, LLC. Start-up health insights Q1 and mid-year reports. 2015. https://www.start-uphealth.com

Woolhandler S, Campbell T, Himmelstein DU. Costs of health care administration in the United States and Canada. N Engl J Med. 2003;349:768–75.

Dr. Razouki   has over 15 years of experience in venture capital and private equity investment with a focus on healthcare and technology, shifting from an excellence in clinical practice and research to the management and financing of healthcare and education systems. A graduate of **Columbia Business School**, Dr. Razouki is the first ever Arab national to receive an MBA with a focus on Healthcare Management and Finance. Dr. Razouki is a member of the **Hermes Honors Society** of Columbia Business School, an honor bestowed on the top 1000 global alumni of the university. An Oral and Maxillofacial surgeon by training, Dr. Razouki has completed clinical rotations at New York Presbyterian Hospital of **Columbia University Medical Center**, Harlem Hospital, **Cleveland University Hospital** of Case Western Reserve University, and Mass General Hospital of **Harvard University**. Dr. Razouki graduated with Cum Laude Honors from **Creighton University** with a Bachelor's in Biology (Ethology) and TPP (Theology, Philosophy and Political Science).

In 2007, Dr. Razouki joined the world's largest and oldest strategic consulting firms, **Booz Allen Hamilton**, which at the time was operating in over 100 countries across six continents with four billion dollars in revenue. Dr. Razouki had the honor of working with all six GCC Ministers of health and completed health and public sector projects across the GCC, Lebanon and Egypt.

In 2009, Dr. Razouki was selected to join the Office of Tony Blair to lead the development of the Kuwait 2030 Vision for Health, Education and Entrepreneurship together with the Council of Minister of Kuwait. Dr. Razouki was also selected to head the Prime Minister's Early Warning System Committee on Health and played an integral part in the establishment of the Kuwait Talent Bank, which would go on to form the backbone of the Kuwait Youth Parliament and the future Ministry of State for Youth Affairs.

In 2011, Dr. Razouki and his partners completed the purchase of a Kuwait based healthcare development company, which was rebranded as Kleos Healthcare. Today, Kleos is widely recognized as a regional thought leader on Middle East healthcare, with a variety of projects in its pipeline ranging from developing a Medical Takaful Insurance company to working on a 750 million USD government PPP.

In 2012, Dr. Razouki co-founded Dubai based Glambox.me, one of the region's leading e-commerce platforms that later on completed a ~1.4 million USD Series A funding round (which at the time was the largest Series A round in the history of Middle East entrepreneurship) with notable MENA VC firms including STC Ventures, MBC Ventures, and R&R ventures.

Dr. Razouki has also invested in multiple digital platforms in New York and Silicon Valley, including most notably Instavest.com, a global leader in personalized FinTech valued at 12 million USD that manages over $250 million worth of assets, and ShiftSmart, a leading San Francisco start-up focusing on improving employee development and retention for the growing Sharing Economy valued at 5 million USD.

In 2015, Dr. Razouki was the first ever Kuwaiti doctor to complete the *"Reforming of Public Systems: Health, Higher Education and Finance"* Executive Education course at the prestigious Grande École, **Paris Institute of Political** Studies ("Sciences Po").

Dr. Razouki believes that the future of healthcare is approaching the singularity of coalescing the physical world with the digital. As a result, Dr. Razouki has incubated, funded, and developed multiple local, regional, and international digital health platforms including the **2014 LTE MENA winner** for best mobile application—AbiDoc—the region's first online appointment booking platform and call center and Kuwait's largest network of private hospitals, clinics, and doctors; MEDtrip—the world's top medical tourism platform with offices in Denver, Colorado, and Cebu, Philippines; Sihatech—Saudi Arabia's largest digital health application company, Nabta Health— the MENA region's first women's health application; and Cera Care—a London based digital health company focused on excellence in elder care across Europe, which was awarded the Healthcare Startup of the Year 2016 at the Healthcare Startup Awards, from over 1000 entries.

In 2015, Dr. Razouki was presented with the **Kuwait e-Award** for best eHealth application by His Highness Sheikh Sabah Al Ahmed Al Sabah, the Emir of Kuwait. Dr. Razouki was also selected by **Stanford Medicine** as part of a group of 20 global authors to write a chapter on digital health investing in the upcoming Springer published book: *Digital Health: Scaling Healthcare to the World.* He is the only author from the Arab World.

During 2015, Dr. Razouki was also an **Industry Expert Board Member** at Al Ayadi Al Baytha Health Company, a 50 million USD fully owned company of Al Khabeer Capital, which is one of Saudi Arabia's largest and most active private equity investors with over **three billion dollars of assets under management**. Dr. Razouki worked together with the turnaround team at Al Khabeer and the asset management to unlock unrealized value in one of Saudi Arabia's fastest growing medical services companies.

In 2016, Dr. Razouki was selected by the Abdul Rahman Al Sumait Award Executive Committee to represent the science community in Kuwait and present at the first ever meeting of the committee. The Committee is co-chaired by His Excellency Sheikh Sabah Khalid Al Hamad Al Sabah, Kuwait's Minister of Foreign Affairs, and Mr. Bill Gates. At one million USD it is the largest science prize awarded for scientific achievement in Africa. Dr. Razouki was also nominated as one of the top five venture capital investors in the Middle East and North Africa by Arabian Business. Dr. Razouki also won two awards at the seventh annual **Middle East Healthcare Leadership Awards** for both **Middle East Public Private Partnership of the Year** for the Jaber Hospital PPP Sustainable Hospital Project and **Healthcare Entrepreneur of the Year**. Dr. Razouki also won the prestigious Best Startup Award at the 2016 ArabNet Riyadh StartUp Battle Field competition as well as the winner of the 2017 Startup Championship MENA, for Sihatech.

In 2016, Dr. Razouki was also selected to participate in the prestigious World Economic Forum Global Health and Healthcare Community Meeting as part of the Future Trends in Health Task Force which was Chaired by Dr. Melanie Walker, Advisor to the President of the World Bank, Dr. Jim Young Kim. Dr. Razouki was the only participant from Kuwait and had the honor of having **seven out the 10 final key technological trends and themes** accepted in the final outcome report of the forum. Dr. Razouki was also selected by the World Economic Forum and the International Finance Corporation (IFC) as one of the 100 top entrepreneurs shaping the fourth Industrial Revolution in the MENA region.

In 2017, Dr. Razouki was appointed to the Advisory Board of *Popular Science* Magazine. An outlet for eminent scientists such as Charles Darwin and Thomas Edison's writings and ideas in the nineteenth century, *Popular Science* is the most prestigious science magazine in the world and was first launched in 1872.

Dr. Razouki was also appointed by the Kuwait Foundation for the Advancement of Sciences to the Board of Trustees of the Jaber Al Ahmed Center for Molecular Imaging and Nuclear Medicine (JAC), the MENA region's first center of excellence and Type II facility dedicated to the production of common radiopharmaceuticals for applications in positron emission tomography. Dr. Razouki is also Chairman of the Executive Committee.

Dr. Razouki is also the Principal Author of the annual **Middle East Science Report**, the region's premiere publication on the state of science in the MENA region capturing the progress of scientific thought and research across 50 of the region's top universities and research institutions as well as interviewing over 100 of the region's top scientific minds.

In 2017, Dr. Razouki and his partners also closed the largest successful Series A in the history of technology entrepreneurship in the Kingdom of Saudi Arabia by securing 5 million Saudi Riyals to support the growth of the **Saudi Internet Health Application Technology Company** (www.Sihatech.com) from Waed Aramco Entrepreneurship and existing strategic investor Waseel ASP.

Dr. Razouki is the current Chief Business Development Officer of Kuwait Life Sciences Company (KLSC) where he is part of a team that manages over 100 million dollars in assets under management including local, regional, and international investments on behalf of the Kuwait Investment Authority (KIA), the sovereign wealth fund of the State of Kuwait. Dr. Razouki is the youngest ever chief executive at a KIA owned company.

Dr. Razouki is also considered regional thought leader within the Middle East life sciences industry and has championed the building of strong pillars of the local life sciences ecosystem including the region's premiere pharmaceutical licensing and distribution platform: NewBridge—a 50 million USD revenue company operating across all 22 MENA countries including Iraq, Iran, and Turkey as well as South Africa, Clinart—the region's top Clinical Research Organization (CRO) and host of the first ever Phase II Clinical Trial in the history of Kuwait at the Dasman Diabetes Institute, eCore—the region's top active pharmaceutical ingredients licensor and distributor, the Life Sciences Academy—the region's first ever training and development company focused on the healthcare and life sciences industry as well as Innomedics—one of Kuwait's top medical device distribution companies that pioneered the distribution of personalized digital health products in the region.

At KLSC, Dr. Razouki and his team have invested and co-invested with some of the world's top life science venture capital funds including New Leaf Venture Partners in New York, Wellington Partners in Munich, and Kearny Venture Partners and Presidio Partners both of which are based in San Francisco. Notable direct and indirect investments include: CRISPR Therapeutics—a leading personalized genomic medicine company based in Cambridge, Massachusetts (NASDAQ: CRSP); iRhythm Technologies, based in San Francisco, which closed 56% above its listed stock price on the first day of its IPO (NASDAQ: IRTC); Quanta Fluid Solutions—one of the world's first home hemodialysis manufacturers; Median Technologies—a leading global provider of medical imaging solutions, especially in the field of oncology based in France (EPA: ALMDT); and SuperSonic Imagine—a leading global provider of medical ultrasound solutions also based in France (EPA: SSI).

Dr. Razouki is also a former advisor to the central Kuwaiti government where he worked with senior government leaders during the administration of **HE the Prime Minister, Sheikh Nasser Al Mohammad Al Sabah**, and **Deputy Prime Minister for Economic Affairs, Sheikh Ahmed Al Fahad Al Sabah**, on Healthcare, Education, and Entrepreneurial reforms as part of Kuwait's 100 billion dollar **Development Plan**. Dr. Razouki continues to work closely with the **Council of Ministers of Kuwait** and is currently advising the government on the development of the Sabah Al Ahmad National Genome Center together with the Kuwait Foundation for the Advancement of Sciences, a National Pharmaceutical Quality Control Laboratory, and the 1 bn USD Jaber Hospital project, a 1168 facility which will be the largest single healthcare structure in the Middle East.

Chapter 21
An Education in Digital Health

Carlo V. Caballero-Uribe

Abstract The use of social networks as educational platforms is continually grow-ing through a combination of formal and informal methods. This paper describes the concept of *digital health* and the benefits and limitations of certain digital plat-forms, specifically those related to social media, and explains the rise of "informed patients" and a new digital environment for patients and physicians. Additionally, useful resources providing free open-access medical education are explored, with special focus on the benefits available to medical students using Web 2.0 platforms as an accessory tool for learning.

Keywords Digital health • e-Patients • Medical education • Participatory medicine Social media

21.1 The Concept of *Digital Health* and Social Media

We may do whatever we want with new media, except ignore them—Marshall McLuhan

Digital Health is an emerging field of knowledge that combines informatics and its uses to organize health services through the Internet and related technologies, with an emphasis on collaborative work involving global, regional, and local healthcare scenarios through the use of communication and computer technology (ICT) (Van De Belt et al. 2010).

In other words, medical treatment in cyberspace uses the Internet and global communication networks of healthcare and public health providers to enable access to medical information *for healthcare consumers.*

Ready access to information allows obtaining, selecting, and classifying required topics in addition to easing communication among different specialists of all areas

C.V. Caballero-Uribe, M.D., Ph.D(c).
Associated Professor of Medicine, Universidad del Norte, Barranquilla, Colombia
e-mail: carvica@uninorte.edu.co

© Springer International Publishing AG 2018   329
H. Rivas, K. Wac (eds.), *Digital Health*, Health Informatics,
https://doi.org/10.1007/978-3-319-61446-5_21

of medicine. The modernization of education and knowledge diffusion processes force health professionals to submit to this new way of approaching their roles regarding science and medical developments.

The *current best practices* using social media in medicine allows for dynamic, practical, and up-to-date knowledge as well as sharing information and establishing a new form of communication and follow-up with patients.

Medicine is an area of great potential impact in the use of social media as it is increasingly used in the learning process. To the extent that the use of these tools for the acquisition and spread of information is understood, interest in their proper use increases (Hughes et al. 2008).

Social media (SM) has allowed patients to take on an essential role in the healthcare process, which has been improved with important notions such as the "E-patient" concept (Jadad et al. 2003). The growing number of SM applications has improved and favored many people's natural tendency not to cede control over their health to the traditional system, and has enabled them to actively participate in decisions pertaining to their treatment. SM have grown into key channels of patients' active participation in different levels of the healthcare system.

One of the first authors to refer to *E-patients* was Ferguson, who in a seminal paper (Ferguson and Frydman 2004) referred to this kind of patient as a proactive one, properly educated in technology, actively involved in keeping his/her own health, and interested in contributing not only to the treatment and investigation of specific health conditions, but also to the improvement of medical attention processes. A paper published in 2007 dealt with what today we call *E-patients* (Ferguson n.d.), where the letter *e* refers to *equipped, enabled, engaged, empowered*, and *expert meaning new skills for patients to learn (equipped, enabled) to share (engaged), to contribute (empowered) and to add value (expert).*

Several scenarios occur that must be reflected in digital health education (see Chart 21.1).

Chart 21.1 Instigators of Digital Health
- Availability of many information sources
- Patients active in the search for knowledge
- Changes in the role of healthcare professionals

21.2   Medical Education Through Social Media

The strategic use of SM seems to have a multitude of benefits, from keeping updated in a practical and dynamic manner through to sharing and spreading information quickly and efficiently, thereby establishing this as a new way of communication and follow-up with patients. The changing and progressive qualities of these new forms of technology lead to unimaginable reach in the world of medicine, as has already occurred in other fields. SM clearly develop more complex relationships and interactions, i.e., online between patients, physicians, and the general public to the point where we could be discussing the emergence of safe or unsafe relationships and public and personal interactions, or combinations thereof. Some consider that the public nature of social networks hinders physicians' scope of work and affects the doctor–patient relationship (George et al. 2013). This is partly explained by the fact that medicine has traditionally valued privacy, confidentiality, one-on-one interaction, and formal conduct, whereas SM have fostered different principles, such as openness, outreach, connection, transparency, and informality, which seem to antagonize all that we have learned and apparently affect the concept of medical professionalism (Pereira et al. 2015).

To date, there are few serious studies supported on theoretical models that prove the usefulness of SM in medicine. McGowan et al. (2012) studied the elements that influence the use of SM by doctors, specifically to determine what causes medical information to be shared. The study involved defining social media tools, subjecting them to a model based on Davis' for technology adoption (Davis et al. 1989), and assessing the use of SM by 485 specialists (186 oncologists) and general practitioners (299). Results yielded that one-quarter (24.1% or 117/485) use SM on a daily basis or several times a day to search for medical information and over half (57.7% or 279/485) considered SM useful to obtain high-quality information and reach out to peers. Additionally, 57.9% (281/485) stated SM helped them care more effectively for patients and improve the quality of medical attention. Factors favoring the use of SM to share information with other colleagues were, according to the technology acceptance model, ease of use and perceived usefulness. Those with a positive attitude toward social media tools were the ones with the highest percentage of SM use. Neither age nor gender had a significant impact on the use of social media by these physicians. The authors specifically noted the amount of information a doctor must learn, understand, and apply to their clinical practice and how this overload of information surpasses our cognitive skills as a factor in the use of SM and social learning models to help handle the information overload, albeit only if used effectively.

It is generally accepted that more studies are required to examine the impact of the significant use of social tools on physicians' knowledge, attitudes, abilities, and behavior in practice (Cheston et al. 2013).

21.2.1 Benefits and Drawbacks

The growing use of social media has led to the emergence of user guides that acknowledge the tendency to use social media for communication in the healthcare sector. At the same time, these guides warn of the inappropriate use and of the possible ethical and professional implications for the practice of medicine.

A recent review throws some light upon the possible uses, benefits, and drawbacks of SM for communications between the general public, patients, and health professionals as well as the most relevant aspects of their use in the healthcare sector (Moorhead et al. 2013). Six clear benefits were identified:

1. An increase or improvement in interactions.
2. Increased availability of shared information adapted to particular needs.
3. Improvement in access and extension of health information.
4. Social and emotional support from peers.
5. Public health surveillance aspects.
6. Potential to influence health policies.

A systematic review of over 108 references in a qualitative study of medical professionalism focused on the benefits and challenges set forth by the use of SM (Gholami-Kordkheili et al. 2013) found evidence of changes in traditional values, which suggests an inter-professional and inter-generational dialogue, as well as a more precise definition of challenges and benefits obtained through the professional use of social media. Also identified were 12 drawbacks

Lack of reliability	✓	✓	✓
Quality concerns	✓	✓	✓
Lack of confidentiality and privacy	✓	✓	✓
Often unaware of the risks of disclosing personal information online	✓	✓	
Risks associated with communicating harmful or incorrect advice using social media	✓	✓	
Information overload	✓	✓	
Not sure how to correctly apply information found online to their personal health situation	✓	✓	
Certain social media technologies may be more effective in behavior change than others	✓		
Adverse health consequences	✓		
Negative health behaviors	✓		
Social media may act as a deterrent for patients from visiting health professionals		✓	✓
Currently may not often use social media to communicate to patients			

relating basically to the quality of information and its confidentiality and privacy aspects. The study highlighted concerns over the quality and reliability of information and the fact that e-mail is not an official registry of clinical histories and is vulnerable to security breaches. It also suggested training on the use of technology in order to increase trustworthiness and visibility. The study concluded that SM are important tools for developing possibilities in the health sector, but that a more profound and robust investigation on behalf of academia is needed to determine its capability of generating change in communication practices in the short- and long-term.

The American College of Physicians (ACP) published a position document including guidelines on online medical professionalism (Farnan et al. 2013). The ACP recognizes *"that emerging technology and societal trends will continue to change the landscape of social media and social networking and how websites are used by patients and physicians will evolve over time,"* as well as the fact *"social media has transformed communication and is on its way to do so with healthcare.*

As clinical use grows, doctors must be aware of its implications for ethics, professionalism, relationships, and the profession."

These recommendations acknowledge the importance of new media and also identify the absence of user policies or guides for best practice, including areas of concern such as use for matters not pertaining to clinical practice, implications for confidentiality, conflicts of use for social media as a tool for educating patients, and the ways these could affect patients' trust in doctors or the doctor–patient relationship. The recommendations also suggest strategies toward preserving confidentiality.

As a position document for the most important medical association in the United States, with global influence, it points to concerns over professional ethics due to possible transgressions of limits imposed in the doctor–patient relationship. It advises to "separate online personal and professional profiles from requests to register medical histories through e-mail, which are both aspects that seem to affect widespread acceptance of social media in spite of reported benefits".

Additionally, the American Medical Association has stated its position regarding the educational benefit for patients, ethical challenges, establishing limits with patients, rules for the use of social media, online monitoring guidelines, and managing identity and digital reputation (http://www.ama-assn.org/ama/pub/physician-resources/medical-ethics/code-n.d.):

1. The use of online media may bring significant educational benefits to physicians and patients, but also poses ethical challenges. Keeping trust in the profession and in the doctor–patient relationship requires that health professionals consistently apply ethical principles to preserve the relationship, confidentiality, privacy, and respect of persons in online environments and in their communications.
2. Limits between social and professional spheres may be blurred online. Physicians should keep separate cyber-spheres and behave professionally in both.
3. E-mail and other electronic communication should be used by doctors exclusively in a well-established doctor–patient relationship and always under consent from the patient.
4. Doctors should consider periodic self-auditing to assess the exactitude of online information available to them in professional ranking sites and other online venues.
5. A vast and permanent reach characterizes Internet and online communications. Doctors and students shall be aware that whatever they upload may have consequences for their future professional lives.

Several studies show we do not take full advantage of the web's potential and that until recently, healthcare sites barely fostered doctor–patient interaction or lacked health content or information. In general, the Internet represents a content platform for health professionals to a greater extent than a social or professional communications space. Factors such as a lack of time due to excess work, low safety when sharing data, reluctance to engage patients outside of a medical consultation, or being questioned on their knowledge, affect physicians' use of this technology (Chrétien and Kind 2013; Chou et al. 2009).

21.2.2 Medical and Healthcare Resources in Social Media

So-called Web 2.0 platforms enable access to complementary resources in medical teaching. This section deals with some of them and with my experience and that of others with these media:

1. Health social networks: There are networks specifically designed for healthcare professionals, such as Doximity, Sermo, etc., as well as others designed exclusively for researchers, such as Research Gate and Academia.edu, which have steadily grown through peer-to-peer collaboration. Excellent continuing education material is available on blogs or slideshares, as well as open-access books and documents on Scribd.

2. Online courses: Initiatives such as the Khan Academy feature multiple videos and have given rise to the concept of "flipped" or inverse classes, which include a collection of exceptional videos that make learning and teaching fun. The health and medicine collection has steadily grown (https://es.khanacademy.org/science/health-and-medicine n.d.). An additional free online initiative is the Coursera University courses (www.coursera.com n.d.). Coursera offers free online courses in the MOOC (Massive Open Online Courses) modality. Some of the best universities participate with a growing number of high-quality offerings.

3. Medical hashtags: Social media have opened access to medical information. Twitter has been cited as a tool to increase the engagement of residents and medical students, share scientific information, and continuing medical education (http://www.nature.com/polopoly_fs/1.15711!/menu/main/topColumns/topLeft-Column/pdf/512126a.pdf n.d.). There are signs that medical students who use social media improve their knowledge, attitudes, and skills. Any type of hashtag (#) may be followed on Twitter, which of course includes medical hashtags. To participate in chats, first observe and then place a hashtag in your tweets to see and be seen by others. Usually, members of a community define a weekly topic for a certain date. Some of the most notable are Medical Education (#MedEd) every Thursday for an hour, which includes global educators, and Healthcare Leaders (#hcldr); however, there are many more. The same is true for hashtag #FOAMed, created for Free Open Access Medicine. Conference hashtags may also be followed. Symplur (www.symplur.com n.d.) enables following all content generated under these hashtags. Twitter is an interesting case in that in a study of 5156 tweets from doctors with over 500 followers, 49% were related to medicine, 21% to personal communication, 58% included a link, and 12% were considered self-promoting (Chetrien et al. 2011). Interestingly, Twitter is the least used social network in the United States, although it has the strongest professional emphasis of any social network. Differences in uses and platforms may indicate changing cultural trends in the adoption of different tools (Choo et al. 2015).

4. YouTube videos: YouTube is a wonderful source of all types of videos, including medical. YouTube features an education channel where any topic may be studied under the guidance of top global educators.

21.2.3 Is Digital Health Part of the Medical School or Other Health Allied School Curriculum?

In spite of significant advances, the use of these platforms is far from consolidated. There are some pioneers, such as:Bertalan Meskó (@Berci), who teaches an elective course as part of the official medical curriculum in two of his country's top universities (Debrecen and Semmelweis, Hungary), which may be reviewed online (The Social Media Course n.d.); Ryan Madanick (@RyanMadanickMD) (gastroenterologist, head of the Chapel Hill residency program, USA), who directs a seminar at the end of fourth year;Bryan Vartabedian pediatrician from Baylor College of Medicine, USA) (@Doctor_V), who teaches undergraduate students for a year; and the Canadian Medical Association (CMA). Although just a few, the people, schools, universities, and institutions who engage in this work are of great relevance given the rising number of people who search online for information on medical conditions (over 71% according to a recent survey) and who have growing needs for appropriate and credible information.

In our case, for years we have used the hashtag #Rotreuma in our rheumatology rotation. Our preliminary experience was recently published (http://journals.lww.com/jclinrheum/Citation/2016/04000/PANLAR_2016_Abstracts.2.aspx?trendmd-shared= n.d.).

A total of 1576 tweets were analyzed. Original tweets numbered 970 (61.4%), 606 (38.45%) were retweets, and 227 influencers generated content. Of the total number of tweets, 71.9% were produced by undergraduate medical students, 4.8% by internal medicine residents, 2.6% by professors, 1.6% by rheumatologists, 1% by institutions, 3.8% by specialties different to rheumatology and 13.9% for other users. Original tweets of topical interest in rheumatology numbered 726 (74.86%). For tweets with topics of interest, 42% included hashtag #HoyAprendí (*Today I learned*), 84.3% had appropriate content, 97% were written in Spanish, 33.37% featured images, and 232 had sources where 75% of the sources were in Spanish, 24.5% in English, 87% were external, and 50% were formal.

The use of Twitter helps acquire skills that we consider useful for the future (Chart 21.2):

Chart 21.2 Skills Potentially Stimulated in Social Media (e.g., Twitter)
- Mastering ICT (tools).
- Learning another language (communication skills).
- Learning how to best assess academic and non-academic resources (searching skills).
- Practicing how to share information through journals or blogs (research and writing skills).
- Understanding what our patients feel and need (compassionate care).

The following shall improve skills related to:

1. Public thinking and behavior
2. Writing concisely and focusing an idea in 140 characters
3. Learning to use ICT as a natural part of their future medical practice
4. Using words such as openness, collaboration, crowdsourcing, and sharing instead of closeness, individualism, and keeping information
5. Practicing the concept of global networking
6. Learning from real patients through blogs from *e-patients*

The following is advice obtained from years of using these tools in teaching medicine to undergraduate students: This was from a presentation at Doctors 2.0 in 2015. This is the link https://www.slideshare.net/carvica/caballero-final-d20-day2-16-9-2015-2

- Ask or show interest in digital skills or experiences and hobbies of every young person entering rotation to know them better and stimulate their areas of interest.
- Present digital matters as an option while respecting students not comfortable in the digital field and not "bullying" them. Procuring a "digital coach", usually one of his or her own classmates, if difficulties are detected.
- Explain how rotations work and make clear that technology is an accessory to the main purpose of rotation: learning the bases of rheumatology.
- Enjoy, be open with students, and allow them to express their creativity. I frequently give them a general idea to develop and let them do it according to their skills or tastes. Feedback is important. I will periodically make adjustments, try new things, and discard what seems not to be working.

21.2.4   Conclusions and Suggestions

As the use of social media is increasingly being considered a social expectation, plenty of questions remain from an academic point of view (Grajales et al. 2014). What are appropriate relationship norms? What happens when geographical boundaries are transcended and affect specifically local advice? Will professionals have time to participate or get involved, to have different online personalities for personal or professional cases, as current advice suggests? Is the growing number of user guides constraining and restrictive? Should user guides be local or global? Should they be left to the discretion of physicians? Should hospitals favor the use of social media? What is the quality of information shared online?

While we find appropriate answers to these questions, we offer some final guidance to reflect on how to introduce innovative concepts in medical teaching as discussed below.

Promoting innovation: In a changing world, we improve things by the ability to think differently, challenge the establishment, and most importantly because of the belief that everything can be improved.

Acknowledging the power of informal information: Formal communication through magazines and conferences will not be the only ways of conveying or endorsing scientific knowledge. Scientific information shall and will be distributed by even more mass media, not only for a reduced circle of peers, but for a general public that will increasingly demand precise knowledge and justification of studies.

Adjusting the teaching of medicine to the new context: Tasks that will support our future will be those related to the ability to solve problems. Everything mechanical, repetitive, or entailing memorizing tends to become obsolete in a world where it is no longer necessary to have all information in our hands, but rather to know where to find it. We shall develop early critical thinking, introduce contact with patients early on, promote self-learning, and accept the temporality of knowledge by stimulating new skills throughout life.

Actively improving digital skills: We shall occupy ourselves in understanding digital trends to gain better communication skills with patients, the general public, and also with our families. It is impossible to understand the world without comprehending its languages and symbols.

Rethink professional performance: To improve our areas of performance, we should think long-term, visualize all forthcoming changes, and analyze scenarios that allow us to better define what it is that we want and can do.

References

American Medical Association's Opinion 9.124 – Professionalism in the use of social media. 2010. Available at: http://www.ama-assn.org/ama/pub/physician-resources/medical-ethics/code-medical-ethics/opinion9124.page.

Cheston CC, Flickinger TE, Chisolm MS. Social media use in medical education: a systematic review. Acad Med. 2013;88:893–901.

Chetrien C, Azar J, Kind T. Physicians on Twitter. JAMA. 2011;305(6):566–8. doi:10.1001/jama.2011.68.

Choo EK, Ranney ML, Chan TM, Trueger NS, Walsh AE, Tegtmeyer K, et al. Twitter as a tool for communication and knowledge exchange in academic medicine: a guide for skeptics and novices. Med Teach. 2015;37(5):411–6.

Chou WS, Hunt YM, Beckjord EB, Moser RP, Hesse BW. Social media use in the United States: implications for health communication. J Med Internet Res. 2009;11(4):e48.

Chrétien K, Kind T. Social media as a tool in medicine. Circulation. 2013;127:1413–21. Available at: http://circ.ahajournals.org/content/127/13/1413.full.pdf+html

Davis FD, Bagozzi RP, Warshaw PR. User acceptance of computer technology: a comparison of two theoretical models. Manag Sci. 1989;35(8):982–1003.

Farnan J, Sulmasy L, Woster B, Chaudhry H, Rhyne J, Arora V. Online medical professionalism: patient and public relationships: policy statement from the American College of Physicians and the Federation of State Medical Boards. Ann Intern Med. 2013;158(8):620–7. Available at: http://annals.org/article.aspx?articleid=1675927

Ferguson T. How they can help us heal health care. E-patients. Available at: http://e-patients.net/e-Patients_White_Paper.pdf

Ferguson T, Frydman G. The first generation of e-patients. BMJ. 2004;328(7449):1148–9. Available at: http://www.ncbi.nlm.nih.gov/pmc/articles/PMC411079/

George DR, Rovniak LS, Kraschnewski JL. Dangers and opportunities for social media in medicine. Clin Obstet Gynecol. 2013;56(3), 10.1097/ GRF.0b013e318297dc38. http://doi.org/10.1097/GRF.0b013e318297dc38

Gholami-Kordkheili F, Wild V, Strech D. The impact of social media on medical professionalism: a systematic qualitative review of challenges and opportunities. J Med Internet Res. 2013;15(8):e184. Available at: http://www.ncbi.nlm.nih.gov/pmc/articles/PMC3758042/

Grajales FJ 3rd., Sheps S, Ho K, Novak-Lauscher H, Eysenbach G. Social media: A review and tutorial of applications in medicine and health care. J Med Internet Res. 2014;16(2):e13. doi:10.2196/jmir.2912

Hughes B, Joshi I, Wareham J. Health 2.0 and Medicine 2.0: tensions and controversies in the field. J Med Internet Res. 2008;10(3):e23.

Jadad A, Rizo C, Wenkin M. I am a good patient, believe it or not. BMJ. 2003;326(7402):1293–5. Available at: http://www.ncbi.nlm.nih.gov/pmc/articles/PMC1126181/

McGowan BS, Wasko M, Vartabedian BS, Miller RS, Freiherr DD, Abdolrasulnia M. Understanding the factors that influence the adoption and meaningful use of social media by physicians to share medical information. J Med Internet Res. 2012;14(5):e117.

Moorhead A, Hazlett D, Harrison L, Carroll J, Irwin A, Hoving C. A new dimension of health care: systematic review of uses, benefits, and limitations of social media for health communication. J Med Internet Res. 2013;15(4):e85. Available at: http://www.jmir.org/2013/4/e85/

Pereira I, Cunningham AM, Moreau K, Sherbino J, Jalali A. Thou shalt not tweet unprofessionally: an appreciative inquiry into the professional use of social media. Postgrad Med J. 2015;20:1–4.

Scientists and the social networks. http://www.nature.com/polopoly_fs/1.15711!/menu/main/topColumns/topLeftColumn/pdf/512126a.pdf.

The Social Media Course. http://thecourse.webicina.com.

Use of Twitter in medical education: an analysis of the rotation of Rheumatology. http://journals.lww.com/jclinrheum/Citation/2016/04000/PANLAR_2016_Abstracts.2.aspx?trendmd-shared=.

Van De Belt TH, Engelen LJ, Berben SA, Schoonhoven L. Definition of Health 2.0 and Medicine 2.0: a systematic review. J Med Internet Res. 2010;12(2):e18.

www.coursera.com.

www.symplur.com.

Chapter 22
Future Directions of Digital Health

Bertalan Mesko

Abstract The technological revolution has brought structural changes to medicine and healthcare. With truly disruptive innovations such as artificial intelligence or advanced robotics, these changes will be more dramatic. All stakeholders of healthcare must prepare as their roles will be different too. The quest is finding a balance between using new technologies and keeping the human touch in care.

Empowering patients, telemedicine, deep learning algorithms, whole-genome sequencing are all driving forces that will democratize healthcare and make care affordable, accessible and augmented. This will require breaking down the ivory tower; making patients manage their health and disease; as well as creating a regulatory framework which welcomes innovation in a way that products and services remain safe.

While disruptive technologies can offer never-seen solutions in healthcare, we need to solve the ethical challenges first.

Keywords Future • Digital health • Future technologies • Medical technology • Healthcare technology • Artificial intelligence • Robotics in medicine • Bioethics

22.1 A New Era of Medical Technologies

A swarm of disruptive technologies has reached healthcare and the practice of medicine since the early 2000s. Getting in touch with peers through social media, accessing medical information anywhere using smartphones; or receiving care via telemedicine have become common elements of healthcare. The challenge is not whether such technologies will become a major part of care, but how the traditional structures will be able to change when everything else changes around us.

Disruption means a new solution is many times faster, more efficient and cheaper than any solution before that. Artificial intelligence-driven algorithms can help

B. Mesko, M.D., Ph.D.
Semmelweis University, Budapest, Hungary

The Medical Futurist Institute, Budapest, Hungary
e-mail: berci.mesko@gmail.com

© Springer International Publishing AG 2018
H. Rivas, K. Wac (eds.), *Digital Health*, Health Informatics,
https://doi.org/10.1007/978-3-319-61446-5_22

diagnose patients faster than how physicians do it alone. Medical robots can facilitate the jobs of healthcare professionals by moving patients and equipment tirelessly. Virtual reality devices can reduce pain and anxiety for patients staying at the hospitals. Exoskeletons, robotic structures patients can wear, let paralyzed people walk again. Thin sensors, worn as digital tattoos, can alert the patient about alarming changes in their health parameters and vital signs. The opportunities new technologies provide are endless, so as the potential dangers and ethical issues they may cause.

The quest for society today is to prepare in time. This way, we would be able to implement digital health solutions in a meaningful way, prove that the use of technologies makes care more affordable; and patients and their caregivers could work as a team.

The far future of medicine, when the most progressive technologies are part of our everyday lives, should be even more humanistic than it is today. The extensive use of algorithms, robots and sensors should lead to a utopia where everyone receives personalized, accessible, preventive and efficient care. While solving the ethical challenges on the way might become a bigger puzzle than developing the required technologies, this utopia will not arise by itself.

All stakeholders of healthcare today are supposed to change along the way. As their roles have changed over the last centuries, it will keep on changing.

22.2 A Cultural Revolution

Despite the fact that digital health technologies are changing care and the practice of medicine, this is not a technological revolution. Purely technological cannot change lifestyles, habits and methods used for centuries.

Susannah Fox, Chief Technology Officer at Human Health Services of the US thinks that we are living through a time when technology as innovation is a Trojan Horse for change. But this is a cultural revolution rather than a purely a technological change. Cultural revolutions are difficult and take time.

The driving force of that culture change is the democratization of technology development being enabled by the internet. First it was about a greater access to data and easier innovation of software; later easier innovation of hardware too thanks to innovations like crowdfunding and 3D printing.

Four major approaches will ensure democratization of care takes place before healthcare turns into a chaos where patients have quicker access to unregulated technologies than to care in the traditional structure (Table 22.1).

Technology and health care: the view from HHS. The Wall Street Journal. https://www.wsj.com/articles/technology-and-health-care-the-view-from-hhs-1474855381. Accessed 5 Jun 2017.

Table 22.1 The differences between traditional and modern medicine

Traditional medicine	Modern medicine
Point-of-care is the clinic or lab	Point-of-care is where the patient is
Based on populations	Based on the individual
Hierarchy	Partnership
Data owned by institutions	Data owned by the patient
Individual experience	Limitless collaboration
Expensive	Affordable
Ivory tower	Social media

22.3 Embracing Disruption

Currently prevalent changing medical technology is decades old. If you look into a medical black bag, the technology there is obsolete—200 years old stethoscope lying next to 135 years old blood pressure cuff. While the world is growing digital, designing medical technology is still a painfully slow process. In our caution to save lives, we've hobbled our efforts to innovate.

However, disruptive technology is already in development for many problems in healthcare. Hundreds of thousands have access to their genetic data, revealing what medical conditions they are susceptible to. Wearable devices let us measure vital signs and health parameters anywhere, not just the doctor's office. The precision of surgical robots lets doctors perform previously impossible procedures. Exoskeletons let paralyzed people walk again, and smart algorithms help analyze radiology images. News every day make us feel as if we live in science fiction.

But when we walk into the GP's office, it's hard to feel the same. Part of the problem is that disruptive innovations are little known among patients, doctors and even regulators.

1. Medical education is focused on age old, proven technologies, leaving students unprepared to embrace modern ones—there are only a handful of courses world-wide that teach digital literacy to medical professionals.
2. For sure, regulators are simply as much in the dark as the rest of us. Approval processes were designed with twentieth century technology in mind, however, as healthcare is going digital, Moore's Law speeds up medical innovation as well. With massive advances springing up every week, there's simply no time to stick to established methods of regulation.
3. Disruptive medical innovations are often not practical enough to be actually used in the clinical settings or directly by patients. Their creators have focused on research, but the history of computing shows that to truly transform our everyday lives, technological advance must be made useable by a large group of people. Health sensors provide raw data, but rarely give guidance to their users about what it means, and how to act on it, leaving patients frustrated.

The trust in physicians can also be threatened by technology, if healthcare does not embrace it. Even now, patients are using their own skills and technology to make health decisions—Google is already used by over 90% of patients to research medical information. In the meantime, though medical outcomes have never been better, trust in physicians is at an all-time low (34% in the US compared to 73% in 1966)—evident in the popularity of alternative therapies and the anti-vaccine movement. Algorithms, apps and services like IBM Watson, smart health trackers and cheap genome sequencing will hand even more power to patients who will be able to make medical decisions without consulting doctors. But without the expertise of physicians, patients can fall prey to misinformation or faulty technology.

Disruptive medical innovations could change healthcare for the better. Technology in the clinic has been shown to help doctors spend more time with each patient. What's more, with telemedicine, smart algorithms and health trackers making it possible to stream medical data from every home, patients wouldn't have to wait weeks for a doctor's appointment or have to diagnose themselves, but would get the help they need near instantly. Studies have shown that medical outcomes increase and costs go down when technology like artificial intelligence is combined with the human touch of physicians.

If we do not embrace disruptive technology, the doctor-patient relationship may change forever—for the worse. Patients who are entrepreneurial and skilled enough can hack their own health which might lead to biological differences because of financial and resource disparities. Matthew James, born with deformed limbs, offered to put the logo of a company on his prosthesis if they support him, and received the prosthetics he needed. If the potential of medical technology is denied for most of the population, a new social divide will open up in how healthcare is delivered that we cannot tolerate. The future of healthcare must be equally available to all, not even more segregated than it is now.

To embrace disruptive medical technologies, the following steps must be taken:

1. Improving medical training, combining digital and health literacy to prepare a generation of physicians who are open to technology and innovation. Courses such as the Social MEDia Course can teach doctors how to use social media to engage with patients and peers.
2. We need to educate patients to make most of new technologies, and take the reins of their own health.
3. Healthcare agencies and regulators like the FDA must understand the coming changes—both the dangers and the value that can be gained. Passing the GINA Law to protect sensitive patient data and organizing a Patient Advisory Board to include patients in designing healthcare are promising steps forward. Only understanding can arm regulators to walk the narrow tightrope between opening up space innovation and protecting all healthcare stakeholders from the dangers of rampant technological change (Azevedo et al. 2012; Blendon et al. 2014; The Social MEDia Course (n.d.); https://www.fda.gov/advisorycommittees/committeesmeetingmaterials/patientengagementadvisorycommittee/default.htm).

22.4   Putting Patients in the Center of Care

Disruptive technologies are leading to huge structural changes in the traditional healthcare system. For thousands of years, only physicians have been able to acquire and access medical data and make medical decisions. This "ivory tower" of medicine was built on the firm knowledge that physicians know best what's good for the patient, and can't benefit from patient input. Patients were just the subjects of healthcare, not partners. Today, health innovation allows patients almost the same opportunities as physicians, but they're not yet equipped to use it responsibly. For the sake of both, physicians must learn to work with patients and treat them as equal partners, while patients must assume more responsibility for their health. This new equilibrium will lead to improved effectiveness and motivation for patients to better managing of their condition (Fig. 22.1).

Access to health data has leveled the playing field, arming patients to make informed decisions about their health. More health information is available via Google and crowdsourcing through social media communities than even the most trained physicians possess.

Thanks to direct to consumer genomics and sophisticated health trackers, patients can acquire more detailed data than their clinicians. Patients are finding new ways to take advantage of this data. Doug Kanter measured every aspect of his life relevant to his diabetes.

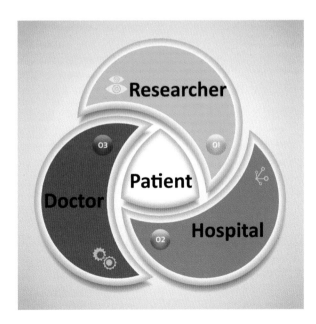

Fig. 22.1 The new structure of healthcare

He realized that his average blood sugar levels became lower due to self-management. Other patients will follow, and they are sure to get more encouragement. Studies show that involving patients in medical decisions brings greater clinical benefits and decreases costs—something that regulators looking to keep runaway healthcare costs in check are sure to pick up on.

But before patients can take control, medicine and health technology need to accommodate them. Current digital health technology like health trackers provides raw data that needs the expertise of trained physicians to be actionable. Instead of raw data, innovators should be focusing on helping patients make decisions about lifestyle. Even more important is that though vast amounts of information are available online, much of it is biased or faulty. Patients searching online can as easily stumble upon pseudo-scientific rambling as find helpful resources. Without proper training, it's often hard to distinguish between the two. Finally, most healthcare processes were designed decades ago, "suffering" patients instead of focusing on them. Involving patients in designing the delivery of care was not even considered until Dr. Tom Ferguson published his e-patient white paper in the early 2000s.

Patients also need to change before they can take charge of their health. Patients need to become experts on their own health by being proactive. They need to find digital channels and methods to keep themselves up to date. Online and in-person patient communities offer tremendous support, and a chance to "crowdsource" many health questions. Most importantly, patients need to learn to question medical advice, especially from unreliable sources, distinguishing between biased and reliable medical information. They need to demand personalized care and a say in medical decisions.

The future of care will put empowered patients in the center, who will be ready to take charge of their health. To make this a reality, every healthcare stakeholder needs to do its part. Physicians must be ready to work with patients as equal partners. This will lead to both for increased outcomes, more quality time spent with patients and higher job satisfaction, preventing burnout.

- Patients must step up and take charge of their health. If they demand to have their say in medical decisions while seeking out reliable medical information and becoming experts on their care, doctors will be happy to give them a seat at the table. Building patient communities will further help organize support and channel information to each and every patient.
- Digital health companies must support patient decisions with technology. Moving away from raw measurements and data will lead to improved customer satisfaction and retention, not to mention lasting lifestyle change.
- Regulators and administrators must start designing care with patients, for patients. The Health Design movement has proved that patient centric design results in increased satisfaction and benefits. What's more, patient advisory boards at hospitals, pharma companies and even the FDA show that patients have vital insights into healthcare processes that can fuel innovation and business performance as well (Smith et al. 2013; http://dougkanter.me/Databetes).

22.5   Shifting from Treatment to Prevention

Preventing disease has never before been a realistic goal. We have never before understood medical conditions and their underlying causes like we do now. Complex phenomena like the biology of cancer or the causes of diabetes have been documented for the first time in the past few decades by analyzing the ever growing amount of medical data. But the general population has a hard time sifting through the tons of health advice to find reliable advice on living a healthy life. Many are still unaware of well-understood, unhealthy habits like a mostly sedentary lifestyle, the lack of exercise, or excessive alcohol consumption. Changing behavior has proven difficult. We just need to look at how enduring smoking is in much of the world, even after it has been proven to be a strong cancer-causing habit.

But prevention is finally achievable because of new wearables and other health sensors. Wearable, implanted, and digestible sensors stand to provide access to real time, high fidelity data on each individual's health, helping anyone understand their health. Even more important, this understanding has been shown to fuel behavior change. Gamification can drive healthy habits—like how the Wellapets app changed asthma monitoring for kids by making it a game instead of a chore.

However, for this technology to be truly transformative, it must mature. Quantified health technology is still a fad that few can afford or take advantage of. Only 16% of US adults used some kind of wearable in 2015, and only a fraction of this number use it in less developed countries. Part of the reason is price, but prices are expected to drop over time. The bigger issue is that current technology only provides raw data, often requiring a trained physician to understand and analyze. As it is, wearables cannot drive decision making and behavior change. About half of all FitBit users stop using their device as they don't find it useful enough. But there are promising signs that wearables will grow into a transformative trend if it actively pushes users to live healthily. L'Oréal, for example, released a wearable that alerts its user when exposure to unhealthy radiation from the Sun is too high.

To truly shift focus to prevention, regulators and employers must start subsidizing it at least as heavily as they do treatment. With healthcare expenses predicted to grow unmanageable in many developed countries, as 395 million people will live to be 80 worldwide by 2050, this will make prevention a primary area to invest in for health agencies. Today, being proactive by using health sensors to generate more data is not rewarded in the healthcare system. A great example for a country taking prevention seriously is Norway where the medical association is pressing the government to back its proposal for a ban on tobacco sales to citizens born after the year 2000. Others could follow. Employers or insurers could also save serious resources by subsidizing prevention and healthy living. Omada Health provides a service to employers that helps employees live a healthy life, cutting diabetes-related health costs in half in just 2–3 years for the employer.

We need to make prevention popular by promoting the idea of quantifying health. Millions of preventable deaths are caused by lifestyle choices such as tobacco smoking, poor diet, and physical inactivity, and alcohol consumption. Having measured my health data like vital signs and stress levels for over a decade has opened new possibilities in my life. I wish to make patients and physicians aware of these; and push both innovators and regulators to make sure health trackers are accurate, using them is rewarded and algorithms deliver quality information (The Verge 2017; http://www.who.int/ageing/about/facts/en/).

22.6 Digitizing Care

Disruptive technologies must transform the current healthcare system, but to get there, we need to digitize the delivery of care. The World Health Organization estimates that there is a worldwide shortage of around 4.3 million physicians, nurses, and allied health workers. And care is often unavailable where it is most needed. Worse, with civilizational diseases like diabetes and obesity on the rise, healthcare costs are expected to grow even faster. American health spending will reach nearly $5 trillion, or 20% of gross domestic product by 2021.

The current practice of medicine is simply unsustainable.

Healthcare must transform from paper based to digital and quantifiable. Current healthcare systems are dominated by paper-based processes, which cannot be measured and analyzed as easily as digital ones. And even if a medical system is digitized today, it is fragmented and cannot be simply accessed across systems, platforms and locations. The American Medical Association estimates that over $300 billion is wasted through failures of care delivery and outmoded treatments that don't benefit patients. The United States National Academy of Sciences estimated in 2005 that "between $0.30 and $0.40 of every dollar spent on healthcare is spent on the costs of poor quality.

We can only identify the very individual causes civilizational diseases stem from with large amounts of digitized, quality information. Genomic data, for example, is only available for a handful of people—no wonder that President Obama launched an initiative to combine a database of 1,000,000 patient's genomes. Once healthcare systems are integrated and digital, smart algorithms like IBM Watson can sift through them, looking for patterns in the data, helping us understand, treat, and even prevent disease.

Digitization will enable widespread access to improved healthcare. Many face to face patient-doctor meetings are not necessary, as they could be solved from home by letting doctors access patient data and interact with them remotely. The American Medical Association showed that roughly one billion doctor visits occur each year in the United States, and of those, 70% are unnecessary and could be avoided by consulting with a physician by phone, email or text. What's more, a local GP or clinic cannot treat many complex or rare diseases which require expertise only available hundreds of miles away. The combination of telemedicine services and data from health trackers will make this a possibility in the next few years. The rise of remote diagnosis and medicine would not mean the end of the "human touch" in medicine, as many fear.

On the contrary, with digital data, it's easier to share, consult and crowdsource, opening the way for truly personalized care where it is most needed.

We must do five things to ensure everyone has access to quality, affordable care, while avoiding the threat of ubiquitous access to private health data:

1. Make devices and sensors that record health data widely available.
2. Develop integrated systems that can store and analyze it, growing our understanding of disease and measuring physician performance.
3. Design smart algorithms to support decision-making, prescribe personalized treatment and ensure compliance with therapy.
4. Make access to someone's own health data a basic human right.
5. Protect health data and privacy of patients to avoid misuse of information. (http://www.who.int/mediacentre/news/releases/2013/health-workforce-shortage/en/; http://www.tossc3.com/healthcare-must-digitize-data/; http://www.businesswire.com/news/home/20141218005175/en/Opinion-Raises-6-Million-Increase-Round-the-clock-Doctor)

22.7 Replacing or Extending Us

There is fear around the use of disruptive technologies in healthcare and society. Medical professionals are afraid of getting replaced by robots and algorithms, while patients are afraid to lose control over their lives. The most potential scenario is a healthy balance between keeping the human touch and using technologies. Technologies provide us with a chance to improve ourselves, to extend our capabilities.

When things from robotic hands to novel cancer therapies become mainstream, more people will appreciate their potential to change lives. Economic demand for them will increase. We will have to work out ethical issues and regulations.

Change in healthcare has been occurring for years. We will have access to devices that can measure anything. Wearables, insideables, and digestibles will appear with increasing frequency and people will become more accepting of them. The wearable revolution will have an effect on how we think and socialize. Then home testing becomes reality for simple blood analyses to complicated genome sequencing. A huge amount of data will result, and we must rely on technology to make sense of it. Statisticians and biomedical engineers might rule during these years, when we will be able to customize treatment based on an individual's genomic background. By the 2020s robots and artificial intelligence will probably take center stage. New technology often produces outcomes we can't prepare for. Industrialization prompted in labor unions and climate change. Software caused the need for firewalls and antivirus industries. The list could go on. Even the best technological evolution could lead to a world without privacy, freedom of choice, democracy, or even healthcare. It is not enough to improve technologies constantly; we have to adapt to whatever future we create.

Computers are amazing at completing specified tasks and algorithms of artificial intelligence will make them able to respond to new situations and be creative. We cannot compete with computing power or their speed and scope. We need to find those skills such as creativity or problem solving we can maximally improve to the limits if there are any limits at all. Technology can actually help us in this, and there is no need to see ever-improving technology as a threat to society.

Computers make more efficient decisions if people are re-checking them. IBM's Watson doesn't make a decision by itself even though it checks more information in seconds than a doctor can in years. Surgical robots don't operate without human control in the way depicted in *Prometheus*. They augment what a surgeon can do. Wearable devices do not change our lifestyle, but give us the freedom to change it ourselves. Disruptive technology coupled with the human brain is a winning combination.

The following sub-chapters describe those trends and technologies that have the biggest potential to make care affordable, efficient and humanistic. I chose these trends based on scenario analysis, the status of current research directions and prediction models. The first sub-chapters are focusing on the short-term changes and the most futuristic scenarios are depicted in the last ones.

22.8   Gamifying Health

WellaPets is a smartphone application that can be downloaded for free on the App Store, Google Play or Amazon Appstore. The child adopts, customizes and begins caring for his or her own Wellapet. By regularly visiting their pet, kids are able to play games with them, collect items for their pet's home, and care for their pet's asthma. Developers have worked with pediatricians to ensure that Wellapets teaches kids what they need to know if they, their friend or their sibling has asthma.

"MySugr Companion Diabetes Management App" works as a diabetes logbook providing immediate feedback and rewarding users with points which can be used to tame their "diabetes monster". The goal is to tame the user's monster every day, thus keeping track of their medical condition.

In the future, it is going to be extremely difficult not to fully comply with the prescribed therapy patients agreed upon. Moreover, compliance with medication should be as simple and comfortable for patients as possible. The real goal is to be able to measure health parameters, monitor them and engage when needed. As it is nearly impossible to get everyone motivated about their own health, let's find solutions that trick them into that by implementing methods of gamification seamlessly into their lives.

22.9 Augmented and Virtual Reality

Medical virtual reality (VR) is an area with fascinating possibilities. It has not just moved the imagination of science-fiction fans, but also clinical researchers and real life medical practitioners. Although the field is brand new, there are already great examples of VR having a positive effect on patients' lives and physicians' work.

For the first time in the history of medicine, on 14 April 2016 Shafi Ahmed cancer surgeon performed an operation using a virtual reality camera at the Royal London hospital. Everyone could participate in the operation in real time through the Medical Realities website and the VR in OR app. No matter whether a promising medical student from Cape Town, an interested journalist from Seattle or a worried relative, everyone could follow through two 360° cameras how the surgeon removed a cancerous tissue from the bowel of the patient.

Virtual reality could elevate the teaching and learning experience in medicine to a whole new level. Today, only a few students can peek over the shoulder of the surgeon during an operation and it is challenging to learn the tricks of the trade like that. With a virtual reality camera, surgeons can stream operations globally and allow medical students to actually be there in the OR using their VR goggles.

Brennan Spiegel and his team at the Cedars-Sinai hospital in Los Angeles introduced VR worlds to their patients to help them release stress and reduce pain. With the special goggles, they could escape the four walls of the hospital and visit amazing landscapes in Iceland, participate in the work of an art studio or swim together with whales in the deep blue ocean. Not only can the hospital experience be improved with medical VR, but the costs of care may also be reduced. By reducing stress and pain, the length of the patient's stay in the ward or the amount of resources utilized can both be decreased.

Augmented reality differs from its most known "relative", virtual reality (VR) since the latter creates a 3D world completely detaching the user from reality. There are two respects in which AR is unique: users do not lose touch with reality and it puts information into eyesight as fast as possible. These distinctive features enable AR to become a driving force in the future of medicine.

The response is augmented reality (AR) and the rising interest of people in its use. Pokémon Go is made with exactly this technology: the device (in this case your phone) transmits a live or indirect view of a physical, real-world environment which is augmented by computer-generated sensory input such as sound, video, graphics or GPS data. In the future, augmented reality could be a built-in feature in a glass, headset or digital contact lens.

The start-up company AccuVein is using AR technology to make both nurses' and patients' lives easier. AccuVein's marketing specialist, Vinny Luciano said 40% of IVs (intravenous injections) miss the vein on the first stick, with the numbers getting worse for children and the elderly. AccuVein uses augmented reality by using a handheld scanner that projects over skin and shows nurses and doctors where veins are in the patients' bodies. Luciano estimates that it's been used on more than ten million patients, making finding a vein on the first stick 3.5× more likely. Such technologies could assist healthcare professionals and extend their skills (Tashjian et al. 2017).

22.10   Genetics, Precision Medicine and Bio-Hacking

The first labs of the so-called Do-It-Yourself Biology community, a grassroots movement which was initiated to let students and others interested in biotechnology use professional laboratory equipment for their experiments, was launched in 2008. These enthusiasts seek to popularize biotechnology in the way that programmers popularized computing from their garages in the 1970s. Along with equipment, these labs provide a wellspring of biotech outreach and education. Local groups of DIY BIO are available from the US and Europe to Asia and Oceania.

BioCurious, a hackerspace for biotech, opened in 2011 with the mission statement that innovations in biology should be accessible, affordable, and open to everyone. They are building a community biology lab for amateurs, inventors, entrepreneurs, and anyone who wants to experiment with friends. They provide a complete working laboratory and technical library; equipment from fluorescent microscopes to PCR machines; materials; co-working space; and a training center for biotechniques. Citizen scientists will get a chance to perform experiments and do research.

I envision a day when it will be quite common to have our genomes sequenced. The magic number will be 7,000,000,000 (global population) times 3,000,000,000 (number of base pairs in our DNA) equaling 2.1×10^{19} which is the number of base pairs that should soon be available. Based on trends in other industries such as mobile phones, the cost of sequencing a human genome will be close to zero, while the analysis needed to draw conclusions useful to medical decisions will be expensive.

Such genomics-based precision medicine could bring a new era to cancer care. Cancer diagnosis must be early and accurate. Many cancer types cannot be detected early enough at the moment, while others are detected in time, but treated too severely. This notion requires not only great healthcare facilities and new diagnosis technologies, but also the proactivity of patients. During cancer treatments, re-biopsies are needed many times. It means a new sample from the ever-changing tumour must be obtained to define the next step of the therapy. With the current, invasive biopsy techniques, this is a huge challenge not only for patients, but also for caregivers. Fluid biopsy extracts cancer cells from a simple blood sample. As Illumina, the DNA sequencer giant, announced a spin-off focused solely on making fluid biopsy commercially viable, it might be the next breakthrough in oncology.

By getting a clear knowledge about what genetic and environmental factors lead to the different types of cancers, including the given patient's own genetic makeup, it would be possible to catch cancer in its infancy. This requires process innovation in healthcare, as well as more precise and specific cancer biomarkers supported by better screening technologies. Cancer Research UK's Cancer Grand Challenges feature a call for researchers to discover new, previously unknown carcinogenic events, bringing this trend closer to reality.

Today, we either use chemotherapy to destroy any reproducing cells causing serious side effects; or targeted therapies which show low rates of response due to heterogeneity of the tumour and the poor accuracy of matching treatments to patients. The price of new drugs is going up steeply and personalized drugs cost even more, while effective cancer care be widely available to everyone.

In the case of AIDS, combining drugs with different targets resulted in the treatment that finally put a dent in the disease. Research shows the same applies to cancer, but combining the increasing number of cancer therapies has so far proven difficult due to the sheer number of possible combinations. New approaches in the field of systems biology that use computer models to predict therapy effects are promising to cut through this complexity, and deliver effective combinational therapies in the coming years. All the while, new approaches like immunotherapies put emphasis on making the patient's immune system sensitive to cancer cells again, this way letting the immune system fight back.

Companies like Foundation Medicine are creating customized treatment plans based on the genetic makeup of the patient's tumour. They sequence DNA from the patient's tumor, and try to match the key mutations to drugs on the market or clinical trials already on the way. Over time, this will become the standard for assigning cancer treatment regimes.

22.11 Medical Robots

Medical robots do not only exist in sci-fi movies and the distant future, they are coming to healthcare and all stakeholders must prepare for them. Robots can support, assist and extend the service health workers are offering. In jobs with repetitive and monotonous functions they might even obtain the capacity to completely replace humans.

Thus, medical professionals and caretakers would do well to learn more about medical robots: what they are capable of, how to work with them and in what way they might complement the tasks they perform daily. Otherwise human medical workers might get replaced or grow frustrated if they experience that robots are able to do their jobs and they cannot change their previous tasks into something irreplaceable.

Statistics of the Centers for Disease Control and Prevention show that in the United States 1 in every 25 patients will contract hospital acquired infections (HAIs) such as MRSA (methicillin-resistant Staphylococcus aureus) and C. diff (Clostridium difficile), and 1 in 9 will die.

The Xenex Robot might constitute the next level of hygiene. It allows for fast and effective systematic disinfection of any space within a healthcare facility. This helpful automatic tool destroys deadly microorganisms causing HAIs by utilizing special UV disinfection methodologies. The Xenex Robot is more effective in causing cellular damage to microorganisms than other devices for disinfection, thus the number of HAIs might be more effectively reduced. Westchester Medical Center reported a 70% drop in Intensive Care Unit C. diff with the use of Xenex Robots.

Pepper, the 1.2 m tall humanoid "social robot" will be "employed" as a receptionist in two Belgian hospitals. It's a fascinating idea—because let's be honest: there is not a single person who was not even once greeted by a grumpy receptionist during a hospital visit and got lost in a hospital floor due to information hastily provided by kind but tired nurses at the end of their shift.

Pepper can recognise the human voice in 20 languages and can detect whether it is talking to a man, woman or child. Its skills enable Pepper to "work" as a receptionist in huge hospitals and to accompany visitors to the correct department so they do not get lost while trying to see their loved ones. "Social robots" such as Pepper or the smaller Nao might also be used as assistance in exercise sessions and help children overcome their fears of surgery.

Intouch health and its telehealth network could help in such situations. Through the waste network patients in remote areas have access to high-quality emergency consultations for stroke, cardiovascular, and burn services in the exact time they need it. Moreover with telehealth, medical professionals in such towns and rural areas also have access to specialty services and patients can be treated in their own communities. Through this network, a "telemedical robot" has already established over 750,000 clinical encounters where it was not possible before (https://www.cdc.gov/hai/surveillance/).

22.12   Health Sensors and Portable Diagnostics

When Dr. McCoy grabbed his tricorder and scanned a patient, the portable, hand-held device immediately listed vital signs, other parameters, and a diagnosis. It was the Swiss Army knife for physicians. When our class discussion turned to potential medical uses, a doubtful student asked how such a thing could work in real when it came from science fiction. I then gave him another list to consider. A visual display device from Star Trek is Google Glass now. The heads-up display in Minority Report is air touch technology. Iron Man is currently being developed by DARPA. The self-directed vacuum cleaner from The Jetsons now exists as Roomba. I could go on.

A working tricorder could bring about a new era in medicine. Instead of expensive machines and long waiting times, information would be available immediately. Physicians could scan a patient, or patients could scan themselves and receive a list of diagnostic options and suggestions. Imagine the influence it could have on underdeveloped regions. It should not substitute for medical supervision, but when there is none it comes in handy.

It could be useful when a diagnosis needs confirming or when standard laboratory equipment is not available. A high-power microscope with a smartphone, for example, could analyze swab samples and photos of skin lesions. Sensors could pick up abnormalities in DNA, or detect antibodies and specific proteins. An electronic nose, an ultrasonic probe, or almost anything we have now could be yoked to a smartphone and augment its features.

An in-person doctor visit includes assessing the patient's condition, health parameters, and other data. Much of this could be performed without needing the presence of a medical professional. I'm merely pointing out an absence of medical staff is the case in many regions of the world.

This situation is an impetus behind the Nokia Sensing X Challenge that has called for teams to design prototypes of a working tricorder. It should measure a wide range of biomarkers with a droplet of blood, be able to diagnose malaria, high blood pressure, and similar conditions, as well as monitor epilepsy.

The Qualcomm Tricorder X Prize was announced in 2012 to motivate innovators in this direction. It featured 230 teams from 30 countries, and promised an award of $10 million to the first team to build a working medical tricorder. The device had to correctly diagnose 15 different medical conditions from a sore throat to sleep apnea and colon cancer.

Moreover, a huge army of wearable sensors help patients assess their health and quantify health parameters at home. A 2014 report showed that 71% of 16–24-year-olds want wearable technology. Predictions for 2018 include a market value of $12 billion; a shipment of 112 million wearables and that one third of Americans will own at least a pedometer.

Now a growing population is using devices to measure a health parameter and while this market is expected to continue growing, devices are expected to shrink, get cheaper and more comfortable. At this point, nobody can be blamed for over-tracking their health as we got a chance for that for the first time in history. Eventually, by the time the technology behind them gets better, we should get to the stage of meaningful use as well (Fig. 22.2).

Parameters and habits patients can measure today at home:

- Daily activities (number of steps, calories burnt, distance covered)
- Sleep quality + smart alarm
- Blood pressure

Fig. 22.2 A wearable sensor

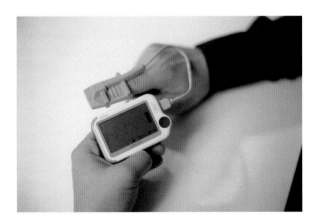

- Blood oxygen levels
- Blood glucose levels
- Cardiac fitness
- Stress
- Pulse
- Body temperature
- Eating habits
- ECG
- Cognitive skills
- Brain activities
- Productivity

The next obvious step is designing smaller gadgets that can still provide a lot of useful data. Smartclothes are meant to fill this gap. Examples include Hexoskin and MC10. Both companies are working on different clothes and sensors that can be included in clothes. Imagine the fashion industry grabbing this opportunity and getting health tracking closer to their audiences.

Then there might be "insideables", devices implanted into our body or just under the skin. There are people already having such RFID implants with which they can open up a laptop, a smartphone or even the garage door.

Also, "digestables", pills or tiny gadgets that can be swallowed could track digestion and the absorption of drugs. Colonoscopy could become an important diagnostic procedure that most people are not afraid of. A little pill cam could be swallowed and the recordings become available in hours.

The end of the product line is probably represented by thin digital tattoos that can be replaced easily and measures all vital signs and health parameters. It could notify the patient and even their caregiver through a smartphone if there is something they should take care of (http://tricorder.xprize.org/).

22.13   Growing Organs in Labs

In the US alone, on average 18 people die every day from the lack of available organs. Every 14 min someone is added to a kidney transplant list.

Technology exists that assists organs in doing their function instead of having to replace them. Impella is the smallest heart pump in use today. It is the size of a pencil and is FDA approved to support the heart for up to 6 h during cardiac surgeries. HeartMate II will act like a pair of cardiac crutches. It is the size of an avocado, and people have been living with it for years. All the recipients have an almost undetectable pulse. When those hearts have to be replaced in the future one hopes that tissue engineering will have matured.

In 2014 they announced the successful printing of liver tissue that functioned like a real liver for weeks. The three-dimensional liver models, known as exVive3D, are only a few millimeters wide. One print head of the 3D bioprinter deposits a support matrix. The other head precisely places human liver cells in it. The tissue contains all cell types normally found in the liver. It can produce proteins such as albumin and fibrinogen, and also synthesize cholesterol. Previous models were two-dimensional. The 3D version can distinguish between toxic and harmless compounds. The long-term goal is to eliminate animal testing by pharmaceutical companies given that such liver tissues could assess the toxicity of potential drugs.

Synthetic skin, a bionic ear, bladder, or cornea might be the first organs to be either bioprinted or grown in the lab on demand. After that, more complicated ones might be engineered to be fully functioning organs. Twenty years from now we might look back at transplantation waiting lists and marvel at what a brutal world it was in the early 21st century.

Organovo just announced that their bioprinted liver assays are able to function for more than 40 days. Organovo's top executives and other industry experts suggest that within a decade we will be able to print solid organs such as liver, heart, and kidney. Hundreds of thousands of people worldwide are waiting for an organ donor. Imagine how such a technology could transform their lives (https://www.kidney.org/news/newsroom/factsheets/Organ-Donation-and-Transplantation-Stats).

22.14 Prosthetics

Creating traditional prosthetics is very time-consuming and destructive, which means that any modifications would destroy the original molds. Researchers at the University of Toronto, in collaboration with Autodesk Research and CBM Canada, used 3D printing to quickly produce cheap and easily customizable prosthetic sockets for patients in the developing world. Basically, they scan a damaged limb using Xbox Kinect, design the parts digitally, and then send the model to the printer which manufactures the socket in a few hours using polylactic acid, a thermoplastic that is easily modifiable with heat. The cost with this method is under $10. If we merge 3D printing with open source templates that anyone can manufacture, distribute, and modify, then a new era of cheaper prosthetics for amputees around the world could begin.

Ekso Bionics was launched in California in 2005 with a brave mission to design and develop powered exoskeletons that could make walking possible again for paralyzed people. A powered exoskeleton is a mobile framework that a person wears. It contains motors or hydraulics that deliver part of the energy needed for limb movement.

Their exoskeletons are used by individuals with various degrees of paralysis and stemming by a variety of causes. By the end of 2012 Ekso Bionics had helped individuals take more than a million steps that would not otherwise have been possible. Boxtel is one of ten Ekso Bionics test pilots who received a customized exoskeleton. According to Boxtel, the project "represents the triumph of human creativity and technology that converged to restore my authentic functionality in a stunningly beautiful, fashionable and organic design."

22.15 3D Printing

Kaiba Gionfriddo was born prematurely in 2011. After 8 months his lung development caused concerns, although he was sent home with his parents as his breathing was normal. Six weeks later, Kaiba stopped breathing and turned blue. He was diagnosed with tracheobronchomalacia, a long Latin word that means his windpipe was so weak that it collapsed. He had a tracheostomy and was put on a ventilator—the conventional treatment. Still, Kaiba would stop breathing almost daily. His heart would stop, too. His caregivers 3D printed a bioresorbable device that instantly helped Kaiba breathe. This case is considered a prime example of how customized 3D printing is transforming healthcare as we know it.

Since then this area has been skyrocketing. The list of objects that have been successfully printed demonstrates the potential this technology holds for the near future.

Tissues with blood vessels: Researchers at Harvard University were the first to use a custom-built 3D printer and a dissolving ink to create a swatch of tissue that contains skin cells interwoven with structural material interwoven that can potentially function as blood vessels.

Drugs: Lee Cronin, a chemist at the University of Glasgow, wants to do for the discovery and distribution of prescription drugs what Apple did for music. In a TED talk he described a prototype 3D printer capable of assembling chemical compounds at the molecular level. Patients would go to an online drugstore with their digital prescription, buy the blueprint and the chemical ink needed, and then print the drug at home. In the future he said we might sell not drugs but rather blueprints or apps.

Tumor Models: Researchers in China and the US have both printed models of cancerous tumors to aid discovery of new anti-cancer drugs and to better understand how tumors develop, grow, and spread.

Bone: Professor Susmita Bose of Washington State University modified a 3D printer to bind chemicals to a ceramic powder creating intricate ceramic scaffolds that promote the growth of the bone in any shape.

Heart Valve: Jonathan Butcher of Cornell University has printed a heart valve that will soon be tested in sheep. He used a combination of cells and biomaterials to control the valve's stiffness.

Ear cartilage: Lawrence Bonassar of Cornell University used 3D photos of human ears to create ear molds. The molds were then filled with a gel containing bovine cartilage cells suspended in collagen, which held the shape of the ear while cells grew their extracellular matrix.

Medical equipment: Already, 3D printing is occurring in underdeveloped areas. "Not Impossible Labs" based in Venice, California took 3D printers to Sudan where the chaos of war has left many people with amputated limbs. The organization's founder, Mick Ebeling, trained locals how to operate the machinery, create patient-specific limbs, and fit these new, very inexpensive prosthetics.

Cranium Replacement: Dutch surgeons replaced the entire top of a 22 year-old woman's skull with a customized printed implant made from plastic.

Synthetic skin: James Yoo at the Wake Forest School of Medicine in the US has developed a printer that can print skin straight onto the wounds of burn victims.

22.16   Physiological Simulation

New drugs are approved through human clinical trials. These are rigorous, starting in animal trials and gradually moving to patients. It typically costs billions of dollars and takes many years to complete, sometimes more than a decade. Patients in trials are exposed to side effects that cannot be predicted or expected. If the trial is successful, it may or may not receive FDA approval.

Online services have helped clinical trials. TrialReach tries to bridge the gap between patients and researchers who are developing new drugs. If more patients have a chance to participate in trials, they might become more engaged with potential treatments or even be able to access new treatments before they become FDA approved and freely available. TrialX similarly matches clinical trials to patients according to their gender, age, location, and medical condition. The number of such services is growing to accommodate an increasing demand from patients.

In the late nineteenth century patients had no protection. Anyone could sell snake oil containing who-knows-what. In 1906, the FDA was born and required every tonic, nostrum, and product to be tested and proven both safe and efficient. While an extremely important element of healthcare today, it puts immense economic pressure to bear on bringing new treatments to market.

If a pharmaceutical company jumps through all the hoops and wins approval, they can sell their new product for a limited time under patent protection. If it does not win approval all their investment goes down the drain. Some patient activists are arguing that the process should be changed. For example, Perry Cohen, a Parkinson's disease patient, has argued for years that the FDA has been using the wrong criteria. As he sees it the question is for whose benefit trials are being done, and who gets to say what that benefit means.

Obviously, we a need a faster and less expensive method that is also safe. What if it's time to use disruptive innovations to change how clinical trials are performed?

We need to mimic human physiology digitally for this which is hard. Fortunately, we are not imitating the end product, and so while mimicking human physiology is extremely difficult it is not totally impossible. A comprehensive system would make it possible to model conditions, symptoms, and even drug effects. To achieve this, every tiny detail of the human body needs to be included in the simulation—from the way we react to temperature changes to the circadian rhythms that influence the action of hormones.

HumMod is one of the most advanced simulations. It provides a top–down model of human physiology from whole organs to individual molecules. It features more than 1500 equations and 6500 variables such as body fluids, circulation, electrolytes, hormones, metabolism, and skin temperature. HumMod aims to simulate how human physiology works, and claims to be the most sophisticated mathematical model of human physiology ever created.

HumMod has been in development for decades and it is still far from completion. By far, I mean perhaps decades still. There are those who argue that human physiology cannot be digitally imitated. Maybe supplementary technologies are needed such as organ microchips. For example, organs-on-chips are engineered to mimic how the lung or the heart works at the cellular level. They are translucent, and so can provide a window into the inner workings of a particular organ.

The Wyss Institute plans to build ten different organs-on-chips and connect them together. Doing this may mimic whole-body physiology better, and thus better assess responses to new drug candidates.

At the very least, the virtual patients must almost perfectly mimic the physiology of the target patients, with all of the variation that actual patients show. The model should encompass circulatory, neural, endocrine, and metabolic systems, and each of these must demonstrate valid mechanism-based responses to physiological and pharmacological stimuli. Probably cognitive computers would be needed to deal with the gargantuan amount of resulting data.

22.17   Artificial Intelligence Engines in Digital Health

With the evolution of digital capacity, more and more data is produced and stored in the digital space. The amount of available digital data is growing by a mind-blowing speed, doubling every 2 year. In 2017, it encompassed zettabytes, however by 2020 the digital universe—the data we create and copy annually—will reach 44 zettabytes, or 44 trillion gigabytes (!).

Usually, we make sense of the world around us with the help of rules and processes which build up a system. The world of Big Data is so huge that we will need artificial intelligence (AI) to be able to keep track of it.

We have not yet reached the state of "real" AI, but it is ready to sneak into our lives without any great announcement or fanfares—narrow AI is already in our cars, in Google searches, Amazon suggestions and in many other devices. Apple's Siri, Microsoft's Cortana, Google's OK Google, and Amazon's Echo services are nifty in the way that they extract questions from speech using natural-language processing and then do a limited set of useful things, such as look for a restaurant, get driving directions, find an open slot for a meeting, or run a simple web search.

The most obvious application of artificial intelligence in healthcare is data management. Collecting it, storing it, normalizing it, tracing its lineage—it is the first step in revolutionizing the existing healthcare systems. Recently, the AI research branch of the search giant, Google, launched its Google Deepmind Health project, which is used to mine the data of medical records in order to provide better and faster health services. The project is in its initial phase, and at present they are cooperating with the Moorfields Eye Hospital NHS Foundation Trust to improve eye treatment.

IBM Watson launched its special program for oncologists—and I interviewed one of the professors working with it—which is able to provide clinicians evidence-based treatment options. Watson for Oncology has an advanced ability to analyze the meaning and context of structured and unstructured data in clinical notes and reports that may be critical to selecting a treatment pathway. Then by combining attributes from the patient's file with clinical expertise, research and data, the program identifies potential treatment plans for a patient.

IBM launched another algorithm called Medical Sieve. It is an ambitious long-term exploratory project to build a next generation "cognitive assistant" with analytical, reasoning capabilities and a wide range of clinical knowledge. Medical Sieve is qualified to assist in clinical decision making in radiology and cardiology. The "cognitive health assistant" is able to analyze radiology images to spot and detect problems faster and more reliably. Radiologists in the future should only look at the most complicated cases where human supervision is useful.

Artificial intelligence will have a huge impact on genetics and genomics as well. Deep Genomics aims at identifying patterns in huge data sets of genetic information and medical records, looking for mutations and linkages to disease. They are inventing a new generation of computational technologies that can tell doctors what will happen within a cell when DNA is altered by genetic variation, whether natural or therapeutic.

Developing pharmaceuticals through clinical trials take sometimes more than a decade and costs billions of dollars. Speeding this up and making more cost-effective would have an enormous effect on today's healthcare and how innovations reach everyday medicine. Atomwise uses supercomputers that root out therapies from a database of molecular structures. In 2016, Atomwise launched a virtual search for safe, existing medicines that could be redesigned to treat the Ebola virus. They found two drugs predicted by the company's AI technology which may significantly reduce Ebola infectivity. This analysis, which typically would have taken months or years, was completed in less than 1 day. "If we can fight back deadly viruses months or years faster that represents tens of thousands of lives," said Alexander Levy, COO of Atomwise. "Imagine how many people might survive the next pandemic because a technology like Atomwise exists," he added.

Ninety-seven percent of healthcare invoices in the Netherlands are digital containing data regarding the treatment, the doctor and the hospital. These invoices could be easily retrieved. A local company, Zorgprisma Publiek analyzes the invoices and uses

IBM Watson in the cloud to mine the data. They can tell if a doctor, clinic or hospital makes mistakes repetitively in treating a certain type of condition in order to help them improve and avoid unnecessary hospitalizations of patients.

I do not think that the situation is so gloomy, but I agree with those who stress the need to prepare for the use of artificial intelligence appropriately. We need the following preparations to avoid the pitfalls of the utilization of AI:

- creation of ethical standards which are applicable to and obligatory for the whole healthcare sector
- gradual development of AI in order to give some time for mapping of the possible downsides
- for medical professionals: acquirement of basic knowledge about how AI works in a medical setting in order to understand how such solutions might help them in their everyday job
- for patients: getting accustomed to artificial intelligence and discovering its benefits for themselves—e.g. with the help of Cognitoys which support the cognitive development of small children with the help of AI in a fun and gentle way or with such services as Siri.
- for companies developing AI solutions (such as IBM): even more communication towards the general public about the potential advantages and risks of using AI in medicine.
- for decision-makers at healthcare institutions: doing all the necessary steps to be able to measure the success and the effectiveness of the system. It is also important to push companies towards offering affordable AI-solutions, since it is the only way to bring the promise of science fiction into reality and turn AI into the stethoscope of the twenty-first century (https://www.emc.com/leadership/digital-universe/2014iview/executive-summary.htm).

22.18   Ethical Issues

With amazing advantages come risks and danger which we have to prepare for in time. It has already been proven that pacemakers and insulin pumps can be hacked. Security experts have warned that vulnerabilities could be used to murder patients on a massive scale—sometime soon. The question is—what can we do to protect wearable devices that are connected to our physiological system from being hacked and controlled from a distance? Companies developing such technologies should make sure they are safe and users should be as vigilant as possible when using them.

We share much more information about ourselves than we think. Check mypermissions.org to see what services and apps you have given permission to access your personal information already. What if, as augmented reality spreads, all this information will be easily available to someone you just met? Kids who are born now represent the first generation whose lives are logged in meticulous detail—either by themselves or well-meaning but clueless relations. While such big data could significantly improve healthcare, how can we prevent companies and governments from misusing these? What if you ate red meat and your insurance company immediately raised your insurance rates because you're not eating healthy enough?

Physicians are worried because patients Google their symptoms and treatments, and they might take the misinformation they find more seriously than what their caregiver tells them. But patients will soon be able to scan themselves, do blood tests and even genetic analysis on demand with other, unregulated companies or at home, then use publicly available algorithms to analyse their data. This will open the way for even more serious cases of misinterpretation, maltreatment or self-medication. Will we able to persuade patients to turn to doctors with this wealth of data and improve their care, and not just put their trust into algorithms? If you think this sounds like science fiction, check the finalist of the Nokia Sensing XChallenge, who have developed just such scanners.

A disruptive technology can provide an unforeseen advantage over others or augment certain human capabilities to an unprecedented level. As a consequence, what if people start asking their doctors to replace their healthy limbs for robotic ones because it would let them run faster? What if they start asking for brain chips to get smarter? If now you can get a new nose or larger breasts, what would prevent you from getting new muscles or brain implants?

Today, societies struggle to fight gender and financial inequality. But once technology can truly augment human capabilities, people will get smarter, healthier and faster only because they can afford to be augmented. What if I can buy an exoskeleton or a personalized drug to live longer and you cannot? How do we prepare society for a time when financial differences lead to biological ones?

Longevity studies have been going on for decades. Several aspects of the secret of long life have been discovered. Sooner or later, we will be able to significantly prolong life. Developed countries with aging populations are already struggling to maintain their health. How will the basics of society shift if a majority of people start living for more than 100 years? Could we support this population financially and medically? Can we ensure that ageing doesn't come with a severe decline in health?

In the wildest futuristic scenarios, tiny nanorobots in our bloodstream could detect diseases. These microscopic robots would send alerts to our smartphones or digital contact lenses before disease could develop in our body. When most human bodies will contain tiny robots, how can we prevent terrorists from hacking these devices to gain direct control over our health?

Evidence based medicine shapes how we deliver healthcare today. It is by definition a lengthy process. Certain solutions such as simulations with cognitive computers instead of long and expensive clinical trials might make them faster but even these won't match the pace of technological development. Over the last few years, technological advances have become so fast, it's really hard to keep track of them anymore. How will doctors be able to keep up to date? When patients start seeing

Table 22.2 Major trends and technologies grouped by their projected time-span needed to become common practice

Today	Short-term future	Long-term future
Gamification	Augmented reality	Artificial intelligence
Telemedicine	Virtual reality	Humanoid robots
Health sensors	Medical robots	Portable diagnostics
3D printing	Whole-genome sequencing	Virtual clinical trials
Cloud-based algorithms	Digital tattoos	Nanotechnology
Medical records	3D bioprinting	Brain-computer interfaces
Smartphones and tablets	Exoskeletons	Cryonics, longevity

the amazing innovations out there that aren't accessible to them in everyday care, will they reach for them outside the healthcare system?

There are movements and philosophies that highlight a narrow concept or approach even though it is highly unlikely that any one solution will lead to a prosperous future. Transhumanism focuses more on the future of science, medicine and technology than on the individuals. Singularitarians believe in a technological singularity but do not give people guidance about what to do. A network of interconnected people, devices, and concepts is the only way to solve global issues. It is advisable not to trust just one movement or philosophy such as transhumanism or singularitarians. The most plausible solution will be a mix of all the concepts trying to describe the coming decades. We should be skeptical and analytical before accepting one major philosophy about the future. The future is going to be interconnected and not a one way ride.

A man named Davecat lives with his wife and mistress, both of whom are Synthetiks—specially designed, life-sized dolls. Accordingly, Davecat calls himself a technosexual. While some will not understand how Davecat thinks about his partners, his story heralds the diversity of concepts surrounding sexuality that will arise in the next couple of years. How can we prepare for all these if we cannot even solve today's issues in sexuality? Our current concepts about sexuality are very much based on biology. But dealing with technology that sneaks into our private lives might be a bigger challenge for people than even the LGBT revolution.

Let's start discussing these bioethical issues at home, at the workplace and on public forums. This way, we can prepare to exploit the advantages technology offers, while keeping the potential dangers at bay (Table 22.2).

22.19 Conclusion

A revolution in the world of technology has a huge impact on the future of medicine and healthcare. It also initiates a cultural change which leads to a new status quo making empowered patients partners with their physicians. In this new system, there is partnership instead of hierarchy; collaboration instead of orders; and data instead of pure experience.

While technology is not the final solution for healthcare's problems today, it certainly provides us with the tools to make change happen.

In an utopistic scenario, artificial intelligence, medical robots and thin sensors could help us stay healthy and prevent diseases from arising. While such innovations will turn the wheels of delivering care, human comfort, empathy and that one supporting word from our caregiver will be stronger and more important than ever.

References

Azevedo MF, de Oliveira VE, da Silva EMK 2012 Access to health information on the internet: a public health issue?. Rev Assoc Med Bras [Internet]. [Cited 2017 Jun 5] 58(6):650–658. Available from: http://www.scielo.br/scielo.php?script=sci_arttext&pid=S0104-42302012000600008&lng=en. doi:https://doi.org/10.1590/S0104-42302012000600008.

Blendon RJ, Benson JM, Hero JO. N Engl J Med. 2014;371:1570–2. https://doi.org/10.1056/NEJMp1407373.

Mesko B. The guide to the future of medicine. 2014. Webicina Kft.

Mesko B. My Health: upgraded. 2015. Webicina Kft.

Smith CW, Graedon T, Graedon J, Greene A, Grohol J, Sands D, collaboration with the SPM Founder's group. A model for the future of health care. J Participat Med. 2013;5:e20.

Tashjian VC, Mosadeghi S, Howard AR, Lopez M, Dupuy T, Reid M, Martinez B, Ahmed S, Dailey F, Robbins K, Rosen B, Fuller G, Danovitch I, IsHak W, Spiegel B. Virtual reality for management of pain in hospitalized patients: results of a controlled trial. JMIR Ment Health. 2017;4(1):e9.

Technology and health care: the view from HHS. (2016) The Wall Street J. https://www.wsj.com/articles/technology-and-health-care-the-view-from-hhs-1474855381. Accessed 5 Jun 2017.

The Social MEDia Course. (2016.) http://thecourse.webicina.com/. Accessed 5 Jun 2017.

Tons of people are buying Fitbits, but are they actually using them? (n.d.) .The Verge. https://www.theverge.com/tech/2015/8/6/9110035/fitbit-fitness-tracker-watch-active-users-sales. Accessed 5 Jun 2017.

Topol E. Patients will see you now.

Topol E. The creative destruction of medicine.

http://dougkanter.me/Databetes. (n.d..) Accessed 5 Jun 2017.

https://www.fda.gov/advisorycommittees/committeesmeetingmaterials/patientengagementadvisorycommittee/default.htm. (n.d..) Accessed 5 Jun 2017.

Index